THE PRINCIPLES AND METHODS IN MODERN TOXICOLOGY

SYMPOSIA OF THE
GIOVANNI LORENZINI FOUNDATION
Volume 6

Other volumes in this series:

Volume 1   Molecular Biology and Pharmacology of Cyclic Nucleotides
            G. Folco and R. Paoletti editors, 1978

Volume 2   Genetic Engineering
            H.W. Boyer and S. Nicosia editors, 1978

Volume 3   Radioimmunoassay of Drugs and Hormones in
            Cardiovascular Medicine
            A. Albertini, M. Da Prada and B.A. Peskar editors, 1979

Volume 4   Drug Assessment: Criteria and Methods
            J.Z. Bowers and G.P. Velo editors, 1979

Volume 5   *In vivo* and *in vitro* Erythropoiesis: The Friend System
            G.B. Rossi editor, 1980

THE PRINCIPLES AND METHODS IN MODERN TOXICOLOGY

Proceedings of the International Course on The Principles and Methods in Modern Toxicology held in Belgirate, Italy, 22-26 October, 1979

Editors:

C.L. Galli
S.D. Murphy
and
R. Paoletti

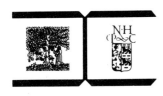

1980

ELSEVIER/NORTH-HOLLAND BIOMEDICAL PRESS
AMSTERDAM · NEW YORK · OXFORD

ISBN for this volume: 0-444-80230-4
ISBN for the series: 0-444-80040-9

Published by:
Elsevier/North-Holland Biomedical Press
335 Jan van Galenstraat, P.O. Box 211
Amsterdam, The Netherlands

Sole distributors for the USA and Canada:
Elsevier North Holland Inc.
52 Vanderbilt Avenue
New York, N.Y. 10017

Library of Congress Cataloging in Publication Data

International Course on the Principles and Methods in
    Modern Toxicology, Belgirate, Italy, 1979.
    The principles and methods in modern toxicology.

    (Symposia of the Giovanni Lorenzini Foundation ; v. 6)
    Bibliography: p.
    Includes index.
    1. Toxicology--Congresses. 2. Toxicology,
Experimental--Congresses. 3. Toxicity testing--
Congresses. I. Galli, Corrado L. II. Murphy,
Sheldon Douglas, 1933-   III. Paoletti, Rodolfo.
IV. Title. V. Series: Fondazione Giovanni Lorenzini.
Symposia of the Giovanni Lorenzini Foundation ; v. 6.
[DNLM: 1. Toxicology--Methods--Congresses. QV600
I626p 1979]
RA1191.I63   1979   615.9   80-14106
ISBN 0-444-80230-4

Printed in The Netherlands

PREFACE

The proceedings of the International Course on "Principles and Methods in Modern Toxicology" organized by the Fondazione Giovanni Lorenzini and by the Institute of Pharmacology and Pharmacognosy, University of Milan, held at Belgirate on October 22-26, 1979, are now presented to the international scientific community.

This Course is the first organized by the Fondazione Giovanni Lorenzini in order to discuss the most up-to-date developments in the field of the environmental toxicology. This Course is therefore general in nature and it will be followed by more focused activities devoted to methods for more specific problems in the area of modern quantitative toxicology. The distinguished group of international experts who have participated in this meeting has been asked to collaborate in planning the future series; they believe that such enterprise is timely. There is an evident need for common methodology, legislation and training for toxicologists in the industrialized countries.

The Fondazione Giovanni Lorenzini is proud to have collaborated with this scientific event in its tradition of interest in continuing education and pioneering activities.

The review and the experimental papers collected in this monography represent the results of a collaborative effort and they are offered to the scientific communities for evaluation as contributions to an emergent science.

We are particularly grateful to the lecturers, to the editors of this volume and to the distinguished audience that has stimulated a most fruitful discussion, and we hope that this monograph may be of use to active toxicologists and scientists training in many countries.

Prof. Rodolfo Paoletti
President, Fondazione
Giovanni Lorenzini

CONTENTS

Preface   V

Toxicity testing: Scope and design
    R. Truhaut   1

Chemical safety evaluations and toxicological decisions
    G. Vettorazzi   9

Legislative action tending to control potentially toxic
    substances: Purposes, means and present achievements
    A. Gerard   35

Chemical analysis in toxicological research
    K.R. Hill   55

Biochemical aspects of tissue change
    J.W. Daniel   71

The metabolism and chemobiokinetics of environmental
    chemicals
    D.V. Parke   85

General principles of genetic toxicology and methods for
    mutagenesis assessment
    N. Loprieno   107

Reproductive toxicity
    I.C. Munro   125

Teratology and safety evaluation
    A.K. Palmer   139

Testing for carcinogenicity
    G. Della Porta and T.A. Dragani   159

Subchronic toxicity studies: Methodology, interpretations
    and problems
    P.S. Elias   169

Chronic studies
    R.L. Baron   191

Short-term tests for carcinogenicity
    C. Schlatter and W.K. Lutz   207

Toxicologic pathology: Issues and uncertainties
    P.M. Newberne and R.G. McConnell   223

The choice of animal species in experimental toxicology
    A. Mondino   259

Assessment of the potential for toxic interactions among
    environmental pollutants
    S.D. Murphy   277

Toxicology of immunity
    A. Nicolin, A. Cosco, O. Marelli and F. Sarra   295

Good laboratory practice
    G. Falconi   311

Interaction between epidemiology of cancer and experimental
    carcinogenesis
    B. Terracini   321

Round Table - Survey on current methods and new approaches
    to the evaluation of mutagenic potential   341

Round table - An example of environmental toxicology:
    The dioxin event   367

Author index   399

© 1980 Elsevier/North-Holland Biomedical Press
The Principles and Methods in Modern Toxicology
C.L. Galli, S.D. Murphy and R. Paoletti, editors.

TOXICITY TESTING: SCOPE AND DESIGN

R. TRUHAUT

Toxicological Research Center, René Descartes University, Paris (France)

GENERAL OVERVIEW

It is a pleasure and an honour to have this opportunity to speak to you all this morning and to talk about one of my favorite topics.

Since the end of the last century, society has entered a new era, the chemical era. This era has been characterized by an extraordinary expansion of industrial development and by a consequent increase in the use of chemical agents in most varied applications. This spectacular progress in the chemical sciences and technology has undoubtedly brought about a great economic and social benefit and, therefore, an indisputable improvement in the living standards of many world populations.

However, the hazards which might result from people's exposure to a considerable and ever increasing number of chemicals in modern life should not be overlooked. Certain products may be hazardous to human health and, therefore, present important problems for toxicologists, hygienists, physicians, engineers, and technologists who are concerned with the protection of public health.

Toxicology focuses on the detection of toxic risks to humans. This is essential for establishing preventive measures since one can only prevent risks which are known and have been identified. The term 'toxic' is derived from the Greek word 'toxon' that means bow which recalls that, unfortunately, humans have always been concerned with finding ways to kill. That may well have been the reason why toxicology or the science of poisons first developed along the lines of legal or forensic medicine.

In the second stage of development of toxicology, interest shifted to drugs and pharmacotherapy; emphasis was given to establishing relationships between effective (medically beneficial) and toxic (side action) effects and the corresponding doses responsible for these effects.

In the course of the chemical era already mentioned the field of toxicology has grown considerably. It includes the study of agents to which workers in industry and agriculture may be occupationally exposed (occupational toxicology), components of air pollution, aqueous effluents of industry, automobile exhaust (environmental toxicology), pesticides used to combat parasites and agricultural pests, intentional and non-intentional food chemicals (food toxicology), multiple chemical agents, material in household ingredients, cosmetics, packaging materials, etc.

Toxicity testing is necessary to establish risks of these chemicals to human population. Experimental toxicology, thus, is concerned with the design of tests which would enable the determination of the potential of a substance to cause injury and with the development of enough data to warrant conclusions that levels of exposure should be so low in relation to harmful doses that there would be a practical certainty that no harm can result. Such information can usually be obtained by studies in animal models; since emphasis is generally on the detection of subtle long-range effects deriving from chronic low level exposure, suitable designed chronic or lifetime studies are the basis for most decisions regarding safety of chemicals.

THE DESIGN OF TOXICITY TESTING

The problem of designing animal experiments includes two sources of uncertainties: a) the uncertainty whether the animals chosen for the toxicity testing are appropriate models from which to extrapolate the results to humans, and b) the uncertainty whether effects that may occur only in very low incidence in the population can be detected with the number of experimental subjects that are practical in laboratory investigations. Since the goal of toxicity testing is to insure the least possibility to harm to humans, the experimental studies should be designed to detect any and all toxic effects. There is no ideal animal available which has the high susceptibility to every possible adverse effect and in which the induced adverse effects are comparable to those observed in humans; thus the inherent limitations of animal studies and the consequent difficulties are evident. These difficulties represent scientific challenges of great practical significance and require that the maximum creative competence be harnessed to solve these problems.

For practical purposes, several national and international groups concerned with toxicity testing have made specific recommendations in this regard.

Essential to the success of toxicity testing are proper experimental design and proper interpretation of results. Essential also is the maintenance of good laboratory management and practice so as to prevent or minimize contamination of air, food, water and equipment, to minimize the incidence of intercurrent disease, and to assure adequate records of, and the preservation of important experimental material.

In designing the studies, basic minimum requirements should include observations on growth, food intake, clinical examination, hematology, blood chemistry, urinalysis, gross pathology and histopathology. Additional observations or tests should be included either as a direct result of observations made during interim sacrifices or as a result of prior knowledge based on structural similarities to compounds studies previously or on earlier screening studies, either acute or subacute.

It is clear that toxicity testing should be done under the guidance of qualified scientists who, by training and experience, are competent to respond to unforeseen toxicological manifestations noted during the course of the study by initiating reasonable additional experimental procedures or modifications of established protocols. An earlier decision to follow a certain protocol cannot in any way obviate the requirement for data to answer new questions raised by the experimental results of the original protocol when these questions are pertinent at the time of the final evaluation for safe use of the chemical in question. For a better understanding of the problem, it is necessary, at this point, to introduce some general notions which are very well established in human toxicology. It is believed that the application of these concepts to the specific field of experimental toxicology would be useful. These concepts are: 1) the various forms of toxicity directly affecting certain living organisms; 2) the adverse effects indirectly affecting humans, caused by direct biological (possibly toxic) effects on other organisms living in the biosphere; 3) the effect of various factors on manifestation of toxicity; 4) the importance of establishing qualitative and, particularly, quantitative dose–effect relationships so that toxicity thresholds and,therefore, allowable limits can be established.

VARIOUS FORMS OF TOXICITY

1. Acute or subacute toxicity

The first form of toxicity that will be considered is acute or subacute toxicity, i.e., toxicity resulting immediately or after a short delay from the absorption of an adequately large single dose or of several rapidly successive doses of a chemical. In humans, for instance, this occurs following the ingestion of many products, for some, by penetration through the skin and, in the case of gases or vapours, such as carbon monoxide, chlorine, or hydrogen cyanide, following inhalation.

The manifestations of this form of toxicity are spectacular since they may even be expressed in sudden death. That is the reason why the belief that poisons are substances which kill violently is so widespread. Experimentally, for the matter, the estimation of the acute toxicity of a given substance is currently carried out in the laboratory by determining the lethal dose and particularly the lethal dose 50, i.e., the dose which produces death in 50% of the treated animals. This dose may vary widely, depending on the species of experimental animals as well as on diverse factors, particularly the route of the administration. In the case of gases and vapors, when the lethal concentrations is determined, the time of exposure is always specified.

2. Long-term toxicity from absorption of repeated small doses

It cannot be emphasized enough that toxic effects do not only result from absorption of relatively high doses in a short time. Quite often, they also result form the repetitive absorption of even minute doses, or of doses too low to cause acute toxic effects. This repetitive administration leads to intoxications which are much more insidious because they generally appear without any signal. This, then, is a matter of long-term toxicity resulting in the phenomena of cumulation of doses and cumulation of effects. Cumulation of doses occurs particularly in the case of so-called cumulative poisons, e.g., elemental derivatives of arsenic, fluorine, heavy metals (lead, mercury, cadmium, etc.) and halogenated aromatic compounds such as polychlorobiphenyls or inseticides of the DDT-type. These poisons are retained in living organisms due to their physical nature (much greater solubility in lipids than in aqueous liquids; adsorption, etc.), due to their chemical nature (fixation to certain cellular components), or due to their harmful effects on excretory organs which hamper their elimination (heavy metals). The absorption of small doses of such cumulative products which, if normally eliminated, would have no discernible consequences, brings about disorders at the level of the receptors when, after certain time, toxic concentration thresholds have been reached. Cumulation of effects is exemplified by substances with an inherent carcinogenic action. From results obtained in rat studies with paradimethylaminoazobenzene (butter yellow), a hepatoma-producing azo-dye stuff, Druckrey and Kupfmuller in 1949 forwarded the a priori paradoxical concept of addition of effects from each individual dose over the entire lifetime of the experimental animal, whatever the rates of elimination and metabolic degradation. There would not only be a cumulation of doses but a total summation of absolutely irreversible effects. Thus, carcinogenic substances would occupy a separate place among agents of long-term toxicity, because in their case, it would not be possible to establish threshold doses, since, due to persistence of the effect after elimination of the product, no dose, however small, would be without danger if the dose would be repeated and if a sufficiently long period would permit the manifestation of their activity. More recently, however, various considerations made one wonder whether the concept of absolute irreversibility of effects is not an exaggerated presentation of the facts. Certain observations in the field of molecular biology, for instance, make one admit the possibility of a repair of lesions at the level of nuclear macromolecules, lesions which precede the development of malignant proliferation. This involves very important problems which are currently being discussed with great interest on an international level and which prompted research on dose- effect relationships of carcinogenic agents, both physical, like X-rays or radiations emitted by radioactive elements, and chemical,

3. Long-term effects resulting from absorption of a single dose

It should be emphasized that in addition to immediate acute or subacute toxic effects and more or less long-term toxic effects resulting from the repeated absorption of small doses, there are also more or less long-term effects which may result from a single dose or from a single exposure. During the last few years, various examples have been given of products capable of causing serious effects in humans and laboratory animals after a more or less prolonged latency period during which the products themselves had already disappeared from the organism. It is in this way, for instance, that the herbicide Paraquat, derived from bipyridinium, produces, several weeks after ingestion of a certain dose and having caused only a minor gastrointestinal disorder, a proliferation of fibroblasts at the level of the pulmonary epithelium which may become fatal by inhibition of oxigen diffusion. Another example is the delayed neurotoxic action of certain organophosphorus compounds, expressed as axon degeneration in the central nervous system, with demyelination leading to paralysis. These are the so-called 'hit and run poisons'. Research is currently being carried out to discover the biochemical lesions which are at fault.

In certain cases, the effects of a single dose may manifest themselves after a very long time. This has been shown, in experiments with laboratory animals, to be the case with carcinogens like nitrosamines and related substances (nitrosamides). Thus, the administration to a pregnant rat half-way in the gestational period, of N-nitroso-N-methylurea, at a dose which does not cause any apparent toxic effect in that animal, produces cerebral cancers in the offspring when they reach adulthood (transplacental carcinogenesis).

4. Special forms of toxicity: teratogenic and mutagenic effects

The hint at an attack in utero directs attention toward effects on functions of reproduction and, particularly embryotoxic effects. This leads to the examination of teratogenic effects which represent a particular type of embryotoxicity.

Mention should also be made of mutagenic effects, i.e. the production of mutations giving rise to substances with genotoxic properties. Their identification, at least in higher mammals, is difficult, and, currently, work is very actively being carried out in specialized laboratories in an attempt to establish an adequate experimental method. Other very specific effects also deserve attention, for instance, immunosuppressive effects, behavioral effects, sensitizing effects, and many other, perhaps more subtle effects. It is believed that, by simply mentioning these various categories of effects, attention may be drawn to the multiple and multidisciplinary methodological approaches that come into play in the testing for possible toxicity of chemical agents.

CONCLUSION

This paper tried to put into perspective the general principles which should guide the scope and the design of toxicity testing.

We are, however, fully aware that because of the multiplicity and of the complexity of the problem, the approaches taken are far from being ideal in every case. Consequently, we understand the necessity to keep an open mind to new develoments permitting to correct and to improve the toxicological methodologies. Further research in this typically pluridisciplinary field must be encouraged and supported. Nevertheless looking at the situation as it presented itself some 20 years ago, we feel that the toxicological approaches so far followed were very useful in giving, on as much as possible scientific basis, guidance to the regulatory authorities to cope with the difficult task of protecting public health from the impact of the chemical era.

GENERAL REFERENCES

1. Truhaut, R. (1962) Additifs aux aliments: les risques de nocivité pouvant résulter de leur emploi inconsideré. Les méthods de prévention. Bull. Soc. Hyg.Aliment.50 (No.4-5-6), 77-185.

2. Truhaut,R. (1963) Toxicité à long terme et pouvoir cancérogène. Act.Pharmacologiques, 15 Série, Masson Edit. , Paris, 256-306.

3. Truhaut, R. (1966) Problèmes toxicologiques posés par l'emploi des pesticides en agriculture. Bull. de l'I.N.S.E.R.M., 21, 1063-1120.

4. Truhaut, R. (1969) Aperçus sur les dangers de l'ère chimique. Pure and Applied Chem., 18; 111-128.

5. Truhaut, R. (1969) Quelque remarques sur l'evaluation toxicologique des agents chimiques pouvant être incorporés aux aliments. Ann.Hyg.L.Fr.Méd. et Nutrition, 5, 33-44.

6. Truhaut, R. (1970) Observations récentes dans le domain de la toxicologie dit alimentaire. Bull. Acad.Nat.Med., 154, 789-800.

7. Vettorazzi, G. (1979) International Regulatory Aspects for Pesticide Chemicals. Vol. I, Toxicity Profiles, CRC Press Inc., Boca Raton, Florida, U.S.A.

8. Vettorazzi, G. (in press) Handbook of International Food Regulatory Toxicology. Vol. I. Toxicological Methodology and Principles of Interpretation of Experimental Findings. Spectrum Publications Inc., Jamaica, New York 11432, U.S.A.

9. World Health Organization. Principles and Methods for Evaluating the Toxicity of Chemicals. Part I, W.H.O.,Geneva, Switzerland.

© 1980 Elsevier/North-Holland Biomedical Press
The Principles and Methods in Modern Toxicology
C.L. Galli, S.D. Murphy and R. Paoletti, editors.

CHEMICAL SAFETY EVALUATIONS AND TOXICOLOGICAL DECISIONS

G.VETTORAZZI

Scientist,World Health Organization,Geneva,Switzerland, and

Professor of Experimental Toxicology,University of Milan,Italy

INTRODUCTION

Safety evaluations as they relate to chemical substances may
mean different things to different people. For example, to the drug
toxicologist safety evaluation is the process by which therapeutic
effects are related to the lethal effect by establishing a margin
of safety or 'therapeutic index'. This practice has been a common
procedure in pharmacology with regard to drug development for many
years; it should be, however, noticed that the same practice has
become more complex since the drug toxicologist today wishes to
develop drugs that have not only a high therapeutic index but also
a high index regarding all undesirable side actions and all undesi=
rable effects of the drug.

To the occupational toxicologist safety evaluation indicates the
process of identifying and interpreting data on uptake/response
relationship with the aim of establishing permissible levels of
occupational exposure. Similarly, to the environmental(including
food) toxicologist safety evaluation, as currently practised, re=
presents the determination, for a given compound, of the dose that
is without detectable effect in the experimental animal of choice
and then, by application of 'safety factors' to that dose, the
estimation of the amount that can safely be consumed by man.

At first sight carrying out a safety evaluation on a chemical it
may appear a relatively simple process whether the toxic material
is a drug, industrial chemical, environmental contaminant or a

natural product. In reality, safety evaluations are anything but
simple, particularly when concepts such as risk estimation and so=
cially acceptable risk are brought to bear.

There seemsto be general consensus that a sound safety evalua=
tion should be based on sound toxicological considerations and
decisions. These decisions, by their very nature, belong in the do=
main of technical and scientific decisions rather than in that of
political and administrative ones, and they should, therefore, be
based solely on technical and scientific knowledge. In turn, poli=
tical and administrative decisions as to whether the use of a
substance presents a socially acceptable risk are based on the
toxicological decisions that have been taken after exhaustive scru=
tiny of scientifica facts. It follows that the availability of
scientific data when a toxicological decision is taken is crucial
to the whole process of safety evaluation of a chemical. The qua=
lity of the decision will reflect the quality and the quantity of
the data on which it has been based.

Safety evaluations and toxicological decisions are commonly car=
ried out by individuals operating in 'expert committees' and very
rarely by one individual or by computer; in a matter which requires
broad representation of many disciplines and vast partecipation of
solid experience, society feels better protected when it relies
upon collective judgements rather than upon whims of individuals.
At present, there are many of these 'expert committees' at the
national, regional and international level. In addition to carrying
out safety evaluations on a great variety of chemical substances,
these groups have also been operational in fostering the development
of requirements for testing procedures, which, over the past
several decades, have become more complex and elaborate. In the
1940's, for example,it was not uncommon to call a study of thirty
days' duration a chronic toxicity study. Total testing of safety
of food chemicals and drugs was commonly conducted in a few rats,

a few rabbits and a few mice; this was considered an adequate to=
xicological data base at that time. By the late 1950', safety
testing had become more elaborate and more formalized. A 1958
World Health Organization(WHO) report distinguished between three
types of toxicity studies: acute, short-term and long-term(chronic).
In 1959, the staff of the U.S. Food and Drug Administration Divi=
sion of Pharmacology published a major review of the then existing
requirements for toxicity testing of chemicals. This review incor=
porated the principles of the WHO report of the prior year and
provided additional information on the techniques used in the
interpretation of toxicological findings in animals. It was a ma=
jor milestone in toxicological testing and served as a guideline
for such testing for a number of years. Throughout the 1960' and
1970's further elaboration of toxicological testing has taken pla=
ce. Chronic toxicity testing sometimes included both rodent and
non-rodent species, and the period of observation in non-rodents
frequently extended for half a decade or more. Further attention
was directed toward appraisal of teratogenic, mutagenic and embryo
toxic effects. A National Academy of Science (U.S.) report gives a
good summary of the status of the general requirements for toxico=
logical testing of chemicals as of 1970.

It is clear that the past thirty-five years have seen a major
change in the accepted requirements for toxicological testing of
chemicals in general and food chemicals in particular, from rela=
tively simple testing to a very complex battery of testing procedu
res. These current procedures are designed to elicit not only the
conventional adverse reactions that can occur from a chemical, but
also the more subtle and complex expression of toxicity that may
only be observed over the entire lifespan of the experimental ani=
mal, for example, in carcinogenicity testing or in multigeneration
reproduction studies. It is anticipated that the next thirty-five
years will produce similar improvements in toxicity testing. Toxi=

cology is, of course, a very dynamic field, and there is little
doubt that new types of testing procedures will ever cease to be
proposed.

THE PROCESS

There are two main stages in the toxicological assessment of a
chemical. The first is the collection of relevant data, which are
usually derived from experimental testing in laboratory animals
and, whenever possible, from observations in humans. The second is
the interpretation and assessment of the data in order to arrive
at a decision about the limits of acceptability that will protect
humans without, possibly, hampering the proper use of the chemical.
The whole process includes the following major steps: The toxico=
logical methodology (1) leads to the design of appropriate investi
gations (2), which ought to supply adequate information (3) which,
given proper interpretation (4), could assist in the formulation
of toxicological decisions (5), which should provide a reasonable
basis for regulations (6) on the safe use of a chemical substance.

Steps (4) and (5), may not, or may only partially be combined
since the interpretation of the results obtained experimentally by
the scientist who conducted the investigation would have to be ta=
ken into consideration by the group of individual experts charged
with the task of formulating a decision.

ASSESSMENT (the concept of Acceptable Daily Intake)

The expression 'Acceptable Daily Intake' has become part of the
terminology concerning the safety evaluation principally of food
chemicals and it has been condensed into an acronym (ADI). This
expression has been extensively used to denote either a concept or
a figure expressed in terms of milligrams per Kilogram of body
weight. The concept of the ADI is based on the widely accepted
opinion that all chemicals are toxic but that their toxicity vary

markedly, not only in nature, but also in the amount that is requi_
red to produce signs and symptoms of toxicity. The figure(mg/kg
body weight) is derived from experimental data in laboratory ani=
mals and/or appropriate observations in humans. It is defined as
the amount of a chemical that could be ingested daily without ap=
preciable risk to the person, in the light of all information avai_
lable at the time of the evaluation. 'Without appreciable risk' is
taken to mean the practical certainty that injury will not result
after a lifetime of exposure. From the above discussion it appears
that the ADI figure is intended to represent an index of safety for
chemicals, serving as a basis for assessing the health hazards of
chemicals in the diet.

How are the ADI figures arrived at during the process of evalua_
tion? In general, the interpretation of toxicological data rests
on the judgement of experts and involves the identification of a
no-effect level based preferably and when available, on long-term
toxicological studies. This level should be the daily dose that
produces no indication of toxicity in the test animal. When the
toxicity data available on a specific chemical is abundant, the
selection of a no-effect level from a particular investigation may
require time-consuming efford on the part of experts.

It may be useful at this point to indicate one of the general
principle of experimental toxicological methodology. This princi=
ple states that there will be some quantity of each chemical below
which there will be no detectable effect on biological systems
(threshold limit), and that there will be some greater amount at
which a significant effect will be observed on essentially all bio_
logical systems (effect limit). Between that amount of each chemi=
cal which produces no effects and that amount which produces a
significan effect, there will be a range of amounts that will pro=
duce significant effects on some types of biological systems. It is
generally among this range of amounts that a level is chosen

for extrapolating safe levels in humans. This is generally done by
applying a safety factor to the no-effect level established in
experimental animals.

SAFETY FACTORS

It has been observed that the most uncertain aspect of any sa=
fety evaluation is the relevance of animal data to humans. This
uncertainty originates not only from the problem of species dif=
ferences, but also and principally from the very nature of the ty=
pe of safety index that one wishes to derive from the maximum dai=
ly dose of a chemical which could be fed continually to an appro=
priate animal species without ill-effect. For food chemicals this
index of safety is the ADI.

Extrapolation to humans is accomplished by dividing the no-
effect level in animals by an arbitrary factor. The degree of sa=
fety thus obtained will vary with the size of the factor chosen as
well as with the slope of the log dose-response curve.

For the sake of clarity, however, it should be pointed out that
the safety factors used in safety evaluations of food chemicals
and the margin of safety obtained by this process, are not to be
confused with the connotations that are given to these terms by
either the experimental toxicologist of the drug toxicologist. For
the experimental toxicologist the margin of safety is the magnitu=
de of the rage of doses involved in progressing from the non-effec
tive dose to a lethal dose when comparing relative toxicities. If
for compound X the range is less than for compound Y, compound Y
is said to have a greater margin of safety than compound X. Simil
arly, for the drug toxicologist, the margin of safety is the dosa
ge range between the dose producing the lethal effect and the dose
producing the desired effect.

In contrast, the margin of safety employed in toxicological
evaluation of food chemicals is one which allow for facts such as

any differences in sensitivity between the animal species used in
the experiment and humans, the wide variations in sensitivity among
human population, the fact that the number of animals tested is
small when compared with the size of the human population that may
be exposed as well as the greater variaty of complicating disease
processes in the human population, the difficulty of estimating the
human intake and the possibility of synergistic action among chemicals.
A discussion on the size of arbitrary factors may lead to further
appretiation of this pragmatic solution. The safety factors propo=
sed by some methods relative to risk assessment take account of the
slope of the log dose-response curve and its standard deviation so
that the acceptable daily intake for humans should be the threshold
daily dose found in the most appropriate animal species minus six
standard deviations. Other authors suggest to extrapolate to the
acceptable daily intake by means of an arbitrary shallow probit
slope of one normal deviate per log, giving 1 in a 100 million
'safety'. The simple method, however, is to divide the maximum no-
effect level from animal experiments by an arbitrary factor of 100.
The only reason for 100 and not 101 is merely because 100 has been
widely used. However, the size of this safety factor can be varied
according to the case dealt with and based on the opinionated
experts' judgement. In practice, the margin of safety has varied
from 10-fold to 500-fold, based principally on the scope and compre
hensiveness of the data available. Examples of reasons for varia=
tions: the case of a chemical for which an adequate amount of toxi=
cological data is not available; situations where temporary ADIs are
recommended; wide variation in daily intake of foods particularly
popular with children; the nature of the toxic effect produced by a
chemical at very high levels of intake; in the case of an intentio=
nal food chemical being a beneficial constituent of the diet or
being a normal body constituent, or a normal intermediary metaboli=
te or converted by digestion or metabolism to a normal constituent

of the diet; when a substance is not absorbed from the gastrointes=
tinal tract and when the toxicological data derived from experiments
in humans are available which would obviate the need for interspe=
cies extrapolation.

In summary, it can be said that the 100-fold margin of safety is
a useful general guide which should not be rigidly applied and its
magnitude is technically a factor of the adequacy of available
toxicological data.

Biological scientists generally agree that for every biological
effect there can be demonstrated in each individual experimental
system, humans, mouse, or in vitro preparation, a threshold level
where the effect will not be evoked. This threshold level will vary
from one individual to another, but it may be impractical to estima
te the level at which the most susceptible indivisual in a popula=
tion will not respond. Nevertheless, safety evaluations until now
have been founded on the concept of determining the maximum no-
effect dose. The unique difficulties inherent in safety evaluations
arise from this unusual goal of attempting to prove scientifically
that no deleterious effect can take place, i.e. to prove the nega=
tive. On the one hand, experimenters are concerned with establish=
ing that phenomena apparently resulting from their experiments are
real and not artifacts that have occurred simply by chance. On the
other hand, the concern is also to ensure that the absence of posi=
tive findings, assuming adequate protocols and procedures, is not
due to chance or to the inadequancy of sample size. It should, how=
ever, recognized that the usual practice of concluding 'no-effects'
when statistically significant changes have not been observed tends
to encourage poor experimentation if the ultimate goal is only to
demonstrate 'no-effects'. Nevertheless, the 'no-effect' approach
with the 100-fold margin of safety has been a practical approach to
a difficult problem. This approach has usually worked well but its

acceptance should not obscure the fact that it has no experimental or theoretical basis. When followed blindly, as some author have pointed out, it can lead occasionally to rather irrational experi= mental practices which should not be uncritically accepted.

ESSENTIAL DATA REQUIREMENTS

The type of information required for the assessment of the to= xicity of a chemical is a complex matter. The matter is further complicated if the assessment of toxicity relates principally to chronic rather than acute effects. Representative examples of this order are the carcinogenic, mutagenic and teratogenic effects, which are insidious, hard to predict and for which the levels of exposu= re are generally very low but sometimes of very long duration. It can, therefore, be appreciated how the design and the suitabili= ty of a specific toxicological testing procedure could have been, and still may be, the object of controversy among workers in the field.

In general, the type of information and the procedures that ge= nerate it, should be designed to permit the estimation of a maximum no-effect dose using laboratory animal models. The extrapolation of findings and observations from these animal models to humans for assessing human health hazards is then accomplished based on a generally agreed assumption that if a particular effect is observed in several species of animals, there is a good possibility that this effect will also be observed in humans; at least, this pos= sibility should not be excluded without some sound specific reasons.

The following type of information is usually considered neces= sary for safety evaluation of chemicals:

a) Chemical profile

Adequate chemical specifications for identity and purity of the substance under testing are extremely important in toxicological assessment. This tends to be the most neglected aspect and at

18

times it may deceive scientists by its apparent simplicity. The na=
me of a substance by itself is totally useless without an accompa=
nying definition of what is intended by that name. A chemical pro=
ducts is not a single compound but a commercial product that may
contain perhaps only 70% of the pure compound after which the pro=
duct is named; it may contain 90% or 95% but never 100%. For the
purpouse of the toxicological evaluation the purity of a substan=
ce could be irrelevant, the important consideration being only
whether the purity of the material used is consistent with the pu=
rity of the material that was toxicologically tested. This aspect
presents a number of difficulties. For example, materials that were
tested many years ago may not have had adequate specifications and
this may call into question the acceptability of the toxicological
data because its relevance to the material manufactured at the pre=
sent time is unknown. Furthermore, materials of different specifi=
cations may have been used for different parts of the testing pro=
gram. These may be materials of different grades prepared by the
same manufacturer or materials of similar grade but produced by
different manufacturers using different processes. It follows that
it is highly irresponsible to carry out new toxicological tests on
chemicals that are already in use without ensuring that the mater=
ial used complies with the appropriate specifications.

Before toxicity tests are undertaken, the investigator must be
certain that the material supplied for testing has the same speci=
fications as that which will subsequently be used commercially. He
must also know the nature and quantity of the more important impu=
rities, since these may represent a greater health hazard than the
chemical itself. The chemical nature and physical properties of
the substance under test may guide the investigator in the design
of his experiments since they may indicate possible pathways of
absorption and metabolism, as well as likely biological effects.

It should be emphasized, however, that the toxic or other bio=

logical effects of the test material cannot be predicted solely
from considerations of its chemical and physical properties.
Specifications for chemicals produced commercially should be broad
enough to include all the variations in the composition that, ac=
cording to current knowledge, do not significantly affect their
biological properties. Tests for impurities such as lead, arsenic
and other metals as a measure of good manufacturing practice
should be maintained, unless and until a better measure becomes
available. These tests are needed, irrespective of the high stan=
dards usually maintained in manufacture, in case where inexperien=
ced and less well-equipped manufacturers may produce the same
chemicals.

It is therefore essential that adequate specifications for
identity and purity should be available before toxicological work
is initiated. Toxicologists and regulatory bodies need assurance
that the material to be tested corresponds to that to be used in
practice. Ideally, the specifications should be such as to define
a material that will give reproducible biological results.

b) Metabolic and biochemical profile

A number of types of studies are included under this heading.
Significant biochemical aspects include mode, rate and degree of
absorption, level of storage in organs and tissues, metabolic
transformation, and mode and rate of elimination. Modifications
of substances during metabolism may significantly affects their
toxicity. Knowledge of whether or not a chemical is rapidly me=
tabolized into innocuous degradation products, rapidly excreted or
accumulated in certain organs and tissues may be of great value in
assessing potential hazards. Studies of the metabolism of the
material, together with the identification of the metabolites,
might be extended to include balance experiments in which an at=
tempt is made to account for the administered dose as metabolites
excreted or material stored in the body. These studies would be

done in the first instance with high dosage levels and should be
extended to include doses nearer the levels proposed for use and
the study of the effects of continuous administration. Other in=
vestigations might include the examination of enzymic processes
which may be affected, the effect on the nutritive value of the
diet, and the possibility of the formation of toxic substances
during processing, storage and house-hold preparation.

In some cases it may be desirable, in order to learn more
about the mode of action, to carry out certain studies in which
pharmacodynamic techniques are used. Such investigations might
well reveal effects which are not apparent in the short- and
long-term feeding tests, for instance, effects on the cardiovas=
cular, autonomic, nervous or reproductive systems.

There are examples of a major metabolite being inactive and a
minor one being more active than the original material from which
both were derived. Balance studies in which all the metabolites
have to be accounted for are much more difficult than the usual
study in which the identification of one or two metabolites is
all that is accomplished.

As stated above, most metabolic studies must be done at high
dosage levels in the first instance, if the experimenter is to
have any chance of isolating the metabolites. Metabolic processes
are influenced by the size of the dose, and the proportion of the
dose excreted as a particular metabolite may vary at different
dosage levels.

Biochemical studies are long-term projects involving basic
research and they are unlikely to replace the chronic toxicity
tests in the foreseeable future. However, an adequate knowledge of
the metabolism and biochemical effects of a chemical has provided
in some cases a satisfactory basis for recommending its use or
rejection. Furthermore, some compounds may be converted into
substances already present naturally in the body in much greater

amounts. If the biochemical evidence shows that the sole effect of
the chemical is to make a small contribution to existing metabo=
lic loads from natural components, there is no need for detailed
toxicological studies.

In addition, it may be possible to dispense with elaborate
long-term studies if it can be convincingly shown that the subs=
tance is not absorbed or it is broken down completely before abs=
ortion into well-known substances that are generally recognized
as having no deleterious action. In any case, a proper understan=
ding of the changes that the chemical may undergo in the gastro=
intestinal tract or in the body is necessry for the full inter=
pretation of the biological and toxicological data.

Finally, it is highly important that information about the me=
tabolism and distribution of a substance undergoing testing should
be obtained at an early stage since it may then be possible to
make similar investigations in humans. The information from such
investigations will make it possible to choose, for further expe=
rimentation, the animal species corresponding most closely to
the human body in the absorption and metabolism of the chemical,
and thus to obtain data on animal toxicity that will enhance pre=
dictive value.

c) Acute toxicity profile

The term 'acute toxicity test' implies the study of the effects
Produced by the test material when administered generally in a
single dose. The acute toxicity tests should give sufficient in=
formation to enable comparisons of the toxicity of related mate=
rials to be made and to provide the necessary information for the
planning of further studies. Acute toxicity tests may indicate
variation among species and yield some information on the signs
of intoxication and pathological effects. Observations should in=
clude the onset, nature and duration of toxic signs, as well as
mortality. It is important that autopsies be performed on some

animals that die and on some of the survivors. Microscopic examina=
tions of tissues should be carried out if the macroscopic observations indicate that they are needed.

d) Short-term studies

These studies include all investigations other than those conti_
nued for most of the animal lifespan; they are commonly carried
out over 10% of the lifespan or less. As a rule, a number of
different species are used. It is probable that the majority of
toxic effects can be demonstrated in such studies. The dosage level
at which deleterious effects occur, the time taken to cause them,
and the nature of the effects produced are all of interest and of
potential importance. relevant observations in humans may be use=
ful in revealing gross species differences.

The purpose of the short-term tests are to examine the biolo=
gical nature of toxici effects, to assess possible cumulative
action, the variation in species sensitivity, the nature of macro-
and microscopic changes and the approximate dose level at which
these effects occur. They may also provide guidance for the selec=
tion of dosage for long-term tests and indicate special studies
that may be necessary.

e) Long-term studies

Different opinions have been expressed regarding long-term
toxicity studies. By and large, the designation 'long-term studies'
implies the study of the effects produced by the test material
when administered in repeated doses over a long period of time,
usually the major portion of the expected lifespan of short-lived
animal species, sometimes covering the entire lifespan and more
than one generation of such species.

Long-term toxicity tests are carried out to ascertain the ma=
ximum dosage level which produces no discernible ill-effects when
administered over the major portion of the lifespan of the experi=
mental animal, and to reveal effects which are not predictable

from short-term tests.

One of the most important test in the category of chronic stu=
dies is that carried out over the greater part of the animal's
lifespan. Such tests are essential for the assessment of the car=
cinogenic risk and they are also important for the evaluation of
the acceptable or tolerable levels of the chemical under testing,
since it may be ingested daily for the whole lifespan.

f) Special studies

While this heading is rather confusing, it has been customary to
include under it all investigations designed to detect a specific
effect.

I. Reproduction,embryotoxicity and teratogenicity
Studies

If, during the course of short- or long-term studies or in a
pilot experiment there is any evidence to suggest that reproduction
may be affected, specific studies should be undertaken. Reproduc=
tion studies must be carried out in a suitable species over at
least two generations and may have to be continued over three or
more. They should be designed to provide relevant information on
fertility, progress of pregnancy, post-partum condition and pro=
gress of mothers and offspring. Reproduction studies may be de=
signed to include investigations on embryotoxicity and teratogeni=
city (by teratogenicity is meant a toxic effect on the embryo or
the foetus resulting in a congenital abnormality).

Alternatively, it may be more convenient to conduct separate
investigations on these aspects. Many suggested procedures for the
se studies have been published, but no one particular design has
yet emerged as being universally acceptable.

II. Mutagenicity studies

Mutagenic action of chemicals represent a problem since,although
exposure to chemicals in the external environment is increasing,
there is little information on their possible mutagenic action.

This problem cannot be ignored, since it represent one of the poten tial risks from chemical exposure. However, this possible risk must always be considered in the context of toxicological hazards in general.

No specific tests are recommended for the assessment of mutage= nic risk, however some safeguard is provided by multigeneration studies while stressing the difficulties of extrapolating experi= mental data on mutagenicity of chemicals obtained in bacterial systems, yeasts, or Drosophila to possible hazards of chemicals in humans; these special procedures commonly used to detect mutagenic activity cannot be recommended at this point as part of a decision making process.

Many known mutagenic agents belong to classes of chemicals that need metabolic activation. Lack of metabolic activation has been one of the principal limitations of studies in in vitro and micro= bial systems. Furthermore, the activation process in submammalian systems, e.g. Drosophila, might be different from that in mammals and in humans. The development of in vitro systems, including meta bolic activation systems derived from mammals or humans, may make possible rapid screening of substances. Data from such systems would be of value for setting priorities for more definitive mammalian testing.

No single test system can detect and characterize all mutagenic agents; therefore, the use of several tests is desirable and these should primarily be done in mammals. In addition, a number of in vitro and sub-mammalian test systems might be used to answer specific questions.

III. Carcinogenicity studies

From a review of the specialized literature it is evident that tests on experimental animals cannot provide irrefutable proof of the safety of carcinogenicity of a substance for the human species. It is however at least reassuring that the known carcinogenic

activities of certain chemicals in humans are similar in many
ways to those found in experimental animals. Hence it is only
prudent to determine, so far as it is practicable, the carcinoge=
nicity in experimental animals of chemicals. The results of such
tests should determine to a considerable degree whether or not
these substances should be used. It is therefore necessary to
formulate practical procedures for the determination of possible
carcinigenicity within the limits of our present knowledge, and
it is desiderable that all chemicals be fully investigated. It is
however recognized that the available facilities and experienced
personnel for carrying out such studies are limited and may
remain so for an unpredictable time. Therefore, the proposed tests
should be relatively simple and no more time-consuming than neces
sary to facilitate the testing of as many chemicals as possible
within a reasonable period of time.

Several factors must be taken into account in deciding the
scope of the tests required in the case of any particular substan=
ce, namely, the nature of the substance, impurities present, the
proposed use, the particular medium involved, the amount which is
likely to be ingested, and the age and physical condition of the
main consumers. Such considerations would allow for reasonable
priorities in testing to be established and thus provide broader
safeguards in the shortest possible time.

The view has been generally adopted that the minimum safeguard
must be an investigation of the tumour incidence in a chronic
toxicity test. This should involve the study of an adequate number
of animals of two species(e.g. rats and mice) subjected for a
food chemical to the feeding of a suitable dose range of the subs=
tance under question for the lifetime of the animals. Where addit=
ional safeguards are considered necessary, because of the nature
of the chemical or its proposed use, further tests such as the
use of a suitable parenteral route of administration, or studies in

other species of animals, are commonly recommended.

Recent reports discuss current theories regarding the relation ship between mutagenesis and carcinogenesis, postulate similari= ties between the mechanisms of mutagenesis and the mode of action of major groups of chemical and physical carcinogens.

There is increasing evidence that many chemical carcinogens in their carcinogenically reactive form can induce mutations in mi= crobial and some mammalian test systems. But it is impossible to assess whether or not these common properties of many chemical carcinogens and mutagens also point to common sequences of events resulting in a cancer cell or a mutated cell. Furthermore, some potent mutagens do not appear to be carcinogenic in any of the test systems used and certain carcinogens have not been demonstra= ted to be mutagenic. One major difficulty in the comparison of mutagenic and carcinogenic actions is the use of results obtained from different test systems. Induction of point mutations is repor ted mostly from studies in microbial systems, whereas chromosomal abnormalities have been observed in tissue culture and, more recently, in vivo. Carcinogenicity, on the other hand, is repor= ted largely from in vivo studies in rodents. A second difficulty arises from the need for metabolic activation of many chemical mutagens and carcinogens. Until recently most in vitro systems used in mutagenesis bioassays have lacked this activation poten= tial. It is thought that metabolic activation converting a pre-carcinogen into 'ultimate' carcinogen is analogous to the change from pre-mutagen to the 'ultimate' mutagen.

It can be concluded that the relationship between carcinogene= sis and mutagenesis requires further investigation. However, the association between carcinogenicity and mutagenicity of many compounds is sufficiently great to justify the use of mutagenicity tests as pre-screening procedures for possible carcinogens.

g) Epidemiological profile and observations in humans

It has been recognized that observations in humans are of pri=
me importance because of the differences between one species and
another in reactions to toxic substances and the subsequent un=
certainty when extrapolating data from animals to human beings.

Studies in humans may be carried out by the careful observation
of individuals who have ingested the test compound. Additional da=
ta may be obtained by studying individuals exposed to chemicals
occupationally or through accidental ingestion. Finally, studies
may also be carried out in populations consuming a given substance
at high levels because of ethnic proclivities or for therapeutic
reasons.

The usefulness of these studies when coupled with results ob=
tained in experimental animals for predictive purposes should be
emphasized.

Studies in experimental animals on the biological effects of
chemicals that may be introduced into the environment have as one
of their major objective the prediction of any possible hazard to
humans. One of the greatest problem that arises in these studies
is in the extrapolation of the data obtained from investigations
in animals and to the definition of safe levels of exposure in
humans.

Ethical and legal problems may arise in connection with the
provision of human volunteers for toxicological investigations.
Since the situation differs greatly from country to country, it
should be left to the appropriate authorities in each country to
decide any issue involved.

Studies in human volunteers are useful for confirming predicted
margin of safety. Chemicals intended for use as drugs are subjected
to human pharmacological investigations and to clinical trials
that must, of necessity, involve the use of biologically effecti=
ve dosage levels. In the examination of other chemicals from a

toxicological point of view, it is sometimes necessary to ascer=
tain whether the safety margin predicted from animal data is va=
lid. For this purpose it may be helpful to administer the chemical
to human volunteers.

The importance of the desirability of supplementing animal
studies on chemicals by investigations in humans applies specially
to substances to be used in infant food.

TOXICOLOGICAL DECISIONS

Below are listed and summarized the most important conclusions
and decisions regarding the toxicological aspects of chemicals
with special reference to food chemicals which are presently
used in assessing safety.

Acceptable Daily Intake (ADI). The acceptable daily intake
(ADI) expressed on a body weight basis (mg/kg bw) is the amount
of a food chemical that can be taken daily in the diet, even over
a life time, without appreciable risk to human health. It is
generally allocated only to substances for which the available
data include either the results of adequate short-term and long-
term toxicological investigations or satisfactory information on
the biochemistry and metabolic fate of the compound, or both.
Concerning the question of whether or not an ADI allocated to a
particular food chemical can be applied to both sexes and to all
age classes and health conditions including the newborn, infants
and young children, it can be said that, in principle, the safety
factors utilized for the establishment of an ADI should be suffi=
cient to provide for individual variations in metabolism and
sensitivity to foreign chemicals. Consequently, for most food
chemicals, the ADI should be applicable to all children older
than 12 weeks. The applicability, however, of ADI to pregnant
women or to persons in special health conditions (e.g. the under=
nourished, the chronically disable, etc.) has never been specifi=

cally discussed and there are reasons to consider that this pro=
blem warrants further discussion. In this respect, toxicological
and metabolic studies of food chemicals should always include in=
vestigations that would permit an evaluation of safety for these
particular conditions.

Temporary ADI. An ADI may be allocated temporarily, pending
the provision of additional data within a stated period of time.
This measure implies that the toxicological data are adequate to
ensure the safety in use of the chemical during the time for
which the temporary ADI applies. If the additional data necessary
to ensure safety over life time do not become available within
the stated period of time, the temporary ADI may be withdrawn.

ADI not specified. An ADI without an explicit indication of
upper limit of intake may be assigned to substances of very low
toxicity, especially those that are food constituents or that may
be considered as foods or normal metabolites in the human body.
A food chemical having an 'ADI not specified' must meet the cri=
teria of good manufacturing practice – for example, it should
have proved technological efficacy and be used at the minimum
level to achieve technological efficacy, it should not be used to
conceal inferior food quality or adulteration, and it should not
create a nutritional imbalance. The above expression means that,
on the basis of available data (chemical, biochemical and toxico=
logical), the total daily intake of the substance arising from its
use or uses at levels necessary to achieve the desired effect
and from its acceptable background in food, does not represent a
hazard to health. For this reason, and for the reasons stated in
the individual evaluations, the establishment of an acceptable
daily intake expressed in mg/kg body weight is not deemed neces=
sary.

Conditional ADI. This decision implies that there are circums=
tancies in which provisions are made for special use conditions.

No ADI allocated. This decision is applicable to substances for which the available information is not sufficient to esta= blish their safety or when the specifications for identity and purity are not adequate. The fact that an ADI for a chemical was not established should not be interpreted as casting doubt on its safety nor should it be considered for its withdrawal for use.

Not to be used. This decision is applicable to substances for which there is sufficient information on which to base such deci= sion.

Decision postponed. This expression is applicable to cases when no precise information is available concerning matters re= lated to technological uses.

Acceptable level of treatment. Acceptable daily intakes are expressed in milligram of the substance in question per kilogram body weight. There are, however, certain food chemicals that are more appropriately limited in terms of level of treatment, for example, flour treatment agents.

Acceptable residues. Acceptable residues in human food have been established for antibiotic substances found in food.

Maximum residue limit. A maximum residue limit is the maxi= mum concentration of a pesticide residue resulting from the use of a pesticide according to good agricultural practice directly or indirectly for the production and/or protection of the food commodity for which the limit is recommended. It is expressed in milligrams of the residue per kilogram of the commodity.

Temporary maximum residue limit. A temporary maximum residue limit is a maximum residue limit established for a specified, limited period.

Extraneous residue limit. An extraneous residue limit is, for a particular food commodity, the maximum toxicologically accepta= ble concentration of a residue unavoidably arising from sources other than the use of a pesticide directly or indirectly for the production of that food commodity.

Guideline level. A guideline level is the maximum concentration of a pesticide residue that might occur in food after the officially recommended or authorized use of the pesticide for which no acceptable daily intake or temporary acceptable daily intake is established and that need not to be exceeded if good agricultural practice is followed.

Provisional tolerable weekly intake. This decision is established because it is inappropriate to attempt to set ADIs for heavy metals as mercury, lead and cadmium. In retrospect, it is plain that the concept of the ADI for any substance is based on the assumption that each day's intake is ultimately cleared from the body and that, for the most part, such clearance is rapid and complete (unless the compound gives rise to biotransformation products that enter the intermediate metabolism). Exceptions to this general rule have been encountered and have involved the storage of low levels of lipophilic compounds in the body fat of humans. Furthermore, ADIs are intended to be used in allocating the acceptable amounts of a food chemical to specific intended uses where it will serve necessary technological purposes and will be employed in accordance with good manufacturing or agricultural practices. Such concepts are inapplicable to trace contaminants. In view of the above considerations, a new approach was needed in dealing with heavy metal contaminants of food. The basis for this approach is as follows: a) The contaminants are able to accumulate within the body at a rate and to an extent determined by the level of intake and by the chemical form of the heavy metal present in food. Consequently, the basis on which intake is expressed should be more than the amount corresponding to a single day. Moreover, individual foods may contain above-average levels of heavy metal contaminant, so that consumption of such foods on any particular day greatly enhances that day's intake. Accordingly the provisional tolerable intake is expressed on a weekly basis. b) The term 'tolerable', signifying permissibility than acceptability, is used in those cases where intake of a contaminant is unavoidably associated with the consumption of otherwise wholesome and nutri= tious foods, or with inhalation in air. c) The use of the term 'provisional' expresses the tentative nature of the evaluation, in view of the paucity of reliable data on the consequences of human exposure at levels approaching those with which concern should be expressed.

CONCLUSION

Chemical safety assessment is today an important activity which often represent a challenge to public health departments with more traditional emphasis on known health risks to human populations. The chemical era into which the world has entered at the beginning of the century had posed toxicological problems of a different character to those encountered in other histori= cal periods. Correspondingly, the field of toxicology has consi= derably grown.

With the advent of chemical safety assessments toxicology has become linked with regulatory attempts to control toxic chemicals in the total environment, food, water and air. It has thus evolved from an experimental science to a science with a clear social character. The food we eat, the water we drink, the air we breath can be contaminated by potentially toxic chemicals. Toxicology today is concerned with the study of toxic effects evoked by the chemical agents we become in contact in our every day life; furthermore, once the risk factor has been identified, toxicology tries to minimize such a risk by establishing guide= lines for prevention of exposure, safe or tolerable levels and, wherever possible, to indicate treatment in case of overexposure.

Since the continuous release of chemicals into the environment will not be easily stopped, toxicological assessments and safety

evaluations are measures in our hands to foster the knowledge
of the toxic effects produced by these chemical agents on the
human body and to minimize their impact on human health.
The implications for preventive medicine are obvious. The causes
of many degenerative diseases in the human population are unknown.
To the extent that environmental chemicals, for example, are
involved in the cause of human cancer, identifying and control=
ling carcinogenic chemicals could have a major impact.

Finally, the societal need must be balanced against the
estimated risks to society, for this is the only way any
rational decision can be made. With so many chemical compounds
present in the environment today, to develop the data base to
allow risk assessments it will be a major undertaking. But it
must be done, for how can society intelligently regulate
chemicals which pose human benefits and human risks at the same
time without having an estimate of the risk?

GENERAL REFERENCES

Galli,C.L., Paoletti,R. and Vettorazzi,G. (Eds.) Chemical
   Toxicology of Food. Elsevier/North-Holland, 1978

International Agency for Research on Cancer. IARC Monograph
   Programme on the Evaluation of the Carcinogenic Risk of
   Chemicals to Humans. Internal Technical Report No.77/002,
   Lyon, France, 1977

Magri,G.E. (Ed.) Mutagenesis Ambientale. Metodiche di Analisi.
   Vol.I. Test in vitro. AQ/1/18-34. Consiglio Nazionale delle
   Ricerche, Roma, 1979

Ministro della Sanità Italiana (Commissione di Esperti Costi=
   tuita dal). Criteri Guida per la Valutazione degli Effetti
   Mutageni, Cancerogeni e Teratogeni di Composti Chimici.
   Roma,1977

Paget, G.E. (Ed.) Quality Control in Toxicology. MTP Press
   Limited. Lancaster,1977

Vettorazzi, G. International Regulatory Aspects for Pesticide
   Chemicals. Volume I. Toxicity Profiles. CRC Press, Inc.
   Boca Raton, Florida 33431, U.S.A. 1979

Vettorazzi,G. Handbook of International Food Regulatory Toxico=
   logy. Volume I. Toxicological Methodology and Principles
   of Interpretation of Experimental Findings. Spectrum
   Publications, Inc. Jamaica, N.Y. 11432, U.S.A. (in press)

World Health Organization. Principles and Methods for Evalua=
   ting the Toxicity of Chemicals. Part I. WHO,Geneva,
   Switzerland,1978

© 1980 Elsevier/North-Holland Biomedical Press
The Principles and Methods in Modern Toxicology
C.L. Galli, S.D. Murphy and R. Paoletti, editors.

LEGISLATIVE ACTION TENDING TO CONTROL POTENTIALLY TOXIC SUBSTANCES:PURPOSES, MEANS AND PRESENT ACHIEVEMENTS

Alain GERARD
Lecturer at the Brussels University, Director of the Food Law Research Centre ("E.J. Bigwood Centre") at the "Institut d'Etudes européennes".

1. PURPOSES AND BASIC ORIENTATIONS OF LAWS TENDING TO CONTROL THE PRODUCTION, TRADE AND USE OF CHEMICALS

1.1. Purposes

The production of chemicals, either extracted from nature or artificially created, as well as their distribution and their use by industry, agriculture, or even by individual consumers, are not by themselves an innovation. Nevertheless the tremendous development of applied chemistry during the second half of this century has increased considerably the number of chemicals, their use, their presence in the environment and the risk of adverse effects for human beings. Such an evolution, which is spectacular by its nature and by its consequences, requires from public authorities to guarantee by appropriate regulations a sufficient level of protection, both of individuals and of the environment.

The concern for the latter has motivated, in fact, a typical change as to the aims of the related legislation. Legal action in that field commonly tended to protect consumers or users of such products that contain chemical substances likely to cause a damage to health or to affect safety. These regulations, therefore, focus mainly on the use of chemicals, even if particular provisions tend to restrict the discharge of chemicals into water or the atmosphere, to regulate the trade of products containing such chemicals, or to control the exposure of workers to toxic substances at the working place. In the most recent legislations a significant tendency consists in protecting not only consumers' health or users' safety, but also the environment as such, since adverse effects of chemicals can affect human health through water or air as well as they can cause damage through the food chain (food additives) or through medical use (drugs).

Progressively most industrialised countries have set up specific legislations concerning special categories of chemicals according to the intended use, such as substances used as additives in food, drugs, pesticides or fertilisers, etc. It appears, however, that a number of chemicals are excluded from legal control where no comprehensive legislation has been enacted (which is still the common case).

Although legal action relating to chemicals has been, in the past, directed mainly at poisonous or hazardous products that could cause immediate or acute damage to human beings, there is now a systematic tendency of preventing, as far as possible, adverse effects of chemicals on the human health or the environment by anticipating these effects, through appropriate toxicological and eco-toxicological evaluation, before such chemicals are manufactured on industrial scale or imported into the country.

1.2. Possible approaches

At the occasion of a recent colloquium (January 1979) organised in Brussels by the European Environmental Bureau, two basic approaches have been distinguished. The first one has been referred to as the "environmental approach", based on the principle that "new substances must be adequately screened before they are allowed to be commercially produced"[1]. The other approach of toxic substances regulations was called the "commercial" one, characterised by the fact that "industry will always remain responsible for the substances they produce : therefore, governments should not take decisions themselves but only correct the decisions of industry in those cases were they are utterly inacceptable ... At best, governments can claim that some basic information is produced at the moment the substance enters the market"[1].

These antinomic approaches - which are rather two different "philosophies" likely to condition positive legislation on chemical substances - cover several possible regulatory systems which can be summarised as follows , according to their respective legal implications.

1.2.1. The "abuse" principle

The "abuse" principle - corresponding to the "commercial" approach mentioned above - is characterised by the freedom of production or of marketing with the only reservation that governmental authority is entitled, by specific provisions, to restrict or correct possible "abuse" constituted by the manufacturing or marketing of such products that are proved to endanger consumers' health or users' safety. Since there is no limitation to the free distribution of all chemicals which have not been previously prohibited, the legal protection comes only "a posteriori". In the field of regulations governing the use of additives in food, such approach is called the "negative list" system.

In most industrialised countries such a system is being abandoned because it involves an insufficient consumer or environmental protection. It can, however, be improved where it is combined with additional requirements tending to provide the authority with previous appropriate information, enabling it to enact such limitations or prohibitions that the protection of public health will require. The said information results normally from a mandatory notification procedure, but it can be completed on specific request of the authority.

1.2.2. The preventive control principle

In this quite opposite situation there is basically a general prohibition to manufacture, import, distribute or use a product which has not been previously considered as legally acceptable, on the grounds of a toxicological and eco-toxicological evaluation tending to anticipate its effects on human health and the environment. Such a regulatory system implies obviously a more effective and complete protection since it is applied "a priori" and since it is conditioned by previous scientific evaluation to be achieved by, and under the responsibility of the manufacturer or importer.

It implies, finally, a mandatory declaration procedure tending to provide the authority with relevant scientific and technical information relating to the concerned substance.

It implies, subsequently, an official clearance procedure prior to the production (on industrial scale) or to the marketing of the said product. Such a clearance can result :

- Either from governmental regulation, corresponding to the concept of "positive list" in the field of food additives control;
- Or from specific authorisation for manufacturing or distributing the product, which can be given explicitly when a formal decision is enacted ("licensing" procedure) or implicitly when no objection is opposed by the authority within a given term.

1.2.3. Theoretical classification of regulatory systems

It can be concluded that the whole range of possible regulatory systems concerning the control of chemicals can be theoretically classified as follows, according to an increasing order of legal requirements (and with possible combination of several of them) :

(a) Specific legal prohibitions or restrictions relating to the production,
    distribution, use, transportation, storage or disposal of certain defined
    substances.
    In that system, the legislation - or the authority entitled to regulate -
    has to enact case by case such additional or amending provisions that
    appear necessary.

(b) General Provisions subject to further specification by governmental
    regulation.
    The situation is nearly similar to the preceding one, but a more flexible
    regulatory procedure has been instituted to enable the authority to update
    prohibitions or restrictions by specific decisions.

(c) General provisions subject to governmental specifications on the basis of
    scientific or technical information that can be requested by the authority.
    The situation is still basically the same, except that the manufacturer
    or importer can be compelled to provide the authority, but only if requested
    with all relevant information concerning the product when already manu-
    factured or distributed.

(d) Mandatory declaration procedure, applicable before the production (on an
    industrial scale) or the distribution of the product.
    Such a procedure, coupled with general and specific regulations, allows
    the authority to foresee the introduction of new substances and to take
    appropriate measures, either by enacting a specific limitation or prohi-
    bition or by requesting additional information from the industry. To be
    efficient, the declaration procedure must give the authority sufficient
    time to take the appropriate decision.

(e) Mandatory declaration procedure coupled with governmental power to prohibit
    or restrict the production, marketing or use of the substance prior to
    its distribution or manufacture on an industrial scale.
    Insofar as the governmental "veto" power must be exercised within a
    certain period of time during which the ability of manufacturing or
    marketing the product is suspended, this system implies that a legal
    clearance is given to the manufacturer or distributor when no objection
    is expressed by the authority within that given term.

(f) Mandatory declaration procedure coupled with governmental power to
    request a pre-manufacture or pre-market screening of the substance before
    taking appropriate decision.

In this system, the authority may compel the manufacturer or importer of a new substance to produce all relevant toxicological and/or eco-toxicological data that will be deemed appropriate for justifying further clearance.

(g) Authorisation procedure leading to clearance through governmental regulation.

This system implies that a request to manufacture market or use a chemical has to be introduced by the manufacturer or distributor. The authorisation is based on complete toxicological information supplied by the applicant and results from a formal regulation ("positive list") enacted by the authority.

(h) Formal "licensing" procedure.

The situation is the same as the preceding one. It differs only by the fact that a formal "licence" is given case by case by the authority on the basis of previous notification and appropriate toxicological and for eco-toxicological evaluation.

1.2.4. Additional regulatory procedures

(a) Special procedures in case - of imminent hazards.

When a defined chemical, although its manufacturing or marketing has been legally accepted, or has not been objected, by the authority, is proved to create an imminent hazard for human health or for the environment, the authority must be vested with appropriate powers for suspending at once the distribution, use or production and for requiring immediate measures necessary for the protection of the public.

(b) Review procedure.

Since anticipating effects and toxicological evaluation are conditioned by scientific knowledge and technological means, they must always be considered as provisional. Therefore a periodical review procedure is generally included in the law with respect to the legally accepted substances (either by regulatory or explicite or implicite clearance). A delay can be imposed on the authority for that periodical review of the existing list or inventory with a mandate for removing all substances that seem no longer justified.

(c) Public participation procedure.

Insofar as environmental protection is concerned, licensing or reviewing procedures can be subject to public information and discussion where

potentially dangerous substances might have significant environmental
impact. In such case the manufacturing or marketing of these substances
is suspended until the "Environmental Impact Statement" is considered
as complete and correct. Although the Environmental Impact Statement
procedure allows for a better balancing of the environmental aspects
against other (mainly economical) aspects, it seems that it could be hardly
included in a comprehensive regulatory system tending to control the manufacture, distribution or use of chemicals, according to its complexity and
the practical difficulties involved.

Nevertheless, the practice of public participation has become usual in
those countries were "hearings" are instituted for collecting comments or
objections from interested persons in a proposed regulation of general
concern. A less sophisticated system which implies also public participation consists in publishing proposed amendments to existing lists of
accepted substances in order to collect written reactions from interested
persons or institutions within a defined term.

1.3 Legal implications and juridical means

1.3.1. Field of application

Where legislation tending to control chemicals is "use-oriented", the law
refers only to a certain type of substances according to the intended use,
e.g. food additives or drugs. In these examples, a food additive should have
a specified legal definition and a drug is generally defined according to its
purpose (in this case, a substance consumed for preventing or curing deseases).

Since specific legislation ordinarily regulates food additives, food
contaminants, drugs, pesticides, fertilisers, etc., all these categories
of substances subject to particular provisions must be excluded from the scope
of a comprehensive legislation tending to control chemicals. Chemicals which
are not intended for industrial production or general distribution (e.g.
substances produced in small quantities for research purposes) can also be
excluded provided that these exemptions are specified.

1.3.2. General principles governing administrative actions

Some general rules determine criteria governing specific restrictions and
justifying limitations or prohibitions to be enacted by authority. Therefore
such general provisions must be included in the law on the control of toxic
substances, e.g. the rule of preventing unreasonable risk for human health
or the environment.

1.3.3. Executive control or regulatory powers

Precise provisions in the law are necessary for investing the responsible authority with appropriate powers in order to issue subdelegate legislation, taking all measures that will be required by the implementation of the law and organise the control of the compliance to legal provisions. There is a general principle of law that no power can be exercised by an authority unless it has been attributed by a law.

1.3.4. Penal provisions

A similar comment can refer to the penal aspects of the law. It is a general rule of all democratic regimes that only the legislative power is entitled to define all legally prohibited acts as well as the relevant penalities and the appropriate penal procedures for prosecution in court. These provisions must, therefore, be defined in detail in the general law on chemicals.

1.3.5. Emergency action

Among all administrative provisions enabling the authority to take action, a legislation tending to chemical control must empower the authority, as already said, to take appropriate measures that will be required by imminent hazards. Since such an emergency action is by nature exceptional, it has to be defined limitatively by the law. Ordinarily immediate action consists in suspending, or prohibiting provisionally, the manufacture or marketing of chemicals likely to cause imminent damage to the public, and in requesting from the juridical authority (courts) appropriate legal measures (seizure, injunction) that the circumstances will justify.

1.3.6. Substances subject to declaration

Where a mandatory declaration procedure is defined, legislation must determine what categories of substances are subject to previous declaration.

In principle, the chemicals to be declared are newly manufactured or newly imported substances. The concept of "new" substance, however, refers necessarily to a defined situation, which results normally from an existing "positive list" or "inventory" listing already accepted substances. Where a first list or an inventory has not yet been established, the law must define appropriate criteria for precising what types of substances shall be declared.

In principle, mixtures composed of several substances are also subject to declaration. An intended "new use" for an already accepted substance can also be assimilated by the law to a "new substance".

1.3.7. Substances subject to pre-manufacture or pre-market testing

In all "licensing" or "pre-clearance" systems ("positive list" system in the field of food additives control), a toxicological evaluation of the concerned substances is required by means of law before they are allowed to be manufactured, marketed or simply used in products intended for consumers. Where the potential risk of the emission of a chemical into the environment is to be evaluated, eco-toxicological testing is also justified.

The pre-market or pre-manufacture report on possible hazards may not require necessarily a complete testing of the substance. In many cases it can refer, partially or wholly, to previous studies published in the scientific litterature (e.g. technical reports issued by specialised international or national institutions).

Where a mandatory notification system is established, the need of pre-market or pre-manufacture testing depends on the potential risk that the chemical is supposed to cause to human health or the environment. Therefore, the responsible authority keeps a certain latitude of judgement. In such a case, the law on chemicals must define general criteria likely to govern the decision of requiring or not pre-manufacture or a pre-market testing of the substance. Additionally, where no formal authorisation or clearance is made compulsory, the law must determine a delay after which the absence of any request for additional information (including toxicological evaluation) can be regarded as an implicite clearance for the manufacture or marketing of the substance.

1.3.8. Financial burden of testing

When pre-manufacture or pre-market testing is required, the financial burden is to be supported by the manufacturer, importer or distributor who will benefit from the marketing of the substance.

It can happen however that an exemption can be claimed by the notifier and recognised by the authority when it appears that appropriate testing has been already achieved by a previous manufacturer or importer. In such case compensation could have to be paid to the first notifier with due consideration of the cost involved and of the proportion of respective commercial interests. The law must then contain appropriate provisions for fixing criteria of an

equitable share of the testing expenses as well as juridical means for
arbitration.

1.3.9. Nature and content of the information subject to notification or involved in clearance or previous procedures

Since the authority is responsible for public health and environmental
protection, it must be provided with all technical and scientific data likely
to condition the decision to be taken concerning the licensing or prohibition
of a new chemical or mixture. Therefore, the declaration must contain all
specifications that will allow the authority to identify the chemical substance or mixture and to have a basic information on the intended uses, the quantity to be manufactured or imported and the probable effects on human health
and environment.

Where a clearance, licensing or previous authorisation procedure is established, the clearance is obviously based on a toxicological and/or eco-
toxicological evaluation of the product. In such case a clear description
of all data required must appear in the subdelegated legislation in order to
allow the applicant to comply with legal requirements. These data must enable
the authority - generally advised by scientific institutions - to evaluate the
potential risk that the concerned chemical or mixture will cause to human
health or to the environment.

Similar considerations can be expressed relating to the pre-manufacture
or pre-market testing required by the authority according to the law.

1.3.10. Destinatories of the information and disclosure of data

Information contained in mandatory declarations as well as in test reports
are primarily intended for the authority and for the scientific bodies
entitled to consider the data and to give appropriate advice.

It implies thus that the confidential character of certain types of data
must be protected by the law, possibly by specific penalties for those of the
officers who will have unlegally disclosed confidential information.

Nevertheless, some general limitations to the confidentiality of data may be
established by law. A general disclosure is ordinary foreseen with respect to
data relating directly to public health protection. This is particularly the
case in those countries (like U.S.A.) where "hearing procedures" are usually
established in order to collect from every interested person possible objections against an intended regulation or another legal decision likely to concern
the general population. In such case some data can be formally published in

an official notice mentioning also a period of time for collecting observations or possible objections.

Whether the disclosure of data will relate to the previous declaration (mandatory declaration system) or to testing reports (pre-market clearance or hearings procedure), consideration must be given to the legitimate concern of industry in having confidential data not disclosed unless the disclosure is really required for public protection. The type of data subject to disclosure and to publication must, therefore, be clearly stipulated in the law. Specific provisions can additionally compel the authority to inform the manufacturer or importer some time in advance on the data that will be disclosed.

1.3.11. Tests methods

When pre-manufacture or pre-market testing is made mandatory by the law or can be required by the authority, it is obvious that specific provisions either have to determine which methods of testing shall be compulsory, or to standardise the technical testing methods available.

1.3.12. Judicial review or appeal procedures

In all cases where a decision is left to the judgement of the authority with respect to the implementation of the law tending to control chemicals, it is a usual democratic principle that the person concerned - who will be of course the manufacturer or importer of a substance - must have a legal right of appeal against the administrative decision. The case can occur in various situations : prohibition or non acceptance of a substance, new limitation, emergency action, notice of disclosure of data, etc. The appeal is ordinarily considered by courts.

1.3.13. Citizens' individual rights

Citizens' individual rights can be of two different natures. Firstly, they can relate to public interest. In this respect most countries have instituted the citizens' petition right, either in general or defined for specific matters, as it can be the case in the field of chemicals control. Another possibility consists in hearing procedures where they are instituted.

Secondly, by a civil action any citizen has a general right to have a personal damage considered by courts and to obtain appropriate compensation insofar as he is recognised as the victim of a specific tort.

In certain countries the "products liability" theory is also to be considered. This is, however, a matter of general private law which is outside the scope of this lecture.

1.3.13. Consumer protection through classification and labelling

Even when chemicals likely to have potential adverse effects on human health, individual safety or the environment can be legally manufactured or marketed, the protection of users or consumers requires that such chemicals to be adequately classified according to the nature and importance of the risk involved. They must be also labelled in such a way that the user or consumer will be rightly informed on the potential danger and on recommended conditions of use.

2. A FEW EXAMPLES OF COMPREHENSIVE LEGISLATION TENDING TO CONTROL POTENTIALLY TOXIC SUBSTANCES

In a descriptive report published in 1976 by OECD[2] relating to legislation tending to control environmental chemicals, a distinction is made between three types of regulations :

(a) Legislation on pre-market assessment of all chemicals;
(b) Legislation providing a pre-market assessment of pesticides and poisons;
(c) Legislation aimed at post-market control of environmental chemicals.

It results from the said survey that only few countries, at the present time, have passed or proposed a comprehensive legislation for the purpose of ensuring that chemicals are assessed, for environmental as well as human effects,prior to their marketing or use.

The examples that follow are limited to an outline of some of these comprehensive regulations, particularly the Toxic Substances Control Act of the United States of America which constitutes probably, for the moment, the most developed and sophisticated regulation in the field.

2.1 U.S.A. Legal system of control of chemicals

The "Toxic Substances Control Act"[3] has been approved by the United States Congress on October 11, 1976 and has taken effect on January 1, 1977.

2.1.1. Scope and purposes

This Act constitutes a comprehensive legislation governing the control of all chemicals and mixtures, with the exception of those chemical substances that are covered by a special legislation (such as pesticides, radioactive substances, food and food additives, drugs, cosmetics, wrapping materials, etc.).

The purpose of the law is "to grant the Environmental Protection Agency (EPA) the authority to obtain production, use and other information concerning both new and existing chemicals, to require tests to be performed, to determine the health and environmental effects of selected chemicals, and to regulate those substances which present or are likely to present an unreasonable risk to health or to environment"[2].

A large latitute of judgement is left to the Agency, particularly for estimating the existence of an "unreasonable risk" raising from the marketing or the manufacturing of chemicals, as well as for deciding what type of action shall be necessary for public health or environmental protection.

2.1.2. Basic principles of the TSCA law

According to the law, the Administrator of EPA must require that testing be conducted on such substances or mixtures to develop data with respect to the health and environmental effects when the said substance, according to Administrator's opinion, can present an unreasonable risk of injury, or when it will be produced in substantial quantities and that there are insufficient data and experience upon the said substances or mixtures. EPA has to establish testing standards for existing chemicals likely to present an unreasonable risk, with respect, particularly, to potential carcinogenesis, mutagenesis, teratogenesis, behavioural disorders, cumulative or synergistic effects. The standards for the development of test data are subject to yearly review in order to have them complying with scientific and technological evolution.

A "priority list" of those substances or mixtures that should be subject to particular consideration is to be established by a consultative body, the "Interagency Testing Committee".

In order to evaluate whether or not a chemical can cause an "unreasonable risk" to human health or the environment, the Environmental Protection Agency is provided with a notification relating to each new substance or mixture, or to each significant new use of already commercialised substances. The notification must be entered prior to manufacturing the substance (and not

only prior to marketing), or prior to importation if it is manufactured in
another country. It must contain specified data, including the name and
structure of the substance, the intended uses, the intended quantities to be
manufactured or imported, the possible by-products, the estimated number
of persons likely to be exposed to its effects at the manufacturing stage,
and all available toxicological data. The declaration of each new substance
is subject to an official notice published in the Federal Register and
mentioning the identity and intended uses of the substance as well as the
nature of the tests that have been conducted.

Nevertheless, such notification procedure of new chemicals implies that a
basic list (inventory) of presently existing substances has been established
by EPA. The TSCA law enables the Administrator to establish such inventory
on the basis of notices provided by all manufacturers, importers or userss
of chemicals produced or used (except in small quantities) during the last
three years in the United States. An "Initial Inventory" must firstly be
published, and will be followed, in a defined term, by a "Revised Inventory".

Consequently, all chemicals or mixtures that do not appear in the
Inventory shall be considered as new substances, subject to pre-manufacture
declaration.

The Administrator of EPA has in principle a 90-days "notice period" for
requiring additional information or testing of these declared substances.
During that notice period - that can be extended by EPA decision - the
Administrator is vested with very large powers of action and inspection with
respect to hyman health or environmental protection : he may regulate the
distribution and labelling, control that adequate testing has been conducted,
or prohibit or suspend the manufacture, commerce and use.

When the notice period (with or without extension) has expired, the manufacture on an industrial scale, or the importation of the product may be
undertaken unless additional required information has not yet been obtained
by EPA. There is thus an implicite clearance which cannot, however, be
considered as a "license" since the situation can always be reviewed by the
Administrator and will be subject at any time to further limitations that
could be deemed necessary for health or environmental protection, or to prompt
EPA action in event of an imminent hazard.

When testing should normally be required by EPA upon a declared substance
or mixture, the Administrator may, however, give an exemption for those
substances which have been subject previously to equivalent testing. In such
case the TSCA law gives the first notifier a right of recovering a part of

research expenditures, the share of which is to be established by common
agreement or imposed by EPA arbitration.

2.1.3. The collecting and treatment of information

Many provisions of the TSCA law allows EPA to collect any scientific,
technical and even commercial information likely to contribute to the
"unreasonable risk" assessment with respect to all chemicals or mixtures
manufactured or imported in the United States. This is the case namely :
- For implementing testing requirements rules to be enacted by EPA;
- For establishing the Inventory of existing substances;
- For evaluating new substances or significant new uses;
- For controlling those chemicals and mixtures that are considered as dangerous;
- For taking appropriate measures in case of imminent hazards.

The TSCA law allows the notifier to require a separate confidential treatment for those technical and economical data that he considers, as confidential.
In such case these confidential data can be disclosed only after a 30 days
period after due notice. When such data relate directly to commercial secret,
they cannot be disclosed in principle, and infringements are punishable by
specific penalties.

Nevertheless, a major exception is foreseen by the TSCA law since all data
that relate - in the Administrator's opinion - to health protection or public
safety shall not be considered as confidential.

2.1.4. Present state of implementation

Although the TSCA law is in force theoretically since January 1977, its
implementation by EPA has been subject to delay and practical difficulties.
The Initial Inventory - which condition the declaration procedure applicable
to new substances - as well as the first testing requirements, have just
been published by the Agency a few months ago. Moreover industries have
been very reluctant as to the mandatory declaration of confidential information,
and a special federal study group the "Subcommittee on Trade Secrets and
Date Confidentiality", has been appointed recently by EPA for considering the
problem . Therefore it is still premature to express any judgement concerning
the feasibility and efficiency of that law, although it appears to be at this
time the most comprehensive and developed regulation intended to pre-market
control of chemicals.

2.2. Other national legislations tending to a comprehensive legal control of chemicals

Legislation aimed at pre-market assessment of all chemicals has been enacted in several other countries, such as (by chronological order) in Switzerland (1969), Sweden (1973), Japan (1973), United Kingdom (1974), Canada (1975), France (1978) and Denmark (1979). Similar proposals are under consideration in Norway and in the Federal Republic of Germany.

We will just outline, hereafter, the main orientations of these national regulations.

2.2.1. Switzerland

Switzerland has been the first industrialised country where a general regulation tending to control hazardous chemicals has been enacted, since its Law on trade in toxic substances is dated 1969[4].

It provides that no toxic substance may be put on the national market until it has been classified, according to its potential danger, in one of the defined five categories of toxicity (class I being the most dangerous). Special prohibition of use may also be imposed, if deemed necessary, after testing. The law contains also provisions for regulating trade in toxic substances as well as manufactured products containing such substances.

The Federal Service of Public Hygiene is responsible for the classification and listing of toxic substances. Such classification has been made feasible through a compulsory notification of all chemicals produced or imported in Switzerland, the result of which has been that the Swiss government has set up the first and most complete register of chemical substances at the present time in Europe (according to the OECD report, up until 1975 about 10.000 basic substances have been classified, on the basis of more than 40.000 declarations).

Specific testing for environmental effects, however, has not yet been developed and is currently under consideration.

2.2.2. Sweden

A comprehensive law on "hazardous products" has been enacted in Sweden in 1973[5].

Additionally to general principles, such as the definition of an "overall rule of prudence", and to provisions enabling the government to impose special prohibitions or restrictions for specified products, the law provides that persons handling certain hazardous products will be submitted to notification. The Government is entitled to promulgate regulations governing the duty of public authorities to define those products that are to be regarded as

50

hazardous.

An Ordinance on hazardous products to health and to the environment contains
provisions tending to classify the concerned products regarding to health
hazards, poisons and dangerous substances, and relating to registration and
limitation of pesticides and other types of chemicals. The Products Control
Board, which is a control governmental body, is empowered to issue further
regulations.

2.2.3. Japan

In Japan, the need for comprehensive measures to prevent environmental
pollution by "persistent" chemicals has been recognised following several
environmental crises such as the Minamata disease (caused by mercury).

The Chemical Substances Control Law[6], dated 1973, provides :
- that all new chemicals shall be submitted to official examination on its
  persistency, accumulative tendency and toxicity to human beings prior
  to their production or importation;
- that chemicals tested and designated as "specific substances" shall be
  subject to prohibition or restriction implying a pre-manufacture authorisation upon the request of industry;
- that provisionally approved chemicals shall be subject to further official
  control.

In execution of the said law, PCB's have been designated in 1974 "specified
chemicals" to be brought under strict control concerning the production,
import and use.

2.2.4. United Kingdom

General regulatory powers are contained in a Section of the Control of
Pollution Act of 1974[7], in force since the beginning of 1976. The said
Section has vested the authority with powers to restrict or prohibit the
importation, commercial use or supply of any substance in order to prevent
damage to persons, animals or plants or pollution of air, water or land.

Additionally, a more recent regulation, enacted in 1978, concerns the
packaging and labelling of dangerous substances[8], implying a classification
of those chemicals which are referred to as dangerous ones.

2.2.5. Canada

In Canada, according to the Environmental Contaminants Act 1975 [9], mandatory
declaration to authorities is required for new chemicals which are to be
manufactured or imported in excess of 500 Kg per year. The same law provides

that prohibitions or restrictions may be applied to any prescribed substance
with respect to its release into the environment, the purpose for which it
may be imported, manufactured or used, or its amount in any product.

Investigation will be conducted for testing environmental effects in co-
operation with the industry. The Federal Government is responsible for
deciding what restrictive action, if any, needs to be taken.

2.2.6. France

The law on chemical controls[10] has been adopted in France in 1977. It
provides for pre-manufacture notification of all chemicals which have not
yet been marketed. Producers or importers have to declare any new risk
that can result from the quantity used, from a change of manufacturing process
or from the emission of the said substances into the environment.

Producers or importers of such new chemicals must also submit to authorities
a technical dossier providing information needed for assessing potential
hazards. The competent authority may classify a substance as a "dangerous
product", request from the manufacturer or importer any relevant information
with respect to potential health or environmental effects, as well as prohibit
or restrict the production, composition, storage, transportation, conditioning,
labelling, marketing, use or disposal of any chemical where deemed necessary
for public protection.

Producers of already marketed substances may be required to provide public
authority with appropriate technical or toxicological data in order to
evaluate potential health or environmental risks.

A recent regulation, enacted in January 1979, has determined the content
of the technical dossier to be joined to the declaration.

2.2.7. Denmark

A framework law has been enacted quite recently (1979) in Denmark in order
to protect human health and the environment from potential adverse effects
of chemical substances[11].

Manufacturers and importers are required to submit information which will
be necessary for risk assessment and for enacting safety measures. For new
substances that will be put on the market after October 1st 1980 as well as
for new uses of old substances, a pre-market notification will become
mandatory.

2.3. EEC directive amending the Council directive relating to the classification, packing and labelling of dangerous substances [12]

By a 6th modification - just approved but not yet published in the Official Journal of the Communities - of its previous Directive on the classification, packaging, or labelling of dangerous substances, the EEC Council has imposed on the Member States to take all necessary measures in order to ensure that new substances are not to be placed on the market unless they have been notified to the competent national authority, packaged and labelled in accordance with EEC requirements.

The notifier shall be required to carry out a study prior to marketing a new substance in order to allow health and environmental effects assessment.

Therefore, notification shall be mandatory prior to marketing a new substance (instead of prior to manufacturing for commercial purpose, as it is the case in France and in the United States). Declaration shall be accompanied by a technical dossier containing such characteristics of the substance that are listed in an Annex attached to the directive.

The EEC Commission shall receive copies of all notification dossiers and will keep an inventory of notified substances at the disposal of the Member States. Member States and the Commission, however, shall ensure that any information concerning marketing or manufacturing shall be kept secret.

It can be precised, finally, that informal contacts have been undertaken between the EEC Commission and the Environmental Protection Agency of the United States tending to harmonise future application of both (EEC and USA) legislations as to preliminary control of chemicals .

REFERENCES

1. Dr. G. VONKEMAN, introductory speech, Information day on the regulation of toxic substances, Brussels, 12 January 1979, European Environmental Law Bureau, Brussels.

2. "Regulations relating to Environmental chemicals pre-market and post-market controls", Organisation for Economic Co-operation and Development (Environment Directorate), Paris, 1976.

3. Toxic Substances Control Act (Public Law 94-469), October 11, 1976.

4. "Law on Trade in Toxic Substances", of 21st March 1969.

5. "Act on Products Hazardous to Man or the Environment", of 1st July 1973.

6. "Chemical Substances Control Law", September 1973.

7. "The Control Pollution Act 1974", Section 100.

8. "The Packaging and Labelling of Dangerous Substances Regulations" 1978.

9. "Environmental Contaminants Act" of 1975.

10. "Law on the Control of Chemicals Products" (Law n° 77-771), of July 12, 1977.

11. "Law on Chemical Substances and Products" (Law n° 212) of May 23, 1979.

12. Directive of the Council : "6th modification of the Council Directive of 27 June 1967 on the approximation of the laws of the Member States relating to the classification, packaging and labelling of dangerous substances" (adopted by the Council in September 1979, to be published in the Official Journal of the European Communities).

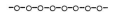

© 1980 Elsevier/North-Holland Biomedical Press
The Principles and Methods in Modern Toxicology
C.L. Galli, S.D. Murphy and R. Paoletti, editors.

CHEMICAL ANALYSIS IN TOXICOLOGICAL RESEARCH

KENNETH R. HILL

Analytical Chemistry Laboratory, Agricultural Environmental

Quality Institute, Science and Education Administration, U.S.

Department of Agriculture, Beltsville, Maryland 20705 (USA)

INTRODUCTION

   Although chemical analysis plays an essential direct role

in all aspects of toxicological research, the relationship

is even more intense in a subtle and somewhat unanticipated

development.   Because of extraordinary advances in analytical

instrumentation and levels of sensitivity over the last two

decades, the requirements for toxicological research and testing

have undergone a virtual revolution and an almost exponential

increase in complexity. The discovery of an ever increasing

number of chemical contaminants in the environment at ng/g

(ppb) or even pg/g (ppt) levels combined with discoveries of

serious biological effects such as oncogenicity and teratogenicity

of chemicals at sub-acute dosages has led to the present situation

where the desired amount of toxicological testing far exceeds

the capacity of existing and projected facilities. It is

important, therefore, to review at this time the major functions

of chemical analysis in toxicological research, since the validity

of the results are completely dependent on them. As Bowman

(1.) states in the preface to his forthcoming book CARCINOGENS

AND RELATED SUBSTANCES, The Analytical Chemical Aspects - "Analyt-

ical chemical control of test substances should begin when

the chemical enters the laboratory and end only after its safe disposal."

CHEMICAL ANALYSIS IN TOXICOLOGICAL RESEARCH

The three major functions of chemical analysis in toxicological research are: 1) the analysis of test chemicals for purity, 2) the analysis of animal feed and water for purity and to verify dosage, and 3) the analysis of test animal tissues, urine, and feces to determine distribution, retention, and the chemical nature of metabolites (terminal residues).

The first function includes the identification of trace components where possible or feasible and scheduled tests of storage stability, since most chemicals must be purchased in sufficient quantities (tens of kilograms) of one lot to last the expected duration of the longest term experiments (2-3 years or more). The need for rigorous purity testing arises because it is, unfortunately, not possible to rely on label statements or vendor specifications. Some specific examples illustrating the possible severity of this problem will be presented later. One interesting aspect of the purity problem is revealed when one considers that a purity of 99.5% or so is commonly acceptable as adequate for some tests. Yet, even if purities of 99.9999% could be achieved and measured, it would still be possible to have many hundreds of thousands of molecules of an impurity present - far below detectable limits. If one subscribes to the so-called "one molecule - one hit" or "no threshold limit" theories of chemical oncogenesis, then it can be argued that no toxicological test for oncogenicity is, was, or probably ever will be valid for establishing absolute

57

cause and effect.

The second function includes not only the analysis of every lot of animal feed (chow) and drinking water but also feeder boxes, bedding, and all other supplies that could bias the bioassay. Some specifications for animal diets currently in effect at the U.S. National Center for Toxicological Research set permissible levels of aflatoxins, estrogenic activity, metals, pesticides and related substances such as PCB's, Vitamins A and B1, fat and protein as shown in the following table.

TENTATIVE SPECIFICATIONS FOR ANIMAL CHOW

Substance	Specifications
Aflatoxins (B_1, B_2, G_1, G_2)	5 ng/g, max.
Estrogenic Activity	5 ng/g - equivalents of DES, max.
Arsenic	1 μg/g, max.
Cadmium	250 ng/g, max.
Calcium	0.75%, min.
Copper	8.0 μg/g, min.
Lead	1.5 μg/g, max.
Mercury	200 ng/g, max.
Selenium	0.05 μg/g, min.; 0.65 μg/g, max.
Zinc	75 μg/g, max.
Dieldrin	20 ng/g, max.
Heptachlor	20 ng/g, max.
Lindane	100 ng/g, max.
Malathion	5 μg/g, max.
Polychlorinated Biphenyls	50 ng/g, max.
Total DDT - Related Substances	100 ng/g, max.
Vitamin A	15 IU/g, min.; 75 IU/g, max.
Vitamin B_1	0.075 mg/g, min.; 0.125 mg/g, max.

Total Fat   4.3% min.; 6.7, max.

Total Protein   21.0% min.; 28.0, max.

   Specifications for bedding and feeder boxes include maximum permissible levels of pesticides individually and by the
class groups organochlorine and organophosphorus), pentachloro-
phenol, PCB's, and moisture as shown in the next table.

SPECIFICATION OF CARDBOARD FEEDER BOXES AND
BEDDING (HARDWOOD CHIPS)

	Feeder Boxes	Bedding
Pentachlorophenol	2.0 µg/g max.	2.0 µg/g max.
Polychlorinated Biphenyls	10 µg/g max.	10 µg/g max.
Total DDT - Related Substances	1.0 µg/g max.	
Diedrin	0.1 µg/g max.	
Lindane	0.1 µg/g max.	
Heptachlor	0.1 µg/g max.	
Malathion	5.0 µg/g max.	
Total Organochlorine Pesticides		1.0 µg/g max.
Total Organophosphorus Pesticides		5.0 µg/g max.
Moisture		8% max.

   Obviously such specifications are always tentative and subject
to revision as knowledge increases. The chemical analyses
conducted under this second function are characterized by the
fact that samples have an unknown history and multiresidue
procedures must be used.

   The third function, analysis of tissues, urine, and feces,
is employed only when information on the distribution, retention,
and/or the chemical nature of metabolites is desired for some
specific purpose. Synthesized compounds containing a radiolabel
as a tracer are generally, but not necessarily always, used

in such investigations. If metabolites are found in sufficient
quantity or of a designated chemical type, then it may become
necessary to synthesize and subject them to further toxicological
testing. If significant toxicity is uncovered then a method of
residue analysis may have to be developed by the analytical chemist. Analyses for the purpose of determining distribution and
retention can be characterized by the fact that the samples have
a known treatment history and therefore specific methods of analysis can usually be employed.

Residue analysis will now be examined in more detail.

RESIDUE ANALYSIS

Once toxicological studies have established the probable degree
of hazard of a chemical, residue analysis is required to regulate
the usage of the chemical to the desired level of safety. Various
kinds of residue analyses are conducted for various purposes, but
they can be roughly grouped into three main types; 1) Food and
Feed, 2) Environmental, and 3) Human Tissues, Plasma, and Excreta.

There are two main purposes for the residue analysis of food
and feed - Regulatory and Research. Regulatory analysis is
carried out to insure and enforce compliance with national and
international laws limiting residue levels in food and feed in
commerce. Enforcement of the previously mentioned specifications
for research animal diets could also be included in this catago-
ry. Since regulatory analysis involves samples of unknown treatment history, multiresidue methods must be used most of the time
and indeed, the existing multiresidue methods were originally
developed just for that purpose. Confirmatory techniques must be
used to verify chemical identity of presumed residues. On the

other hand research residue analysis is conducted to investigate
new chemicals for plant and animal protection or to obtain the
data needed to establish Maximum Residue Limits (MRL's). In either case the expected chemical residue, including any metabolites, is usually a known factor and methods specific to the chem-
ical/sample combination can be used. Confirmation is seldom
necessary.

Analysis of environmental samples generally is performed for
two purposes. One is to survey for chemical pollutants in general
to determine their nature, accumulation trends, and worldwide
distribution and the other, to survey for compliance with regulations on water and air quality by monitoring industrial, urban,
or agricultural effluents. Either multiresidue or specific methods may be used, depending on the objectives of the program. In
the case of general surveys as, for example, the analysis of fat
samples from arctic land and sea animals for organochlorine compounds it is absolutely essential that confirmation by GC/mass
spectrometry be carried out. To an experienced residue analyst,
the scientific literature contains far too many erroneous and
invalid reports of findings of organochlorine pesticides sometimes using methods that could not possibly determine the claimed
chemicals.

The analysis of human tissues, plasma, and excreta can be conveniently divided into four purposes - 1) to detect and monitor
industrial workplace exposure, including toxicological and chemical research laboratories, 2) to determine reentry intervals and
exposure levels for agricultural and forestry workers, 3) to carry
out etiological studies of the nature and distribution of chemicals, and 4) forensic analysis to determine possible chemical

agents involved in deaths arising from suicides, murders, accidents, etc.

SOME IMPORTANT ASPECTS OF CHEMICAL ANALYSES

It will be useful at this point to review certain aspects of chemical analysis that can have an important influence on the interpretation of toxicological data. This review will be divided into statistical aspects including sources of error and a consideration of current analytical procedures such as cleanup techniques, separation techniques, and detection and measurement systems or devices.

It is important to recognize that sampling and subsequent chemical analyses are statistical processes - that is, they depend on replication and statistical treatment of results to approximate the true answer. Due to heterogeneous distribution of a chemical residue within a bulk of material, the true quantity present can never be known since that would require processing and analysis of the entire bulk sample. Rather, representative random samples are taken of bulk material and where possible these are replicated an appropriate number of times so that the final analytical results can be expressed as a mean value plus or minus a standard deviation. Experienced analytical chemists are often distressed to find that their results are treated as "absolute" values in decision making or public debate, especially by administrators or the news media. A consideration of the irreducible errors existing in residue analysis shows that this is meaningless - only orders of magnitude or relative changes have significance. Current best estimates of the sources of error in residue analysis and their magnitudes are given in the following table based on information presented by Horwitz (2) in his paper "The Inevitability of Variability in Pesticide Residue Analysis" presented at the Fourth International Congress of Pesticide Chemistry (IUPAC) in Zurich in 1978.

Sources of Error (Variability)

Source	Estimate of Variance (CV)
1. Sampling	17%
2. Analytical Method	15%
3. Analyst	10%
4. Misinterpretation of results	Not calculated
Total "normal" error	25%

The important thing to note in this table is that even if method and human error were reduced to zero there would still be a variability of approximately 20% due to sampling. For this reason, residue analytical results should never be reported having more than two significant figures and in many cases rounding off to one significant figure will suffice. Just such a policy was adopted by the FAO/WHO Joint Meeting on Pesticide Residues in 1970 (3.).

The distinction between precision and accuracy is sometimes overlooked or confused in interpreting analytical results; more specifically, good precision is sometimes erroneously taken as an indicator of high accuracy. An easy way to keep the distinction in mind is to think of some possible patterns of darts on a dart board target as shown in the following figure.

PRECISION AND ACCURACY

 Prec. - Good
Accur. - Poor

 Prec. - Poor
Accur. - Good

Prec. - Good
Accur. - Good

  Prec. - Poor
Accur. - Poor

Good precision but poor accuracy is illustrated by a tight cluster
that misses the "bulls eye", whereas good accuracy but poor precision is illustrated by a symmetrical pattern of darts around but
not touching the "bulls eye". Both poor precision and poor accuracy (the way most of us play) is illustrated by a loose random
pattern of darts off to one side of the "bulls eye". The desired
combination of good precision and good accuracy is shown, of
course, by a tight cluster centered in the "bulls eye". At the
present time the accuracy of analytical method can be measured
only by interlaboratory collaborative studies of samples fortified
with test chemicals at known levels. It should be recognized
however that even such collaborative studies may not always provide "true" answers due to the possible presence of bound residues
or conjugates in samples containing field-incurred residues.
Whether or not residue analysts should be concerned with bound
residues in food and feed depends on their toxicological significance in the bound state and this question can only be answered
by toxicologists.

Current procedures for residue analysis, whether multiresidue
or specific, generally tend to follow a common routine or sequence
of steps. The initial stage of the analysis, usually referred to
as cleanup, attempts to separate the sought-for chemicals as a
group from all other sample constituents collectively called the
matrix. Following initial preparation such as chopping or

grinding if required, the usual sequence of steps is:
(1) Extraction - either by high-speed blending with an organic
solvent or by Soxhlet extractor. A recent trend in extraction is
to use an apparatus that combines shearing blades with high power
ultrasonic energy to disrupt cell walls. (2) Filtration or centrifugation to physically separate soluble material from insol-
uble. (3) Liquid/liquid partition to remove fats and oils if
present. (4) Column chromatography, thin layer chromatography,
or gel permeation chromatography (if needed) to remove residual
lipids, pigments, and soluble matrix components by selective
adsorption or molecular exclusion. (5) Evaporation to reduce the
volume of solvent to a predetermined level and concentrate the
soluble residues to increase analytical sensitivity.

Following cleanup the sample concentrate is subjected to a
separation technique to resolve, to the highest degree feasible,
the chemical residue components from each other for identification
and measurement (quantitation). Techniques commonly used are
(1) gas chromatography, (2) high performance liquid chromatography, and (3) thin layer chromatography.

The final step -- detection and measurement -- involves the use
of either selective or non-selective chromatographic detectors.
An excellent comprehensive discussion of gas chromatographic
detectors suitable for pesticide residue analysis was recently
provided by Greenhalgh and Holland (4.). Examples of non-selective detectors are the flame ionization (FID) and its photoioniza-
tion variation used with GC, the thermal conductivity (TC) used
with GC, the ultra-violet absorption (UV) used with HPLC and TLC,
and the refractive index (RI) used with HPLC. These detectors
are for general purpose use and will detect almost any organic

compound. That fact limits their use for residue analysis due
to excessive interference from sample matrix components. Examples
of selective detectors are the flame photometric (FPD) (GC), the
electron capture (EC) (GC), the N/P thermionic (GC), the conductivity (GC) which can be used for either chlorine-, sulfur-, or
nitrogen- containing compounds, the microcoulometric (GC), the
microwave plasma emission (GC) which can be selectively tuned for
a wide variety of elements, the moving wire (LC) used for any
carbon-containing compound and its N-and P-selective modifications
(5.), the atomic absorption (LC) used for toxic metal ions, the
thermoelectron (GC, LC) used at present for nitrosoamines, and the
mass spectrometer (GC, LC). These detectors are highly preferred
for residue analyses because they reduce the response to unwanted
compounds and often increase the reliability and sensitivity of
an analysis. They are of maximum benefit when judiciously used to
reinforce each other - that is to increase the degree of confidence in the identification of a compound.

SOME SELECTED EXAMPLES

Because of its extreme importance to valid toxicological research, the need for analysis of test chemicals for purity and
stability will be emphasized by presenting several actual examples
of specific problems that have arisen in toxicological or analytical research.

At the National Center for Toxicological Research in Jefferson,
Arkansas, Bowman (6.) found by analysis that a 10-kg batch of
2-acetylaminofluorene (2-AAF) acquired in 1972 was 85-90% pure and
that the purity could be increased to 99.6% by oven drying. However, due to the extent of the long term testing conducted and

proposed, an additional 10-kg. batch was acquired from the original supplier in 1974. This lot assayed at only 16.2% 2-AAF and
was returned to the vendor for purification. When the purified
material was received it assayed only 1.68% 2-AAF! Had this
material gone untested and been used in the long-term studies,
both the scientific and financial consequences would have been
severe.

A far less critical but nevertheless annoying example of the
unreliability of labels on samples of standards and also of possible storage stability problems occurred at the Analytical Chemistry Laboratory, USDA-SEA-AR, Beltsville, Maryland last summer.
Acetone solutions of manufactuer-supplied standards (labeled
98-100% pure) of the insecticide aldicarb and its primary metabolites aldicarb sulfoxide and aldicarb sulfone were used to investigate the resolving power of different solvent-gradient programs
on an experimental SI-500 silica gel (E. Merck) cleanup column
(5.). The chemical structures of these compounds and their hydrolysis products (oximes) are shown in the next figure.

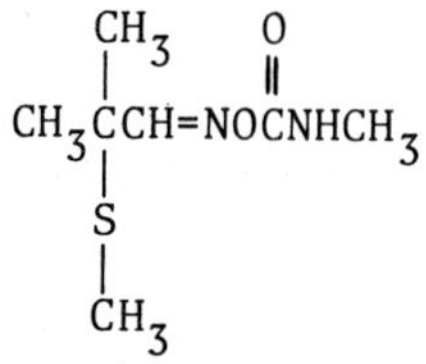

$$CH_3CCH=NOCNHCH_3$$

with CH_3 and O above, S and CH_3 below

Aldicarb

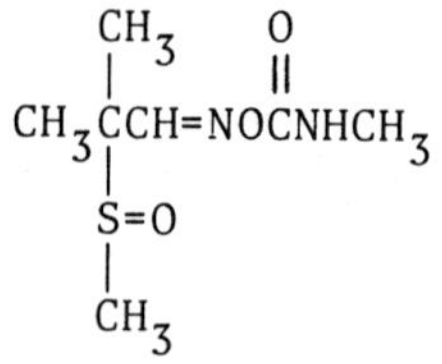

$$CH_3CCH=NOCNHCH_3$$

with CH_3 and O above, $S=O$ and CH_3 below

Aldicarb Sulfoxide

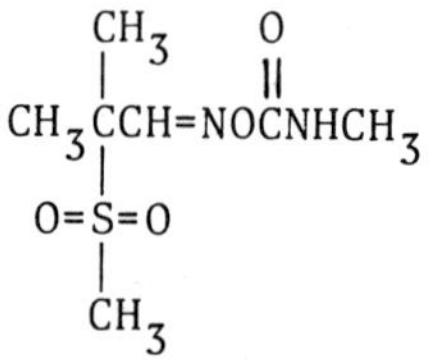

$$CH_3CCH=NOCNHCH_3$$

with CH_3 and O above, $O=S=O$ and CH_3 below

Aldicarb Sulfone

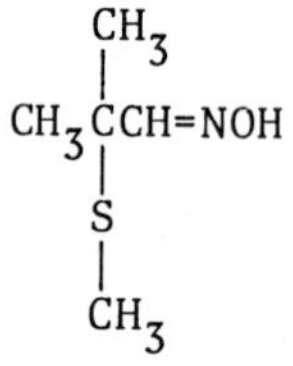

$$CH_3CCH=NOH$$

with CH_3 above, S and CH_3 below

Aldicarb Oxime

$$CH_3CCH=NOH$$

with CH_3 above, $S=O$ and CH_3 below

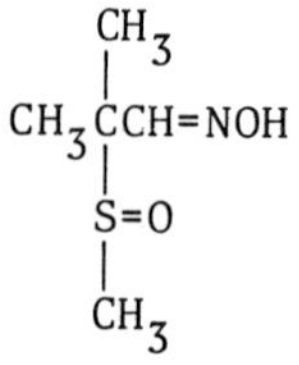

Aldicarb Sulfoxide
Oxime

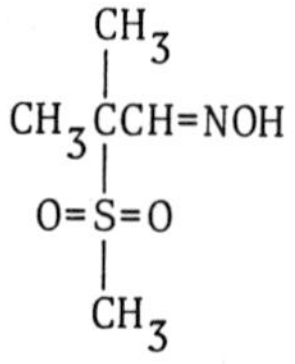

$$CH_3CCH=NOH$$

with CH_3 above, $O=S=O$ and CH_3 below

Aldicarb Sulfone
Oxime

When liquid chromatograms of each of these standards were obtained using an experimental nitrogen-selective detector, the results were surprising as shown in the next three figures.

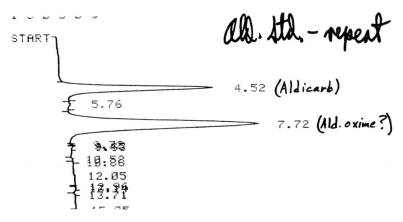

The aldicarb standard contained two components, presumably aldicarb and its oxime, with the latter comprising more than 50% of the mixture.   The aldicarb sulfoxide standard also contained two components in the 80/20 ratio shown.

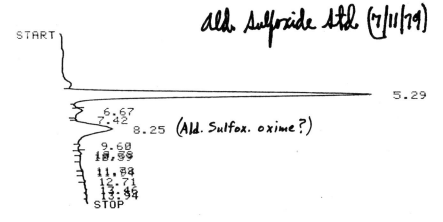

Only the aldicarb sulfone appeared to be reasonably pure.

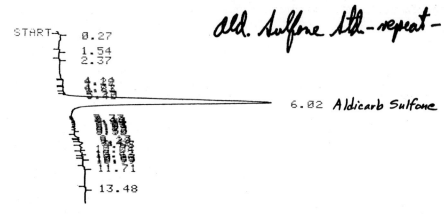

These standards in their original crystalline form had been stored in a refrigerator for slightly more than 2 years and had not undergone any noticeable change in physical appearance. The acetone solutions were less than a week old and had been kept refrigerated when not in actual use. Since the samples had not been assayed when first received it is impossible to say whether the results reflect the purity of the material as received or are due to degradation on storage. Discussions of the problem with other residue analysts indicate similar experiences and shared reservations about the labeled purity as received.

In summary, the best way to emphasize the points made in all of the preceding material is simply to state -- trust nothing, test everything, and take no ones word for the purity of a chemical, except, of course, your friendly collaborative analytical chemist.

ACKNOWLEDGMENT

I wish to give special thanks and acknowledgment to Malcolm C. Bowman, Director, Division of Chemistry, NCTR, Jefferson, Arkansas for his helpful discussions and assistance in supplying reference material and slides.

REFERENCES

1. Bowman, Malcolm C., 1979. CARCINOGENS AND RELATED SUBSTANCES
   - The Analytical Chemical Aspects, Marcel Dekker, Inc.
   publishers, 270 Madison Avenue, New York, New York 10016,
   320 pps.

2. Horwitz, William, 1979. The Inevitability of Variability in
   Pesticide Residue Analysis in Advances in Pesticide Science,
   Symposia Papers presented at the Fourth International Congress
   of Pesticide Chemistry (IUPAC), Zurich, Switzerland, July
   24-28, 1978, Part 3, Pergamon Press Inc., New York, 649-655.

3. Pesticide Residues in Food. Report of the 1970 Joint FAO/WHO
   Meeting, World Health Organization Technical Report Series
   No. 474, Geneva, Section 2.13, page 11 (1971). See also
   Pesticide Residues in Food. Report of the 1973 Joint FAO/WHO
   Meeting, World Health Organization Technical Report Series
   No. 545, Geneva, Section 2.5, page 12 (1974).

4. Greenhalgh, Roy and P. T. Holland. Selection of Gas Chro-
   matographic Detectors for Pesticide Residue Analysis,
   Chemistry and Biology Research Institute, Agriculture Canada,
   Ottawa, Ontario, K1A 0C6.

5. Hill, K. R. and H. L. Crist. A Nitrogen-Selective Detector
   for Liquid Chromatography. J. Chromat. Sci. 17, 395-400,
   July (1979).

6. Bowman, Malcom C., 1978. Chemical Aspects of Toxicological
   Research. Assoc. of Food and Drug Officials, 117-120.

The opinions expressed in this paper are those of the author and
do not necessarily represent official policy of the USDA.

Mention of a pesticide in this paper does not constitute a
recommendation for use by the USDA nor does it imply registration
under the Federal Insecticide, Fungicide, and Rodenticide Act as
amended. Also, mention of a commercial product in this paper
does not constitute an endorsement of this product by the USDA.

© 1980 Elsevier/North-Holland Biomedical Press
The Principles and Methods in Modern Toxicology
C.L. Galli, S.D. Murphy and R. Paoletti, editors.

BIOCHEMICAL ASPECTS OF TISSUE CHANGE

J. W. DANIEL
Life Science Research, Stock, Essex, England

INTRODUCTION

Although it is now possible for toxicologists to detect even the most subtle of effects produced in experimental animals by drugs, food additives, pesticides and industrial chemicals, it is frequently difficult to assess the significance of the observations and their relevance to human health.

The toxicity of most chemicals is known, or presumed, to result from an interaction with a specific intracellular process and significant advances have been made in recent years of the role of 'biochemical lesions' in several pathological and non-pathological conditions. However, the changes that occur are normally complex and it is frequently difficult to determine whether tissue injury is due to a single initiating event or to a concerted action involving several integrated systems. Nevertheless, such investigations are essential to the process of safety evaluation and may provide, in addition, the means of identifying those changes that are related to subsequent alterations in tissue structure and function.

This review summarises some of the biochemical effects induced by hepatotoxic and neurotoxic chemicals and, in addition, the diagnostic value of monitoring the composition of serum and urine.

CELL NECROSIS

Many chemicals are converted in the body to toxic metabolites which are stable chemically and exert their effects by combining reversibly with specific sites in tissues. In some instances, however, metabolism results in the formation of highly reactive electrophilic intermediates which can combine covalently with tissue macromolecules such as RNA, DNA and protein. The formation of such metabolites is now believed to be responsible for the action of many carcinogens and mutagens as well as those which cause cellular necrosis, hypersensitivity reactions, methaemoglobinaemia and other blood dyscrasias.

Studies with bromobenzene[1], acetaminophen[2] (p-hydroxyacetanilide) and carbon tetrachloride[3] have identified some of the events that either precede or may be responsible for the process of cell necrosis. Bromobenzene (Fig. 1) is converted by an $NADPH_2$-dependent microsomal enzyme to the 3,4-epoxide (I) that

combines covalently to proteins, particularly those in the centrilobular region
of liver cells.   Alternatively, it can either re-arrange to the phenol (II),
be converted to the dihydrodiol (III) or react with glutathione to form a conjugate (IV) which is excreted subsequently in the urine as the corresponding
N-acetylcysteine derivative.   The extent to which the epoxide is bound to
tissue macromolecules and the severity of liver necrosis depends, therefore,
upon the rate of formation of the dihydrodiol and the availability of glutathione.

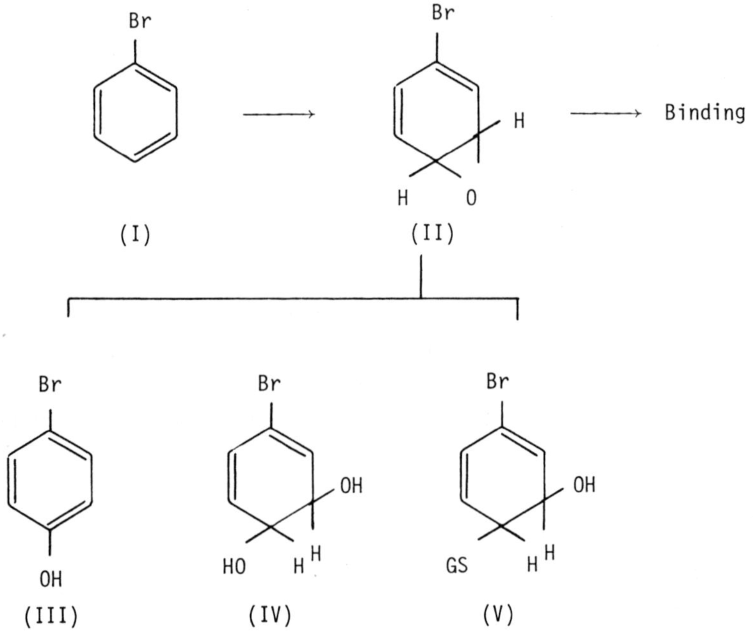

Br

Br

H

→ Binding

H   0

(I)

(II)

Br

Br

Br

OH

OH

HO   H H

GS   H H

OH

(III)

(IV)

(V)

Fig. 1.   Biotransformation of bromobenzene

    Pre-treatment of rats with phenobarbitone stimulates the rate at which the
active metabolite is produced, hastens the depletion of liver glutathione and
increases both the severity of the hepatic necrosis and the amount of covalent
binding of the metabolite.   In contrast, treatment with 3-methylcholanthrene
decreases the toxicity of bromobenzene by stimulating the formation of the non-
toxic 2,3-epoxide.   Dose response studies with bromobenzene in rats have shown
that the proportion of the dose that becomes covalently bound remains low until

a threshold level of 200-350 mg/kg is exceeded.

The formation of an epoxide metabolite is generally considered essential for the mutagenic and carcinogenic activity of polycyclic aromatic hydrocarbons and studies with benzo(a)pyrene[4,5] indicate that the ultimate carcinogen is the trans-7,8-dihydro dihydroxy-9,10-epoxide shown in Figure 2.

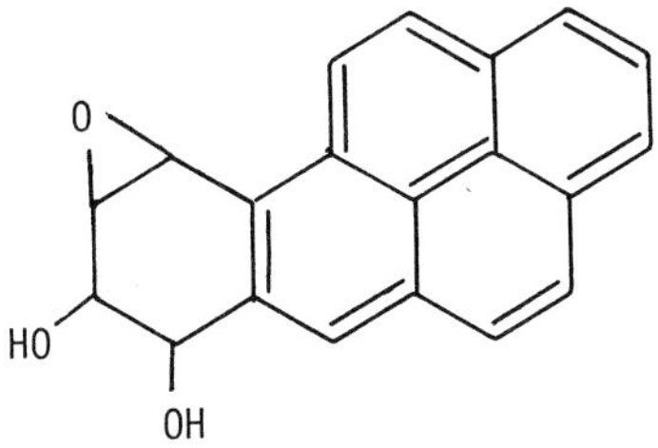

(VI)

Fig. 2.   Trans-7,8-dihydro dihydroxy-9,10-epoxide of benzo(a)pyrene

The hepatocarcinogen, vinyl chloride ($CH_2 = CHCl$) is also converted by hepatic microsomes _in vitro_ to a reactive intermediate that is covalently bound to protein, RNA, DNA and glutathione.   Although the metabolite has not been isolated, it is generally thought to be the epoxide, chloroethylene oxide.   In studies in which male rats were exposed for 6 hours to varying concentrations of vinyl chloride labelled with carbon-14, it was shown that binding to liver proteins was not a linear function of dose, but could be represented by a sigmoid curve that was linear only at concentrations between 50 and 250 ppm[6]. There was little or no increase in the amount of covalent binding at concentrations of 500, 1000 and 5000 ppm, and no radioactivity was found associated with either DNA or RNA.   A dose related depression of glutathione was observed only at concentrations greater than 100 ppm.   More significantly, it was observed that in animals exposed to vinyl chloride at concentrations greater than 50 ppm binding to protein correlated with the induction of hepatic carcinoma.

Acetaminophen (Fig. 3) which is frequently used as a mild analgesic, can at high doses provoke marked centrilobular necrosis in experimental animals[2]. Treatment of mice with phenobarbitone increases the toxicity, whereas the administration of compounds that inhibit cytochrome P-450 mediated reactions decrease the severity of the response.   Necrosis parallels the amount of drug bound to protein and the reduction in glutathione levels, although it has been reported that necrosis does not occur providing the levels of glutathione in the liver are maintained at 15-20% of normal.   The drug is excreted princi- pally as conjugates with glucuronic and sulphuric acids, with only a relatively small proportion being converted to the glutathione conjugate (V).   Studies with microsomes from hamster liver suggest that the epoxide (VI) is not the metabolite that reacts with tissue macromolecules (TM), but that it is probably the N-hydroxy derivative (VII).

The role of N-hydroxylation in the activation of aromatic amino- and nitro- compounds is well documented and accounts for the ability of such compounds to catalyse the formation of ferrihaemoglobin (methaemoglobin)[7].   During the reaction the hydroxylamino-derivatives are converted to the corresponding nitroso-compounds which are reduced subsequently by enzymes, collectively referred to as 'methaemoglobin reductase', present in the red cell (Fig. 4).

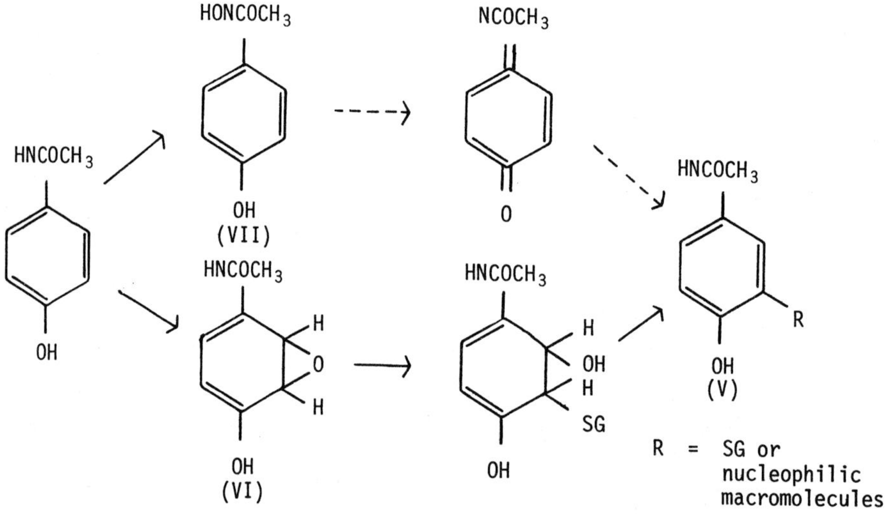

Fig. 3.   Biotransformation of acetaminophen

Few compounds have been as extensively investigated as carbon tetrachloride which produces centrilobular necrosis and fatty infiltration of the liver[3].   A metabolite of carbon tetrachloride is covalently bound to proteins and lipids[8] and, although the reactive intermediate has not been identified, it is gener- ally believed to be the trichloromethyl free-radical which is formed by reduc- tive cleavage of one of the carbon-chlorine bonds.

There is ample evidence to support the hypothesis advanced by Recknagel that the primary event in carbon tetrachloride-induced liver damage is the peroxidation of microsomal lipids initiated by the trichloromethyl radical. The reaction is autocatalytic, leading to disruption of membranes and impaired protein synthesis, and it is the latter that is believed to be responsible for the accumulation of fat by the failure to synthesise the apoprotein required for the excretion of fat from the liver. Carbon tetrachloride also causes the destruction of cytochrome P-450 which may account for the protection afforded by the prior administration of sub-acute doses of the compound. Lipid peroxidation has also been proposed to explain the action of several other compounds including that of oxidant gases on the lung and the pulmonary fibrosis induced by the herbicide, paraquat.

Although glutathione inhibits the binding of carbon tetrachloride to rat liver microsomes, the liver levels are not depleted, presumably because only some 1-2% of the administered dose is metabolised, with most being eliminated unchanged[9,10]. It would appear that one of the roles of glutathione is to protect thiol and other nucleophilic groups in tissue macromolecules from the interaction with electrophilic metabolites.

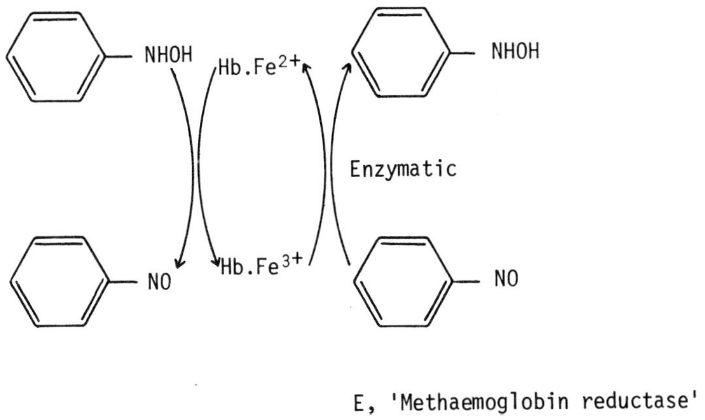

$$\begin{array}{ccc} \text{—NHOH} & \xrightarrow{\text{Hb.Fe}^{2+}} & \text{—NHOH} \\[1em] & \text{Enzymatic} & \\[1em] \text{—NO} & \xleftarrow{\text{Hb.Fe}^{3+}} & \text{—NO} \end{array}$$

E, 'Methaemoglobin reductase'

Fig. 4. Formation of methaemoglobin by phenylhydroxylamine.

LIVER ENLARGEMENT AND ENZYME INDUCTION

A frequent observation in sub-acute and chronic toxicity studies is an increase in the weight of the liver, usually relative to bodyweight, and which is readily reversible when treatment is discontinued. Several hundred compounds

76

are known to produce this response in the rat and, as illustrated by the examples in Table 1, they differ widely both in chemical structure and biological activity.

The histological appearance of the enlarged liver is essentially normal and, apart from an increase in the amount of smooth endoplasmic reticulum, there is little of note in the ultra-structure of the individual cells. The increase in mass is generally attributed to enlargement of the hepatocytes, although there is some evidence to suggest that with some compounds this is preceded by a stage during which synthesis of DNA is stimulated. The induction of liver growth by drugs, hormones, dietary factors and during pregnancy and lactation has been reviewed by Schulte-Hermann[11].

TABLE 1

COMPOUNDS PRODUCING LIVER ENLARGEMENT IN THE RAT

DRUGS	Phenobarbitone Phenylbutazone	Glutethimide Chlorcyclizine	Nikethimide Tolbutamide
INSECTICIDES	Chlordane DDT	Dieldrin α-Hexachlorocyclohexane	Pyrethrum
FOOD ADDITIVES	Butylated hydroxytoluene (BHT) Butylated hydroxyanisole (BHA)		Ethoxyquin
HORMONES	Thyroxine	ACTH	Prolactin

The most notable change associated with this effect is an increase in the activity of those enzymes that catalyse the oxidation of steroid hormones, fatty acids and exogenous chemicals, and which are located in the microsomal fraction of liver homogenates. The electron transfer system in microsomes consists essentially of an $NADPH_2$-dependent reductase and a terminal haemoprotein, cytochrome P-450. The administration of phenobarbitone and related compounds increases the activity of the reductase, the haemoprotein content and that of microsomal protein, while the action of those represented by 3-methylcholanthrene are restricted to the haemoprotein which differs in respect of its spectral properties exhibiting maximal absorption at 448 nm. Compounds in the first group stimulate the rate of metabolism of a wide variety of substrates, whereas those in the second group are more limited in their specificity. This classification may be too rigid, however, for recent observations indicate that anabolic steroids and polychlorinated biphenyl derivatives may act through yet different mechanisms.

Enzyme induction is not confined to the microsomal oxidases, but includes epoxide hydrase and those which catalyse conjugation with glucuronic acid and glutathione.   The activities of δ-aminolaevulinic acid synthetase (δ-ALAS) and ferrochelatase are frequently elevated, leading to an increase in haem synthesis.

Succinyl - CoA + glycine $\xrightarrow{\delta\text{-ALAS}}$ δ-aminolaevulinic acid
$\longrightarrow$ Porphobilinogen $\longrightarrow$ Protoporphyrin $\longrightarrow$ Haem

In phenobarbitone-treated mice it was observed that the increase in the non-microsomal enzymes, malic dehydrogenase, aldolase and the transaminases parallels the increase in liver weight, while glucose 6-phosphate dehydrogenase, isocitric dehydrogenase and malic enzyme showed an initial increase which was not, however, maintained.   The most notable increase, however, was that of $NADPH_2$-oxidase activity[12].   There is, in addition, an increase in the synthesis of DNA which can be prevented by actinomycin D, an inhibitor of gene transcription, and RNA, although there is some evidence that the catabolism of RNA, like that of $NADPH_2$-cytochrome C reductase, is reduced.   Stimulation of microsomal enzymes is not a necessary pre-requisite for the induction of liver growth, butylated hydroxyanisole and allylisopropyl acetamide having little effect on enzyme activity.

Microsomal enzyme induction is also observed with several hepatotoxic compounds and many short-term studies have been conducted to determine whether liver enlargement and the associated effects on microsomal enzyme activity is a toxic, or, in the absence of any demonstrable histological damage, an adaptive response to an increased work-load (hyperfunctional enlargement).   Platt and Cockrill[13] compared the biochemical changes induced in the rat by several hepatotoxic agents (carbon tetrachloride, chloroform, thioacetamide, 1,1,2-trichloroethane, dimethylnitrosamine and ethionine) with those of DDT and halothane (1,1,1-trifluoro-2-bromo-2-chloroethane) and found that the former all markedly reduced the activity of the enzymes glucose 6-phosphatase, aminopyrine demethylase and $NADPH_2$-cytochrome C reductase, while the activity of glucose 6-phosphate dehydrogenase was enhanced.   The protein content of the soluble fraction of the cell, like that of the microsomal component, was also reduced. The response of these parameters to DDT, which is frequently classified as hepatotoxic, was in all respects similar to that obtained with phenobarbitone. In a similar study with a range of pharmacologically active compounds at least five distinct patterns of response were obtained[14] and it was concluded that the measurement of just a single parameter cannot distinguish between a toxic and a physiological response.

Crampton et al[15] compared the biochemical and morphological changes in the liver of female rats fed diets containing either the food-stuff antioxidant, 2,6-di-tert-butyl-4-hydroxytoluene (BHT), phenobarbitone, the food flavouring agent, Safrole, or the food colour, Ponceau MX, for periods of 80-85 weeks.

Both BHT (0.4%) and phenobarbitone (0.25%) increased liver weight and markedly enhanced the activity of the microsomal enzymes catalysing the de-methylation of ethylmorphine and the hydroxylation of aniline and biphenyl. The synthesis of cytochrome P-450 was enhanced as was that of cytochrome b_5 and microsomal protein.   These changes were evident after 7 days of treatment and persisted throughout the entire study of 80 weeks.   The only morphological changes were centrilobular cell enlargement and hypertrophy of the smooth endo-plasmic reticulum.   Histochemical examination revealed a centrilobular depres-sion of glucose 6-phosphatase, while the distribution of lysosomal acid phos-phatase was unaffected.   The changes were in all respects similar to those observed following short-term exposure to these two agents and to be readily reversible once treatment was terminated.

BHT   SAFROLE   PONCEAU MX

Although the initial response to Safrole (0.25%) and Ponceau MX (1%) was similar to that of BHT and phenobarbitone, the activi... of the oxidative enzymes and the levels of cytochrome P-450 returned to control values within 8 weeks following treatment with Safrole, whereas with Ponceau MX the decline was more gradual.   The livers remained enlarged throughout the entire study as were the amounts of microsomal protein and cytochrome b_5.   The synthetic colour had a greater stimulatory effect on the growth of the liver, whereas the influence on microsomal enzyme activity was less than that obtained with Safrole.   Ponceau MX produced a more rapid depression of centrilobular glucose

6-phosphatase activity, while both agents affected the distribution of lysosomal acid phosphatase.   Cell necrosis was apparent after 25 weeks of treatment with Safrole, while liver cell hyperplasia was present in animals fed
Ponceau MX.   Histopathological changes comprising cell necrosis and proliferative lesions which appeared as hepatic nodules were present in all treated
animals at the end of the study.   An initial depression of glucose 6-phospha-
tase is a characteristic response to many hepatotoxins and as such compounds
normally reduce the activity of microsomal enzymes, it is possible that the
effect on glucose 6-phosphatase may reflect damage to the membranes of the
smooth endoplasmic reticulum.   The observations with BHT and phenobarbitone,
however, do not support this interpretation.   Both compounds stimulate the
activity of glucose 6-phosphate dehydrogenase in response to an increased
requirement for $NADPH_2$ and it is possible that there is an enhanced metabolism
of glucose through the pentose pathway.

Golberg[16] concluded that an increase in relative liver weight in the rat
with a reduction in glucose 6-phosphatase activity in the absence of any prolonged stimulation of microsomal enzyme activity was probably indicative of
hepatotoxicity, whereas when microsomal enzyme activity was sustained it represented a physiological response.   While adverse effects may result from the
increased rate of metabolism of physiological substrates, chronic toxicity
studies, particularly with BHT, indicate that such reactions, if they are
present, are not deleterious[17,18].   In contrast, the liver enlargement that
occurs during pregnancy and lactation has several features that could be considered pathological.

NEUROTOXICITY

Many chemicals, examples of which are listed in Table 2, are capable of
damaging the nervous system or produce functional changes which do not involve
alterations in tissue structure[19].

Several organophosphorus compounds, including di-isopropylfluorophosphate
(DFP), Mipafox and tri-o-cresyl phosphate (TOCP), produce delayed neurotoxic
effects both in man and experimental animals and, although treatment with atro-
pine and oximes will protect against any cholinergic response, they are unable
to prevent the development of lesions within the nervous system.   Extensive
damage is observed in the spinal cord and sciatic nerve, while lesions are present in the medulla oblongata, but not in the cerebral cortex or the cerebellum.
The axon is particularly affected with damage commencing at the distal end of
the larger axons.   The delay in the development of the lesion is consistent

TABLE 2

CHEMICALS AFFECTING THE NERVOUS SYSTEM[a]

Organophosphorus compounds
p-Bromophenylacetylurea
Isoniazid
Carbon disulphide; disulphiram; diethyldithiocarbamate
Nitrofurantoin; nitrofurazone; furaltadone
Alkylmercury compounds
Arsenic; lead
Thalidomide
Acrylamide
Thallium salts
Clioquinol
Vinca alkaloids
Trichloroethylene

---

[a] from Cavanagh[19].

with an interaction within some neurones which does not result in immediate
loss of function.   All organophosphorus compounds producing ataxia have a
general capacity to inhibit esterase activity and the possibility that the initial event involves phosphorylation of a particular esterase in nervous tissue
has been examined by Johnson[20] who found that several esters, particularly
phenyl phenylacetate and phenyl phenylvalerate were able to prevent the phosphorylation of the enzyme in vitro by diisopropyl fluorophosphate.   Moreover,
in hens, the species most frequently used to detect the neurotoxic potential of
organophosphorus esters, the enzyme was found to be inhibited by neurotoxic
compounds, but to be unaffected by non-neurotoxic analogues.

Degeneration of peripheral nerves can be readily produced in rats by the
antitubercular drug, isonicotinic acid hydrazide (Isoniazid), involving widespread wallerian-degeneration while both axons and myelin sheaths become frag-
mented.   The mode of action is complex for the compound inhibits the enzyme
pyridoxal phosphate kinase and combines with pyridoxal phosphate (vitamin b_6)
to form a hydrazone that is an even more potent inhibitor of the enzyme.   The
brain has a high requirement for pyridoxal phosphate, a co-factor in both
transaminase and decarboxylating reactions, and is required for the synthesis
of the inhibitory neuro-transmitter γ-aminobutyric acid.   It is unclear how
depletion of vitamin b_6 leads to neuronal degeneration or why other hydrazides
(thiosemicarbazide, isonicotinic acid 2-isopropylhydrazide) produce convulsions
rather than peripheral neuropathy.

Neurochemical investigations in experimental animals have established that
carbon disulphide produces changes in the catecholamine content of both cere-

bral and extra-cerebral tissues[21].   Thus the amount of epinephrine in the
adrenal gland and of nor-epinephrine in brain, heart and adrenals were reduced
when rats were exposed for periods of 4 and 8 hours to carbon disulphide at an
atmospheric concentration of 2 mg/litre.   These changes were accompanied by an
increase in the levels of 3,4-dihydroxyphenylethylamine (dopamine) in brain and
adrenals and it was suggested that the effects were due to inhibition of the
copper-containing enzyme, dopamine β-hydroxylase.   Several amino-acid dithiocarbamate derivatives and diethyldithiocarbamate, but not carbon disulphide,
are effective inhibitors of the enzyme _in vitro_, while the disulphide was inhibitory when tested in the presence of tyramine.   The addition of cuprous
ions reversed the inhibitory activity of glycine dithiocarbamate lending
further support to the hypothesis that the dithiocarbamates bind with enzymic
copper.   It is also possible that carbon disulphide reacts with catecholamines
within the storage granules to produce inhibitory dithiocarbamate derivatives.

It has been proposed that the neuropathy caused by carbon disulphide may be
due to the depletion of vitamin b_6 resulting from the reaction of the compound
with pyridoxamine to produce the corresponding dithiocarbamate.

Thalidomide is known to acylate liver histones, RNA and DNA, as well as the
amines, putrescine and spermidine, both of which are present in nervous tissue.
Since the lesion is similar to that produced by methylmercury compounds, it is
possible that the initial defect occurs in the ribosomes.   Although the morphological changes produced by most neurotoxic chemicals have been characterised, their interaction with cellular processes has not been investigated and
the nature of the biochemical lesion remains obscure.

THE DIAGNOSTIC VALUE OF CHANGES IN THE COMPOSITION OF SERUM AND URINE

Practical considerations restrict the type of studies that can be performed
to monitor changes in tissue function that may occur during sub-acute and
chronic toxicity tests and it is customary to base such an assessment on alterations in the composition of serum and urine.

The most common response involves an increase in enzymes that are normally
absent from the serum or present in relatively small amounts.   Although lactic
dehydrogenase, alkaline phosphatase, glutamic oxaloacetic- and glutamic
pyruvic-transaminases are the enzymes most commonly studied, almost all cytoplasmic enzymes may be studied.   The principle causes of elevated serum enzyme
activity are increased synthesis, including those that are tumour specific
(histaminase), impaired excretion (alkaline phosphatase) and cellular necrosis,
in which there are changes in membrane permeability.   The increased alkaline

phosphatase activity in the serum of female rats treated with ethinyl oest-
radiol[22] has been attributed to enhanced synthesis of the enzyme in liver,
ileum and bone and not to be diagnostic of liver injury.   Similar changes have
been observed in serum and hepatic alkaline phosphatase in beagle dogs treated
with phenobarbitone[23] and in patients receiving prolonged therapy with anti-
convulsant drugs[24].   Elevated serum alkaline phosphate is normally associated
with biliary obstruction for the enzyme is excreted principally in the bile.

Hepatotoxic compounds cause cytoplasmic and, providing the lesion is sufficiently severe, mitochondrial enzymes to leak from damaged cells into the blood
and the nature of the enzymes in serum is frequently characteristic of the
affected tissue.   Sorbitol dehydrogenase, aldolase, arginase, alcohol dehydrogenase, quinine oxidase and ornithine carbamoyl transferase are preferentially
located in the liver, while an increase in creatinine phosphokinase is diagnostic of toxic myopathy.   Plasma γ-glutamyltranspeptidase has been reported
to be a sensitive index of microsomal enzyme induction in man[25], while its
presence in urine was shown to correlate with the morphological damage produced
in rats by mercuric chloride[26].

Alkaline phosphatase, isocitric dehydrogenase and lactic dehydrogenase exist
as several enzymatically active proteins (isoenzymes), differing only in their
physical-chemical characteristics.   The proportions of the individual components are organ specific and analysis of the composition of the isoenzyme pattern in serum provides a method for locating the site of injury.

The determination of the activity of plasma pseudocholinesterase and red
cell acetylcholinesterase is a sensitive index of exposure to carbamate and
organophosphate esters, although the response does not correlate necessarily
with the activity of enzymes in the brain.   Thus a single exposure to the
insecticide 0,0-dimethyl-S-(4-oxobenzotriazino-3-methyl) phosphorodithioate
(Guthion) inhibits brain but not plasma cholinesterase, whereas octamethyl
pyrophosphoramide (OMPA) has the reverse effect for the compound does not
readily permeate the blood-brain barrier.

Lead inhibits δ-aminolaevulinic acid dehydratase that catalyses the formation of porphobilinogen and its determination in red cells provides a sensitive
index of the body-burden of inorganic lead.   Although many of the changes in
serum enzyme activity are non-specific and do not always correlate with the
severity of the induced lesion, they have an important diagnostic role in toxicity studies[27].   This also applies to changes in the ratio of albumin-globulin,
free and esterified cholesterol, bilirubin and serum electrolytes.

Some of the procedures that can be employed for assessing kidney function are listed in Table 3.

TABLE 3

RENAL FUNCTION TESTS IN LABORATORY ANIMALS

Enzymes	:	Alkaline phosphatase	Catalase
		Lactic dehydrogenase	Lysozyme
		Glycosidases	Transaminase
		(Protein)	
Excretion tests	:	Phenol red	
Glomerular filtration rate	:	Inulin; creatinine; (serum urea)	
Renal plasma flow	:	p-aminohippurate (PAH)	
Tubular absorption (TM)	:	PAH; glucose	
Concentration tests			
Dilution tests			

The value of the individual tests under a variety of experimental conditions has been reviewed by Sharratt[28] who concluded that the concentration test, urinary protein and the presence of cells in urine were the only indices which reliably demonstrated functional abnormalities associated with chronic renal lesions.

The presence of microsomal enzyme induction can be inferred in rats by measuring urinary ascorbic acid while D-glucaric acid and 6-β-hydroxycortisol may be used to detect similar changes in man[29].

CONCLUSIONS

Although the problems of interpretation may prove difficult, the integration of such biochemical studies into empirical toxicity tests can only serve to improve the basis upon which the safety of potentially hazardous chemicals is assessed.

REFERENCES
1. Brodie, B.B., Reid, W.D., Cho, A.K., Sipes, G., Krishna, G. and Gillette, J.R. (1971) Proc. Nat. Acad. Sci., 68, 160-164.
2. Mitchell, J.R., Jollow, D.H., Potter, W.Z., Gillette, J.R. and Brodie, B.B. (1973) J. Pharmacol. Exp. Ther., 187, 211-217.
3. Recknagal, R.O. and Glende, E.A. (1973) CRC Crit. Revs. Toxicol., 2, 263-297.
4. Sims, P., Grover, P.L., Swaisland, A., Pal, K. and Hewer, A. (1974) Nature (London), 252-326.

5. Jerina, D.M., Yagi, H., Letur, R.E., Thakker, D.R., Schaefer-Rider, M., Karle, J.M., Levin, W., Wood, A.W., Chang, R.L. and Conney, A.H. (1978) Polycyclic Hydrocarbons and Cancer, Vol. 1, Ed. H.V. Gelboin and P.O.P. Ts'O Academic Press, New York, pp. -73-188.

6. Watanabe, P.G., Zempel, J.A., Pegg, D.G. and Gehring, P.J. (1978) Toxicol. Appl. Pharmac., 44, 571-579.

7. Kiese, M. (1966) Pharmacol. Revs. 18, 1091-1161.

8. Reynolds, E.S. (1967) J. Pharmacol. Exp. Therap., 115, 117-126.

9. Daniel, J.W. (1965) Unpublished observations.

10. Paul, B.B. and Rubinstein, D (1963) J. Pharmacol. Exp. Therap., 141, 141-148.

11. Schulte-Hermann, R. (1974) CRC Crit. Revs. Toxicol., 3, 97-158.

12. Kunz, W., Schaude, G., Schimassek, H., Schmid, W. and Siess, M. (1966) Proceedings European Society for the Study of Drug Toxicity, Excerpta Medica Foundation, Amsterdam, 7, 138-153.

13. Platt, D.S. and Cockrill, B.L. (1969) Biochem. Pharmacol., 18, 445-457.

14. Platt, D.S. and Cockrill, B.L. (1969) Biochem. Pharmacol., 18, 429-444.

15. Crampton, R.F., Gray, T.J.B., Grasso, P. and Parke, D.V. (1977) Toxicology, 7, 289-326.

16. Golberg, L. (1966) Proceedings European Society for the Study of Drug Toxicity, Excerpta Medica Foundation, Amsterdam, 7, 171-184.

17. Daniel, J.W. (1975) Proc. 6th Intern. Cong. Pharmacol., 6, 137-146.

18. National Cancer Institute (1979) NIH Publication No. 79, 1706.

19. Cavanagh, J.B. (1973) CRC Crit. Revs. Toxicol., 2, 365-417.

20. Johnson, M.K. (1975) CRC Crit. Revs. Toxicol., 3, 289-316.

21. McKenna, M.J. and Distefano, V. (1977) J. Pharmacol. Exp. Therap., 202, 253-266.

22. Gopinath, C., Rombout, P.J.A. and van Versendaal, R.G. (1978) Toxicology, 10, 91-102.

23. Litchfield, M.H. and Conning D.M. (1972) Naunyn-Schmiedebergs Archs. Pharmacol., 272, 358-362.

24. Dent, C.E., Richens, A., Rowe, D.J.F. and Stamp, T.C.B. (1970) Brit. Med. J., 4, 69-72.

25. Martin, P.J., Martin, J.V. and Goldberg, D.M. (1975) Brit. Med. J., 1, 17-18.

26. Braun, J.P., Rico, A.G., Benard, P., Burgat-Sacaze, V., Eghbale, B. and Godfrain, J.C. (1977) Toxicology, 11, 73-82.

27. Cornish, H.H. (1971) CRC Crit. Revs. Toxicol., 1, 1-32.

28. Sharratt, M. (1970) Metabolic Aspects of Food Safety, pp. 119-171, Blackwell Scientific Publications, Oxford and Edinburgh.

29. Latham, A.V., Turner, P., Franklin, C. and Maclay, W. (1976) Can. J. Physiol. Pharmacol., 54, 778-782.

© 1980 Elsevier/North-Holland Biomedical Press
The Principles and Methods in Modern Toxicology
C.L. Galli, S.D. Murphy and R. Paoletti, editors.

THE METABOLISM AND CHEMOBIOKINETICS OF ENVIRONMENTAL CHEMICALS

DENNIS V. PARKE

Department of Biochemistry, University of Surrey, Guildford, Surrey, U.K.

Dependence of Toxicology on Metabolism and Chemobiokinetics

This century has seen the development of a major new technology in which selectively-toxic chemicals have been designed and promoted for use as medicines, pesticides, and food additives, by virtue of their ability to inhibit the biological activities of enzymes, micro-organisms, insect pests, and fungi for the medical, social and economic benefit of man. These selectively-toxic chemicals, together with many intermediates and products of the chemical industry, and with the numerous naturally occurring chemicals, may find their way into the living organism where they may elicit toxic effects.

These toxic effects are the biological manifestations of chemical interactions between the ingested environmental chemicals (xenobiotics) and the endogenous biochemical components of the body. Like all chemical processes, these interactions which give rise to toxicity are dependent on, a) the concentration of the environmental chemical, or its reactive metabolite(s), b) the concentration of the biological receptor (e.g. glutathione, acetyl-cholinesterase, cytochrome P-450, DNA), and c) the affinity of the receptor for the environmental chemical or metabolite. This can be represented by the equation:

$$T \propto [C] \, [R] \, A_{Rc}$$

where T is the Toxicity, [C] is the concentration of the environmental chemical or metabolite, [R] is the concentration of the endogenous receptor, and A_{Rc} is the affinity of the receptors for the particular environmental chemical. [C] will depend upon the intrinsic physico-chemical properties of the environmental chemical, C, the route of administration, the dose ingested, and the pathways and rates of metabolism. [R] will depend on the animal species under study, and may also vary with different tissues, age, sex, hormonal status, nutrition, etc. A_{Rc} will be determined both by the nature of the chemical and the animal species, and again will vary according to the tissue studied and to the physiological and environmental conditions of the animal.

This quantitative theoretical approach to toxicology can rationalise the known species differences in chemical toxicity and offers a scientific basis for the extrapolation of animal data to man. A major problem of this kind, which recently occurred, concerned interpretation of the significance to women taking oral contraceptives of the appearance of malignant breast tumours in the beagle dog as the result of administration of synthetic oral contraceptive progestogens. Studies, by a panel of international experts, of the metabolism of the progestogens, of their tissue concentrations and pharmacokinetics, the tissue concentrations of progestogen receptors, and their affinities for these chemicals in both human and dog, enabled the Committee of Safety of Medicines to recommend that "because of differences between the beagle bitch and the human female in the sensitivity to and the metabolism of progestogens, positive carcinogenicity studies in the beagle bitch can no longer be considered as indicative of significant hazard to women".

For similar reasons, the study of the routes and rates of metabolism of a chemical, the study of its 'detoxication' and 'activation', of the kinetics of the ingested chemical itself and of its various metabolites, have long been valued as an integral and essential part of toxicological evaluation. Comparative metabolic and chemobiokinetic studies in experimental animals and man have formed the scientific basis of a) selection of the most appropriate animal species for toxicological studies, b) determination of the chemobio- kinetic equivalent dosage to man, and c) extrapolation to man of animal toxicology data. The undertaking of animal toxicology studies without adequate metabolic and kinetic basis is largely a waste of time, for such empiricism often leads to gross errors in the prediction of toxicity in man, and this occasioned by the false estimate of safety promoted by spurious information may result in exposing human populations to unnecessary dangers or, on the other hand, to establishing excessively high standards of safety and the needless banning of useful chemicals. The importance to toxicology of the factors which comprise the other half of the toxicity equation, namely, the comparative study in animals and man, of the concentration and affinities of the particular tissue receptors concerned with toxic response(s) to the environmental chemical, has only recently been appreciated. However, when it is realized that it was studies of this kind which facilitated the scientific interpretation of questionable animal carcinogenicity data and enabled the various benefits of oral contraceptives to continue to be available to those who required them, such studies will receive the attention they obviously merit.

Metabolism of Environmental Chemicals and Detoxication

The ingestion of an environmental chemical is usually followed by its metabolism which is catalysed by enzymes of the gastrointestinal tract, the

TABLE 1

BIOTRANSFORMATION REACTIONS OF ENVIRONMENTAL CHEMICALS

Oxidations

Microsomal oxidations:

aliphatic hydroxylation	$RCH_3 \xrightarrow{\;O\;}$	RCH_2OH
aromatic hydroxylation	$C_6H_6 \longrightarrow$	C_6H_5OH
epoxidation	$RCH=CHR' \longrightarrow$	$RCH \overset{O}{-} CHR'$

deamination

$$\underset{R'}{\overset{R}{>}}CHNH_2 \longrightarrow \left[\underset{R'}{\overset{R}{>}}C(OH)NH_2 \right] \longrightarrow \underset{R'}{\overset{R}{>}}CO + NH_3$$

dealkylation

$ROCH_3 \longrightarrow [ROCH_2OH] \longrightarrow ROH + HCHO$

(O-, N-, and S-)

$RN(CH_3)_2 \longrightarrow RNHCH_3 + HCHO$

$RSCH_3 \longrightarrow RSH + HCHO$

dehalogenation

$RCCl_3 \longrightarrow RCOCl$

N-hydroxylation	$RNH_2 \xrightarrow{\;O\;}$	$RNHOH$
N-oxidation	$R_3N \longrightarrow$	$R_3N{\to}O$

sulphoxidation

$$\underset{R'}{\overset{R}{>}}S \xrightarrow{\;O\;} \underset{R'}{\overset{R}{>}}S{\to}O \xrightarrow{\;O\;} \underset{R'}{\overset{R}{>}}SO_2$$

desulphuration

$$\underset{R'}{\overset{R}{>}}C=S \longrightarrow \underset{R'}{\overset{R}{>}}C=O$$

$$\underset{R'}{\overset{R}{>}}P\overset{OH}{\underset{S}{\diagdown}} \longrightarrow \underset{R'}{\overset{R}{>}}P\overset{OH}{\underset{O}{\diagdown}}$$

Non-microsomal oxidations:

amine oxidation	$RCH_2NH_2 \xrightarrow{\;O_2\;} RCH=NH \xrightarrow{\;H_2O\;}$	$RCHO + NH_3$
alcohol oxidation	$RCH_2OH \longrightarrow$	$RCHO$
aldehyde oxidation	$RCHO \longrightarrow$	$RCOOH$

Reductions

Microsomal reduction:

nitro reduction

$RNO_2 \xrightarrow{\;2H\;} RNO \xrightarrow{\;2H\;} RNHOH \xrightarrow{\;2H\;} RNH_2$

azo reduction

$RN=NR' \xrightarrow{\;2H\;} RNHNHR' \xrightarrow{\;2H\;} RNH_2 + R'NH_2$

reductive dehalogenation

$RCCl_3 \xrightarrow{\;2H\;} RCHCl_2 + HCl$

metal alkyl dealkylation

$PbR_4 \xrightarrow{\;2H\;} PbHR_3 + RH$

Non-microsomal reduction:

aldehyde reduction

$$\underset{R'}{\overset{R}{\diagdown}}CO \xrightarrow{\;2H\;} \underset{R'}{\overset{R}{\diagdown}}CHOH$$

Hydrolyses

ester hydrolysis	$RCO-OR' \xrightarrow{\;H_2O\;}$	$RCOOH + R'OH$
amide hydrolysis	$RCO-NH_2 \longrightarrow$	$RCOOH + NH_3$

TABLE 2

CONJUGATION REACTIONS OF ENVIRONMENTAL CHEMICALS

Glucuronide conjugations (UDPGA)

O-ether type	ROH	$\longrightarrow$	$RO-C_6H_9O_6$
O-ester type	$RCOOH$	$\longrightarrow$	$RCOO-C_6H_9O_6$
N-glucuronide	RNH_2	$\longrightarrow$	$RNH-C_6H_9O_6$
S-glucuronide	RSH	$\longrightarrow$	$RS-C_6H_9O_6$

Sulphate conjugation (PAPS)

O-sulphate	ROH	$\longrightarrow$	$RO-SO_3H$
N-sulphate (sulphamate)	RNH_2	$\longrightarrow$	$RNH-SO_3H$

Methylations (S-Adenosyl methionine)

O-methylation	ROH	$\longrightarrow$	$RO-CH_3$
S-methylation	RSH	$\longrightarrow$	$RS-CH_3$
N-methylation	RNH_2	$\longrightarrow$	$RNH-CH_3$
	$\geqslant N$		$\geqslant \overset{+}{N}-CH_3$

Acetylations (Acetyl-CoA)

amino acetylation	RNH_2	$\longrightarrow$	$RNH-COCH_3$
sulphamyl acetylation	RSO_2NH_2	$\longrightarrow$	$RSO_2NH-COCH_3$

Amino acid conjugation (Acyl-CoAs)

glycine conjugation	$RCOOH$	$\longrightarrow$	$RCO-NHCH_2COOH$
glutamine conjugation	$RCOOH$	$\longrightarrow$	$RCO-NHCH(CH_2)_2CONH_2$ with $COOH$ branch

Glutathione conjugation (GSH)

alkyl halide

$$RCH_2Cl \longrightarrow RCH_2SG \xrightarrow[-glutamate]{-glycine} RCH_2SCH_2CHNHCOCH_3 \;(\text{with } COOH)$$

aliphatic epoxide

$$RCH\overset{O}{\overset{\diagup\diagdown}{-}}CHR' \longrightarrow \underset{OH}{RCHCHR'}\overset{SG}{|} \longrightarrow \underset{OH}{RCHCHR'}\overset{SCH_2CHNHCOCH_3}{\overset{|}{\overset{COOH}{}}}$$

aromatic epoxide

liver and other tissues, resulting in biotransformation (oxidation, reduction
and hydrolysis) and/or conjugation (biosyntheses with glucuronic acid, sulphate,
acetate, glycine, glutathione, etc.) and yielding a wide variety of metabolites
(see Tables 1 & 2). The biotransformation reactions (phase 1) usually precede
the conjugation reactions (phase 2), e.g. the oxidation of benzene to phenol
and its conjugation to phenylglucuronide and phenylsulphate (see Fig.1), making
the molecule less lipophilic, more polar, and more readily excretable from the
body.

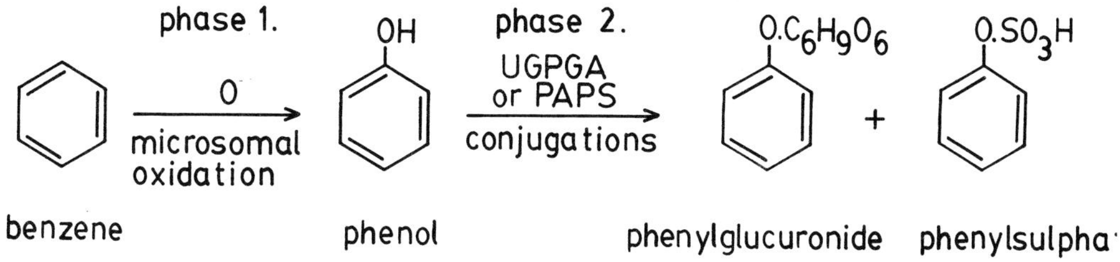

Fig. 1. The biotransformation (phase 1) and conjugation (phase 2) of benzene.

The enzymes which catalyse these reactions are found in many tissues, but are predominantly located in the liver and gastrointestinal tract. Within the cell they may be found in the mitochondria (monoamine oxidase), the cytosol (alcohol dehydrogenase, sulphatase), and especially in the endoplasmic reticulum (mcirosomal oxidases, glucuronyl transferase). The endoplasmic reticulum is a lipoprotein tubular network within the cell which becomes a point of focus for lipophilic environmental chemicals entering the organism. In view of its vital cellular functions it is perhaps not surprising that this organelle is richly endowed with enzyme systems to metabolize environmental chemicals to thus accelerate their removal from the cell and protect itself from their harmful effects. The microsomal mixed-function oxidase system is a membrane-bound, enzyme complex, capable of interacting with molecular oxygen to insert one atom of oxygen into the environmental chemical while the other reacts with 2H to form water[2]. The components of this mixed-function oxidase system are NADPH, cytochrome P-450 reductase (a flavoprotein containing FMN and FAD), and cytochrome P-450, with phosphatidylcholine, cytochrome b_5, and cytochrome b_5 reductase playing secondary roles in the electron transport. A recently proposed version of the reaction mechanism of this mixed-function oxidase is shown in Figure 2[3]. This enzyme system has a number of normal physiological functions, such as the synthesis of cholesterol, corticosteroids and sex hormones, thromboxanes and prostaglandins, and the ω-hydroxylation of fatty acids, so that the metabolism of environmental chemicals could, if excessive, compete with the normal role of the mixed-function oxidases to the detriment of cellular metabolism and the homeostatic mechanisms of the living organism.

The metabolism of environmental chemicals usually leads to detoxication with increased polarity of the molecule and an increased rate of excretion from the living organism. The routes of metabolism can be many, and may include oxidation, reduction and conjugation, but all pathways lead eventually to detoxication and more rapid excretion. For example, nitrobenzene may undergo oxidation to form nitrophenols, reduction to give aniline and aminophenols, and conjugation to the acetamidophenyl glucuronides (see Figure 3).

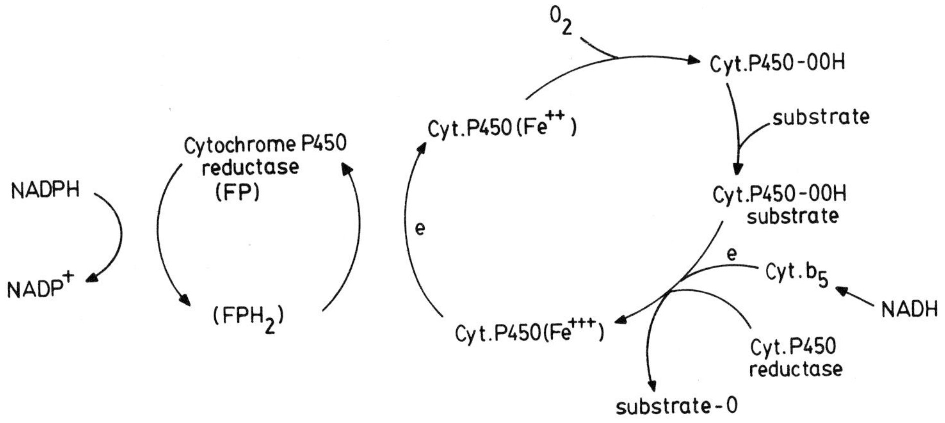

Fig. 2.   The microsomal mixed-function oxidase system.

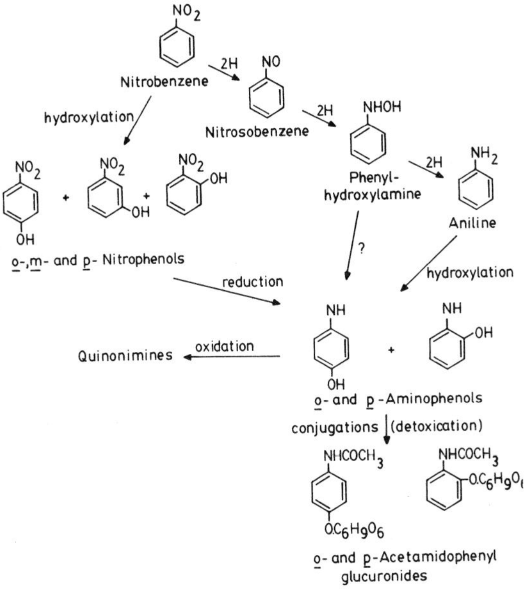

Fig. 3.   The metabolism of nitrobenzene.

Metabolic Activation of Environmental Chemicals

Although metabolism generally results in detoxication and increased excretion, the converse can also occur, and chemicals may be metabolised to yield highly reactive intermediates, such as epoxides, hydroxylamines, free radicals, carbenes, etc. which interact with tissue receptors and other components to initiate toxic reactions. Frequently, of the possible alternative pathways of metabolism, one may lead to detoxication and the other to activation and increased toxicity. Indeed the species differences in metabolic pathways is often the basis of selective toxicity as, for example, in the metabolism of the pesticide malathion, which is detoxicated in man, but activated in insects (see Figure 4).

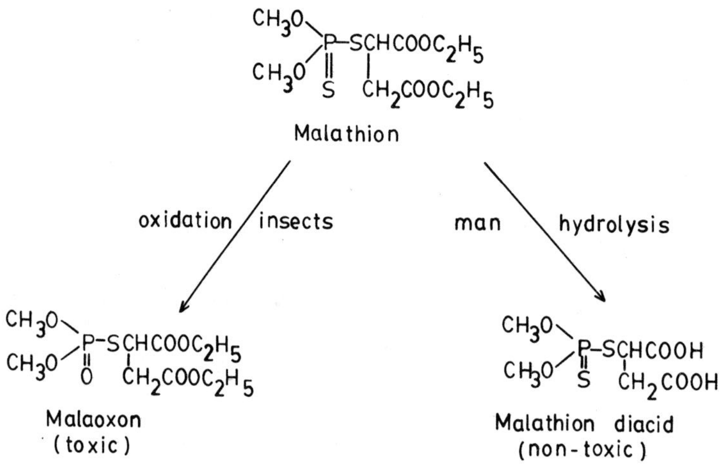

$$CH_3O \diagdown P\text{--}SCHCOOC_2H_5$$
$$CH_3O \diagup \underset{S}{\overset{\|}{}} \quad CH_2COOC_2H_5$$

Malathion

oxidation / insects   man \ hydrolysis

$$CH_3O \diagdown P\text{--}SCHCOOC_2H_5$$
$$CH_3O \diagup \underset{O}{\overset{\|}{}} \quad CH_2COOC_2H_5$$

Malaoxon
(toxic)

$$CH_3O \diagdown P\text{--}SCHCOOH$$
$$CH_3O \diagup \underset{S}{\overset{\|}{}} \quad CH_2COOH$$

Malathion diacid
(non-toxic)

Fig. 4.   Species differences in the metabolism and toxicity of malathion.

The activation of environmental chemicals may involve many of the various metabolic reactions previously described, but especially oxidation, including epoxidation, N-hydroxylation and oxidative dealkylation, as occurs in the activation of the carcinogens, aflatoxin, 2-acetaminofluorene, and dimethylnitrosamine (see Figure 5).

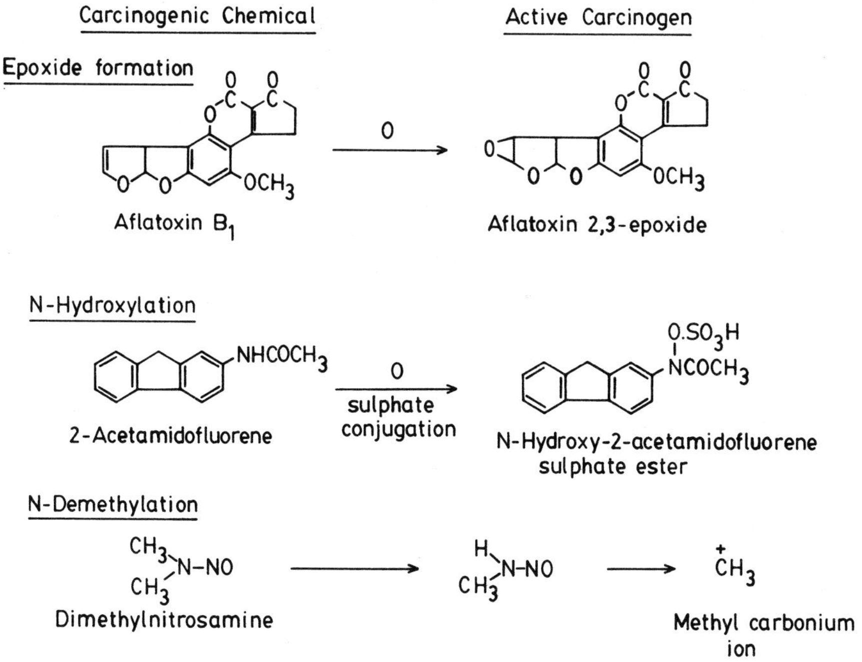

Fig. 5. Activation of environmental chemicals by metabolic oxidation.

Like aflatoxin, many unsaturated aliphatic and aromatic compounds such as tetrachloroethylene, benzene, bromobenzene, naphthalene and benzo(a)pyrene, undergo epoxidation, which is believed to be the basis of their cytotoxicity. These epoxides are highly reactive intermediates; some undergo intramolecular rearrangements to acid chlorides or phenols, others are converted to the less toxic dihydrodiols and catechols by the enzyme epoxide hydrase or are conjugated with glutathione, while yet others escape these tissue defence mechanisms and react with tissue proteins, RNA, or DNA, initiating tissue

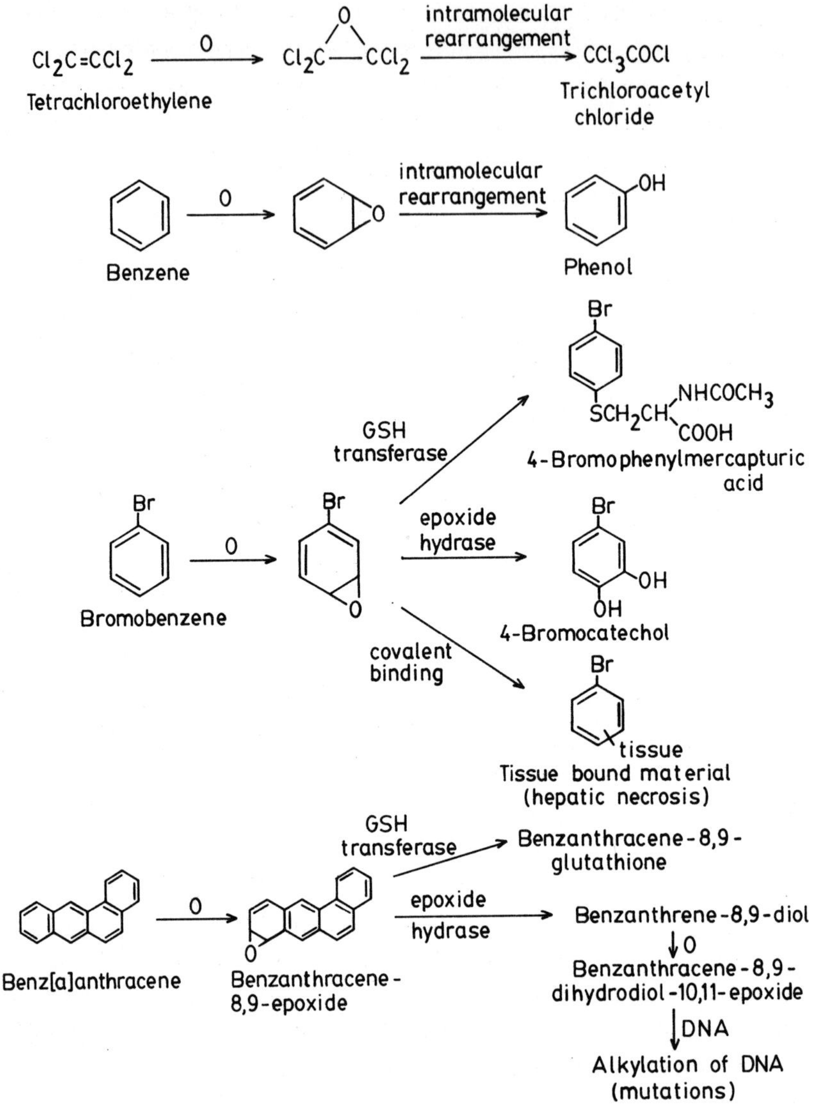

94

Fig. 6. Metabolism of environmental chemicals to reactive epoxide intermediates.

injury and mutations (see Figure 6). The metabolic hydroxylation of aromatic amines leads to the formation of aminophenols which undergo oxidation to ortho- and para-quinoneimines (see Figure 3); these reactive intermediates are potent oxidising agents[4], depleting tissue glutathione, oxidising and covalently binding with other vital tissue components, resulting in tissue necrosis, cataract, diabetes and male infertility .

Metabolism of Environmental Chemicals and Ligand Complex Formation with Cytochrome P-450

Many environmental chemicals, such as halogenohydrocarbons, are resistant to metabolism, especially to oxidation by the mixed-function oxidases. They are, however, dehalogenated by cytochrome P-450, and probably by other haeme proteins, under anaerobic conditions to give carbenes which form stable ligand complexes with cytochrome P-450[2] (see Figure 7).

Similarly, methylene dioxyaryl compounds such as safrole which do undergo hydroxylation, of the methylene group, spontaneously lose the elements of water to form carbenes which again form ligand complexes with cytochrome P-450 (see Figure 7). Many other environmental chemicals, including amines and thiols, similarly undergo metabolic activation to form reactive intermediates which ligand complex to cytochrome P-450. This ligand complex formation inhibits the normal mixed-function oxidase activity of the cytochrome P-450 (biphenyl 4-hydroxylation), but, in contrast, cytochrome P-448 activity (biphenyl 2-hydroxylation) is increased (see Figure 8).

The mechanism of this change of cytochrome mixed-function oxidase activity is not fully understood but, presumably, could be due to one or more of the following: a) cytochrome P-448 is specifically induced, in place of cytochrome P-450, b) cytochrome P-448 activity is in reality catalysed by the flavoprotein (cytochrome P-450 reductase) or c) the cytochrome P-448 activity is due to reactive oxygen species (autoxidation by singlet oxygen, superoxy anion, hydroxyl radical) generated by the cytochrome P-450 ligand complex, which can accept the molecular oxygen and activate it but cannot accept the organic substrate to catalyse its enzyme specific hydroxylation (see Figure 9).

Other metabolism of environmental chemicals has been shown to result in another type of complex formation with cytochrome P-450, namely the desulphuration of thiocarbonyl ($>C=S$) and thiophosphonyl ($\geqslant P=S$) compounds (Table 3) by the microsomal mixed-function oxidase system[5]. In the oxidative metabolism of these chemicals the S is replaced by O to form the corresponding

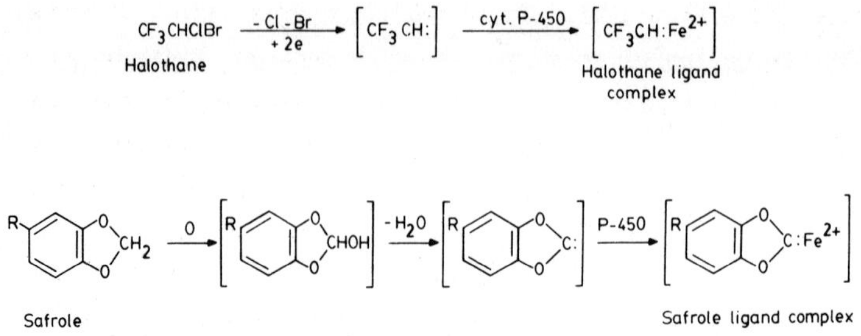

Fig. 7.   Formation of ligand complexes of cytochrome P-450.

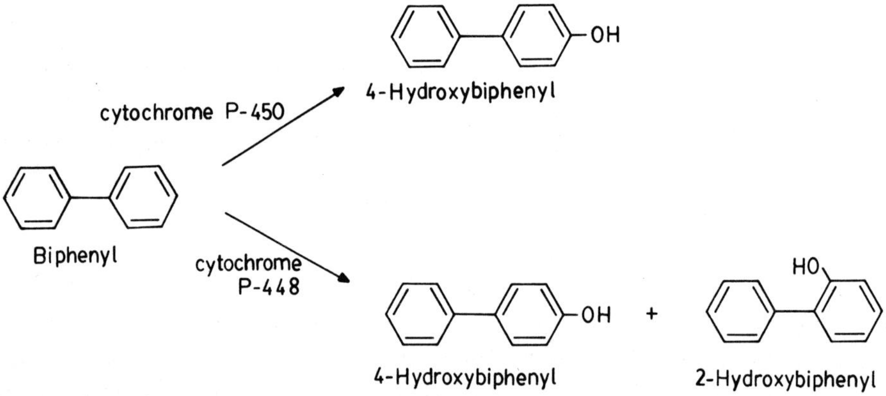

Fig. 8.   Mixed-function oxidation of biphenyl.

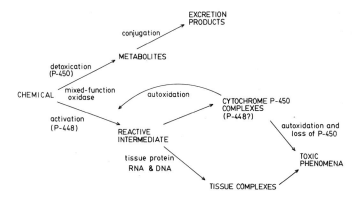

Fig. 9. Cytochrome P-450 complex formation and autoxidation.

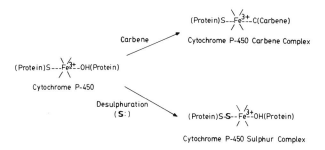

Fig. 10. Possible structure of cytochrome P-450 ligand complexes.

carbonyl ($\geq$C=O) and phosphonyl analogues ($\geq$P=P), and the sulphene S: is transferred to cytochrome P-450, probably at the natural cysteine ligand forming a hydrodisulphide link to the iron of the haeme moiety (Fe$\leftarrow$S-S-R) (see Figure 10). The result of this S-complex formation is that cytochrome P-450 loses its mixed-function oxidase activity, initiating autoxidation and lipid peroxidation, which destroys the cytochrome P-450 and the integrity of the endoplasmic reticulum, resulting in acute and chronic cellular damage.

TABLE 3

SOME ENVIRONMENTAL CHEMICALS METABOLISED BY DESULPHURATION

CS$_2$

Carbon disulphide

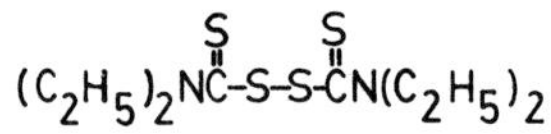

$(C_2H_5)_2N\overset{\overset{S}{\|}}{C}-S-S-\overset{\overset{S}{\|}}{C}N(C_2H_5)_2$

Disulfiram

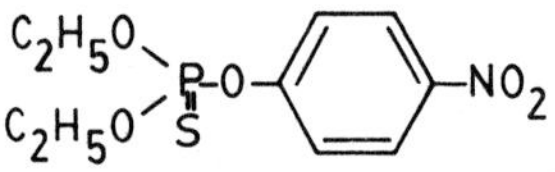

Parathion

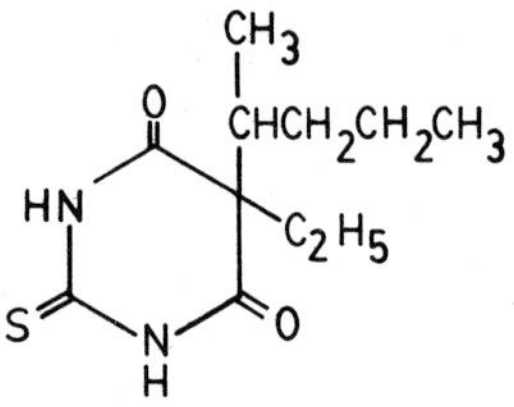

Thiopental

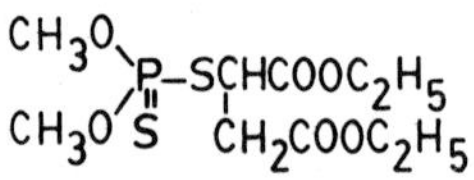

Malathion

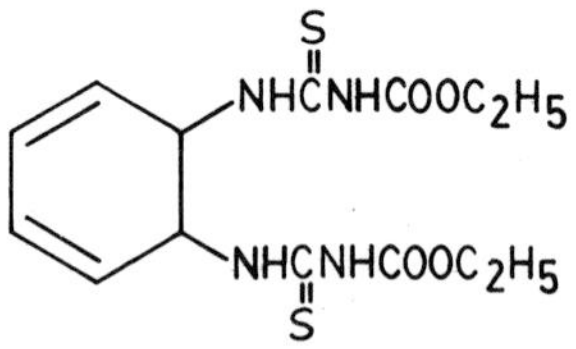

Thiophanate

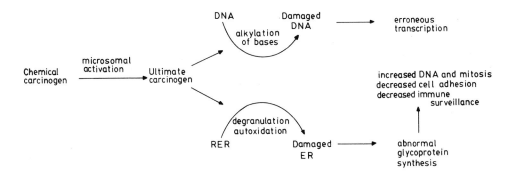

Fig. 11. The role of the endoplasmic reticulum in carcinogenesis.

The cellular autoxidation initiated by this complex formation with
cytochrome P-450 results in increased autophagocytosis and damage to the
structure and function of the cytocavitary network of the cell, which has been
associated with acute lethal injury including carcinogenesis, cardiovascular
lesions, and arthritic disease[6,7]. Injury to the endoplasmic reticulum,
directly by reactive intermediates of environmental chemicals or indirectly by
autoxidation, would be expected to result in changes in glycoprotein synthesis,
in the structure of the cell surface glycocalyx, and in the stability of the
lysosomes and lysosomal enzymes, which would accord with the observed cellular
phenomena of malignancy, namely, changes in mitosis, in differentiation,
proliferation (invasion), and intercellular adhesion (metastases)[7,8]
(see Figure 11).

Detoxication vs. Activation

In summary, the microsomal metabolism of environmental chemicals may result in the following phenomena:

1. Detoxication and accelerated excretion of metabolites.

2. Activation and reaction with cellular components, eliciting toxic reactions.

3. Ligand complex binding to cytochrome P-450, with inhibition or destruction of this enzyme, resulting in autoxidation and non-specific oxidation of environmental chemical substrates.

The outstanding question of toxicology is what are the factors which determine which of these alternative pathways predominate. It has been shown that the final activation of the chemical carcinogen, benzo(a)pyrene, by 9,10-epoxidation (bay region epoxidation) to form the ultimate carcinogen, benzo(a) pyrene-7,8-dihydrodiol-9,10-epoxide, is catalysed only by cytochrome P-448, and that the reconstituted purified cytochrome P-450 does not catalyse this type of epoxidation[9] (Figure 12). Moreover, the 7,8-diol-9,10-epoxide has been shown not to be a substrate for the detoxicating enzyme, epoxide hydrase. Since cytochrome P-448 when purified has been shown to be a complex with the various carcinogenic chemicals (e.g. benzo(a)pyrene) used to induce this cytochrome[10], it is attempting to suggest that the typical P-448 activity may be due to non-specific chemical autoxidation or flavoprotein oxidation, which can activate chemicals by oxidation at positions which are normally inaccessible to enzymic mixed-function oxidation by cytochrome P-450. Apart from the toxicity resulting from the autoxidation, it is possible that the toxicity of bay-region oxygenated environmental chemicals results, at least in part, from the inaccessibility of the epoxide groups to detoxication enzymes such as epoxide hydrase.

Chemobiokinetics of Environmental Chemicals

(i) Species differences - Determination of the rates and extents of metabolism of environmental chemicals to the various detoxication products, or to activated intermediates, is essential to an understanding of the potential toxicity of the chemical and to an evaluation of its safety in man. As the rates of the various alternative metabolic pathways may differ in different animal species, a study of the comparative chemobiokinetics in man and laboratory animals is necessary for the choice of the most appropriate animal species as a suitable experimental model for man. Perhaps, even more important, it is essential for the calculation of the kinetically equivalent dosage for

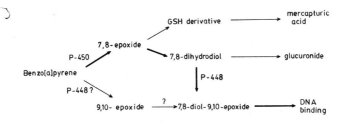

Fig. 12. Alternate pathways of benzo[a]pyrene metabolism.

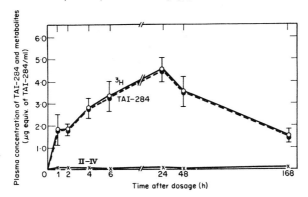

Fig. 13. Plasma levels of TAI-284 and metabolites after oral dosing of ^{3}H-TAI-284 to guinea pigs. (Reproduced with permission of Professor S. Tanayama).

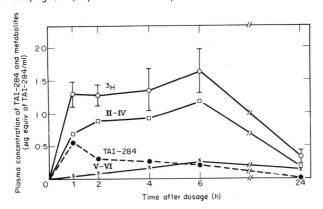

Fig. 14. Plasma levels of TAI-284 and metabolites after oral dosing of ^{3}H-TAI-284 to mice. (Reproduced with permission of Professor S. Tanayama).

the animal toxicity studies. And for extrapolation of the animal toxicity data
to man, comparative kinetic studies in man and the animal species used is at
present the only known scientific basis.

There is now substantial evidence that the rate of microsomal mixed-function
oxidase activity is greater the smaller the animal[11,12]. Those chemicals which
are metabolised primarily by oxidations involving cytochrome P-450 show an
inverse correlation between the rates of metabolism and the body weight of the
animal species under study (see Table 4), so that the ratios of oxidative
metabolism in mouse, rat, dog, primate and man are of the order of 30:20:5:2:1.
This means that where a chemical is primarily metabolised by mixed-function
oxidation the rat will carry out the metabolism at some 20 times the rate
occurring in man. When the chemical is primarily detoxicated by metabolism
this difference in rates of metabolism will often imply similar differences in
acute toxicity, so that for many chemicals equivalent doses calculated on a
body weight basis will be much less toxic to the rat or mouse than to larger
animals such as man. This is a long-appreciated observation of pharmacologists,
and is the reason for calculating dosage for different species on a kinetically-
equivalent basis. Conversely, where chemicals are activated by microsomal
oxidation, the rate of activation and hence the toxicity will be greater the
smaller the species. Unfortunately, much animal toxicology is conducted
without prior calculation of the kinetically-equivalent dosage to man, so that
the assessments of potential toxicity to man may grossly underestimate acute
toxicity and overestimate the chronic toxicity, such as carcinogenicity.

TABLE 4

RATES OF BIPHENYL HYDROXYLATION IN DIFFERENT ANIMAL SPECIES

Species	Bodyweight (kg)	Biphenyl 4-hydroxylation	Biphenyl 2-hydroxylation
		(μmol/g liver per h)	
Mouse	0.04	5.7	2.2
Hamster	0.20	3.8	1.8
Rat	0.25	2.5	0.3
Ferret	1.5	2.0	0.2
Cat	5.0	0.9	0.2

These species differences in rates of metabolic detoxication and metabolic activation seem to apply only to microsomal enzymic hydroxylation reactions. They do not generally apply to conjugation reactions, nor to those non-cytochrome P-450 oxidative reactions, such as bay-region epoxidation and N-hydroxylation, which are effected by non-enzymic autoxidation, by flavoprotein enzymes[13], or possibly by cytochrome P-448. As shown in Table 5, biphenyl 4-hydroxylation (cytochrome P-450) exhibits the general increased enzyme activity with decrease in body weight, but biphenyl 2-hydroxylation (cytochrome P-448) does not follow this trend to the same extent. Indeed, it is well-known that the mouse and hamster are prone to N-hydroxylate chemicals, whereas the rat, guinea pig, man and other species do not so readily effect N-hydroxylation. These species differences in the modes of hydroxylation can result in marked differences in chemobiokinetics and toxicity, as has been demonstrated for the non-steroidal anti-inflammatory drug, 6-chloro-5-cyclohexylindane-1-carboxylic acid (TAI-284), which is metabolised by hydroxylation (see Figures 13 and 14). In the mouse the peak plasma concentration of orally administered drug was 0.5 µg/ml and occurred at 1 hour after dosage; the blood plasma concentration of metabolites was higher than that of unchanged chemical at all times. In contrast, in the guinea pig metabolism is minimal, and no significant concentration of metabolites was found in the blood plasma at any time; the peak plasma concentration of the unchanged compound was 4.5 µg/ml and occurred at 24 hours after oral dosage[14]. The blood concentration of the unmetabolized chemical in the guinea pig 7 days after dosage was three times higher than the peak plasma concentration in the mouse (1 hour after dosage). Little wonder that the pharmacology and toxicology of this drug exhibit wide differences in different species.

(ii) Tissue differences - Just as species differences in metabolism may affect the chemobiokinetics of a chemical, so may tissue differences in metabolism or receptor affinities similarly affect the kinetics. Paraquat, which has an affinity for lung tissue has biological half-lives of 20 hours in the lung and of 1 hour in the blood plasma, in rats given the chemical intravenously[15]. Determination of tissue chemobiokinetics of a chemical are therefore necessary to identify particular target organs and target tissues for toxic effects of the chemical.

(iii) Repeat-dose kinetics, enterhepatic recirculation and accumulation - Much information regarding the absorption, tissue distribution, metabolism and excretion of a chemical can be obtained from a kinetic study following single dosage, but as the physiological and environmental factors governing the animal, and hence governing the chemobiokinetics, may change on repeated dosage, repeat-dose kinetic studies, both in man and experimental animals, are essential to an informed assessment of the potential toxicity of the chemical to man. Many chemicals of high lipophilicity and high molecular weight are excreted in the bile as conjugates of metabolites or conjugates of the original chemical. Some of this biliary-excreted material is eventually voided in the faeces, but some may undergo bacterial hydrolysis in the gut and be reabsorbed to be exposed to a further round of metabolism, distribution and excretion. If exposure to the chemical is continued, the enterophepatic circulation may result in a progressive accumulation of the compound and its metabolites within the body's tissue. This is of special concern with those chemicals, such as DDT, dieldrin, TCCD, PCB's, which are highly lipophilic and resistant to metabolic detoxication because they contain halogen atoms. Chemicals of this type may have biological half-lives measured in years and become permanent components of the body's tissues. Although these chemicals are chemically inert, they are nevertheless often biologically active, and may undergo unusual types of metabolism, such as dehalogenation, carbene formation and ligand complex formation with cytochrome P-450 which result in toxic phenomena.

(iv) Enzyme induction and inhibition - Exposure of animals to high concentrations of chemicals which are readily-metabolized substrates of the microsomal mixed-function oxidases (cytochrome P-450), or to low concentrations of chemicals that are metabolised with difficulty, leads to an increased biosynthesis of these enzymes, known as 'enzyme induction'. This physiological response to a high work load of the enzymes is accompanied by cellular hypertrophy, and is generally considered not to be a manifestation of toxicity. Exposure of animals to certain toxic chemicals, many of which are known carcinogens such as benzo(a)pyrene, 3-methylcholanthrene and safrole, results in a similar phenomenon except that it is cytochrome P-448 which is induced and this is not accompanied by any significant hypertrophy or increase in cytochrome P-450 reductase. As this cytochrome P-448 when solubilised and purified still contains a molecular equivalent of the inducing chemical it is possible that this cytochrome is a ligand or covalent complex, and that its apparent mixed-function oxidase activity may be mediated by the flavoprotein reductase or via activated oxygen species generated by the cytochrome. Whether cytochrome P-448 is a naturally occurring microsomal mixed-function oxidase, as is more generally believed, or a chemical complex of a cytochrome P-450 species with an activated intermediate of an environmental chemical, the effect of cytochrome P-448 on chemical toxicity is not in question.

Exposure of animals to those chemicals which, either directly or indirectly following metabolic activation, can act as competitive or non-competitive inhibitors of the detoxication enzymes, will result in inhibition of metabolism and increased half-lives of other chemicals ingested simultaneously. The irreversible inhibition of the microsomal mixed-function oxidases by ligand complex formation may, by the consequent autoxidation, result in destruction of the cytochrome P-450 and to cytotoxicity. The normal physiological roles of this microsomal enzyme system make this destruction of cytochrome P-450 a major phenomenon of toxicology which may have far-reaching consequences, e.g. metabolic, cardiovascular and arthritic lesions, not always monitored in safety evaluation procedures for environmental chemicals.

REFERENCES

1. C.S.M., 1979. Medicines Act Information Letter, No.25, page 2.

2. Ullrich, V. (1979) Topics in Current Chemistry, ed. F.L. Boschke, Springer-Verlag, Berlin, 83, 68-104.

3. Holtzman, J.L. (1979) Pharmac. Ther., 4, 601-627.

4. Calder, I.C., Williams, P.J., Woods, R.A., Funder, C.C., Green, C.R., Ham, K.N. and Tange, J.D. (1975) Xenobiotica, 5, 303-307.

5. Neal, R.A., Kamataki, T., Lin, M., Ptashne, K.A., Dalvi, R.R. and Poore, R.E. (1977) in Biological Reactive Intermediates, ed. D.J. Jollow, et al., Plenum Press, New York, p.320.

6. Parke, D.V. (1979a) in Drug Toxicity, ed. J.W. Gorrod, Taylor & Francis, London, pp.133-150.

7. Parke, D.V. (1979b) in Regulatory Aspects of Carcinogenesis and Food Additives: The Delaney Clause, ed. F. Coulston, Academic Press, New York, pp.173-187.

8. Apffel, C.A. (1979) Medical Hypotheses, 5, 23-52.

9. Levin, W. et al. (1977) Drug Metabolism Concepts, ACS Symposium Series, No.4, 99-126.

10. Sato, R., Imai, Y. and Hashimoto-Yutsudo, C. (1979) Abstr.L-103, Fourth Int. Symp. on Microsomes and Drug Oxidation, Ann Arbor.

11. Kato, R. (1979) Pharmac. Ther., 6, 41-98.

12. Walker, C.H. (1978) Drug Metabolism Rev., 7, 295-323.

13. Lai, C.-S., Grover, T.A. and Piette, L.H. (1979) Arch. Biochem. Biophys., 193, 373-378.

14. Tanayama, S. (1973) Xenobiotica, 3, 671-680.

15. Smith, L.L., Wyatt, I. and Rose, M.S. (1978) in Industrial and Environmental Xenobiotics, International Congress Series, Exerpta Medica, Amsterdam, pp.135-140.

GENERAL PRINCIPLES OF GENETIC TOXICOLOGY AND METHODS FOR MUTAGENE-
SIS ASSESSMENT

NICOLA LOPRIENO

Laboratorio di Genetica, Istituto di Antropologia e Paleontologia
Umana della Università, Via S. Maria 53, 56100-PISA (Italy).

1. ABSTRACT

Genetic toxicology, a recent branch of genetic and general toxicology, deals essentially with the study of genetic hazards for
man as a consequence of the wide spread use of mutagenic chemicals
in the human environment: this hazard is important for single individuals through the induction of gene - and chromosome - mutations in somatic cells which might cause the development of cancer, and for future generation, through the production of transmis
sible gene - and chromosome - mutations in germinal cells which mi
ght cause genetic diseases.

Genetic research in the last four decades has developed the present knowledge on the cellular process of mutation, the molecular
nature of genetic alteration in the DNA, the mutational nature of
hereditary diseases in man, the mechanisms by which the chemicals
produce alterations in the DNA.

Mutation research developed in the last decade has defined seve
ral in vitro and in vivo methodologies for assessing the mutagenic
and the genetic risks of chemicals. Molecular biology research has
made a convincing understanding of the basic mechanisms which initiate the carcinogenic transformation of a cell, which later on
changes its phenotype into a cancerous irreversible stage: at cellular level several mutation steps are common to both the production of a mutant as well of a malignant cell. Moreover the metabo
lic conversions to which a xenobiotic chemical is submitted when
introduced into the mammals body have been extensively investigated.

During the last four/five years an enormous amount of mutagenic analyses of chemical carcinogens has provided evidence of the existence of a correlation between the mutagenic and the carcinogenic activity of the chemicals at least to a level of 75-80% of all cases analyzed so far.

Genetic toxicology does provide therefore the basic concepts and has made available new toxicological procedures for the analysis of the potential negative interactions between the human population and its present environment.

2. CHEMICAL BASIS OF MUTATION

Mutation theory originated at the time when MENDEL's laws were rediscovered: it received however an experimental basis only after the discovery of the mutagenic effects of X-radiations in 1927 by H.J. MULLER, and a more extensive support after the discovery of chemical mutagens in 1940 by C. AUERBACH in Scotland, F. OELKERS in Germany, and by I.A. RAPOPORT in Soviet Union: in 1947, C. AUERBACH and her coll. stated that "a genetic mutation is a change presumably chemical in nature, in one of the genes which compose the chromosome thread". At that time it was assumed that a simple chemical reaction between the mutagenic compound and the genetic material could be the basis of the mutational event. The extensive series of experimental studies on the genetic effects of chemical mutagens which were developed between 1950 and 1960 has led to the development of mutagenesis theories elaborated by E. FREESE and later by S. BRENNER et al. These theories offered interpretations of the possible molecular alterations that take place in the DNA molecule after treating a cellular organism with a chemical mutagen (Table 1)

TABLE 1

DIRECT ACTIONS OF ENVIRONMENTAL MUTAGENS ON THE GENETIC MATERIAL

A. THE ACTION OF MUTAGENS ON "RESTING DNA"

---

1. DEAMINATION OF BASES

2. ALKYLATION OF BASES

3. CROSSLINKING OF DNA CHAINS

B. THE ACTION OF MUTAGENS ON "REPLICANT & RECOMBINANT DNA"

---

1. INCORPORATION OF BASE ANALOGUES

2. INTERCALATION BETWEEN BASES

3. INTERACTION WITH MEMBRANES

At the present the "mutational process" is no more regarded as the effect of a single and simple chemical reaction (table 2). It is true that a change in the information carried by DNA is a neces

TABLE 2

INDIRECT ACTIONS OF ENVIRONMENTAL MUTAGENS ON THE GENETIC APPARATUS

---

1. MUTATION AS A RESULT OF MISTAKES OF DNA REPLICATING ENZYMES

2. MUTATION AS A RESULT OF MISTAKES OF DNA REPAIR ENZYMES

3. MUTATION AS A RESULT OF DIFFERENT EVENTS DURING RECOMBINATION

---

sary condition for mutation, but it is not a sufficient one, as it is preceded as well as followed by secondary steps which make the mutational process a complex cellular series of events: between the contact of a cell with a chemical mutagen and the production of a mutant cell several steps have been identified (table 3).

TABLE 3

RELATIONSHIPS BETWEEN A CHEMICAL MUTAGEN AND THE PRODUCTION OF MU-
TANT CELLS

---

1. A CHEMICAL MUTAGEN ENTERS INTO THE CELL AND UNDERGOES METABO-
   LIC REACTIONS WHICH DEPEND ON : (A) STRAIN, (B) CELL STAGE,
   (C) METABOLIC STATE.
2. ITS REACTIONS WITH DNA DEPENDS ON: (A) THE BASIS OF ITS CHEMI-
   CAL STRUCTURE, (B) THE COILING OF CHROMOSOMES, (C) THE GENE STA
   TE, (D) THE AMOUNT OF CHROMOSOMAL COMPONENTS.
3. THE INDUCED DNA LESIONS ARE REPAIRED AND THEY DEPEND ON : (A)
   THE AMOUNT AND THE TYPE OF DIFFERENT ENZYMES, (B) THE TIME AVA
   ILABLE BEFORE NEXT DNA REPLICATION, (C) THE REPLICATION OF DNA
   SEGMENTS, (D) EXTERNAL FACTORS (LIGHT, pH, ETC.), (E) GENETIC
   FACTORS.
4. THE MUTATIONAL CHANGE IS THEN : (A) STABILIZED IN THE DNA MOLE
   CULE, (B) TRANSCRIBED INTO A NEW mRNA, (C) TRANSLATED INTO A
   NEW PROTEIN.
5. A NEW MUTANT, RECOMBINANT, CONVERTANT CELL IS PRODUCED WHICH
   GROWS INTO A NEW POPULATION OF CELLS.

This has been the result of a series of studies which have elucidated the role played of several cellular factors beside the
chemical mutagen and the DNA in the establishment of a mutational
phenotypic change.

3. HEREDITARY DISEASES AS A CONSEQUENCE OF MUTATIONS IN MAN

Extensive epidemiological studies have attempted during recent
years to evaluate the incidence of abnormal genotypes in the human
population: the analysis of the frequency of birth disorders due
to mutant genotypes has indicated that 1-2% of the newborns present one of the several genetic anomalies which are of the type
of autosomal dominant/recessive or X-linked factors. Cytogenetic
studies have concluded that a high proportion of the spontaneous

abortion in the human population are represented by freshly occur
red chromosomal mutations; moreover about 6 per thousand live
birth do present an altered phenotype as a consequence of their
chromosomal numerical or structural anomalies.

The types of mutations which have been experimentally produced
in the laboratory are well characterized (table 4); the types of
mutations which can be produced on a mammalian cell grown in vitro,

TABLE 4

THE TYPES OF MUTATIONS

A. POINT OR GENE MUTATIONS

---

1. SUBSTITUTION OF ONE OR SEVERAL BASES (TRANSITION & TRANSVERSION)
2. INSERTION OR DELETION OF ONE OR SEVERAL NUCLEOTIDES (FRAME SHIFT)
3. REMOVAL OF A SEGMENT OF THE POLYNUCLEOTIDE CHAIN (SMALL DELETION)

B. CHROMOSOMAL MUTATIONS

---

1. A SEGMENT MAY JOIN THE DNA MOLECULE IN A DIFFERENT SITE OR ANO
   THER MOLECULE (TRANSLOCATION)
2. A SEGMENT MAY JOIN THE DNA MOLECULE AT THE SITE OF REMOVAL BUT
   ROTATE BY 180°C. (INVERSION)
3. AN ANOMALOUS SEGREGATION OF DNA MOLECULES DURING THE MEIOTIC
   PROCESS (NON-DISJUNCTION).

---

or in mice when they are exposed to chemical mutagens (figg. 1 and
2) and which might represent the different types presented in table 4, reflect those genetic alterations which have been observed
also in human.

The total genetic load of the human population, chromosomal and
genic, has been estimated of the order of 0.4 : about 0.2 prenatal
(0.1 = chromosomal; 0.1 = genic) and 0.2 postnatal (0.005 = chromo
somal; 0.2 = genic): on this grant, and on the basis of recent stu
dies developed in mammals and other organisms with chemical mutagens, we should consider the present amount of altered genotypes

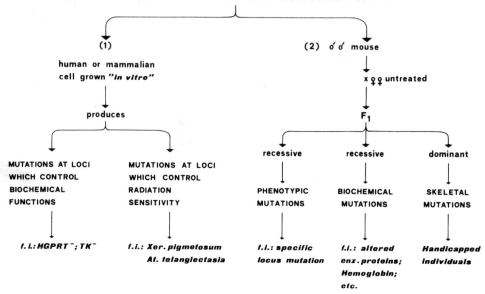

GENETIC RISKS FROM POINT MUTATIONS

AN EXPOSURE TO A CHEMICAL MUTAGEN OF:

(1) human or mammalian cell grown *"in vitro"*

produces

| MUTATIONS AT LOCI WHICH CONTROL BIOCHEMICAL FUNCTIONS | MUTATIONS AT LOCI WHICH CONTROL RADIATION SENSITIVITY |

f.i.: HGPRT⁻; TK⁻ — *f.i.: Xer. pigmetosum At. telangiectasia*

(2) ♂♂ mouse

x ♀♀ untreated

F₁

recessive — recessive — dominant

PHENOTYPIC MUTATIONS — BIOCHEMICAL MUTATIONS — SKELETAL MUTATIONS

f.i.: specific locus mutation — *f.i.: altered enz. proteins; Hemoglobin; etc.* — *Handicapped individuals*

Fig. 1

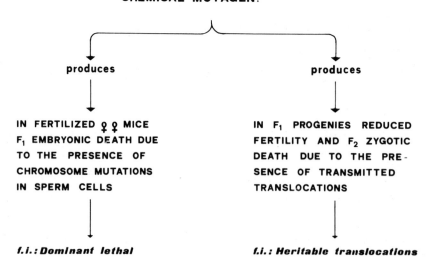

GENETIC RISKS FROM CHROMOSOME MUTATIONS

EXPOSURE OF ♂♂ MICE TO A CHEMICAL MUTAGEN:

produces — produces

IN FERTILIZED ♀♀ MICE F₁ EMBRYONIC DEATH DUE TO THE PRESENCE OF CHROMOSOME MUTATIONS IN SPERM CELLS — IN F₁ PROGENIES REDUCED FERTILITY AND F₂ ZYGOTIC DEATH DUE TO THE PRESENCE OF TRANSMITTED TRANSLOCATIONS

Fig. 2   *f.i.: Dominant lethal* — *f.i.: Heritable translocations*

in the human population as a possible direct consequence of mutations which could have been occurred spontaneously or under the action of chemical mutagens to which the human population might have been exposed (environmental contaminants, drugs, industrial chemicals, food additives, agricultural products, etc.) (table 5).

TABLE 5

N° OF CHEMICALS IN COMMCN USE

1. CHEMICALS IN EVERY DAY USE	50,C00
2. ACTIVE INGREDIENTS IN PESTICIDES	1,500
3. ACTIVE INGREDIENTS IN DRUGS	4,000
4. COMPOUNDS USED AS EXCIPIENTS	2,000
5. FOOD ADDITIVES	2,500
6. CHEMICALS USED TO PROMOTE LIFE	3,000
TOTAL N°	63,000

4. METABOLIC ACTIVATION AND MUTAGENESIS

Recent studies have described the complexity of metabolic reactions (activation and/or detoxification) to which foreign chemicals are submitted in human tissues: the membranes of the liver cell endoplasmic reticulum hydroxylate numerous exogenous compounds by a multimolecular system known as the mixed function oxidase, which carries out several metabolic reactions. Several of the metabolites produced during these metabolic reactions are electrophylic agents which may react with DNA molecule: many environmental contaminants have been shown to be subjected to liver mixed-function oxidase systems, and to be transformed into reactive metabolites. They include haloalkanes, haloalkenes, haloaromatic compounds, nitrosamines and many polycyclic aromatic hydrocarbons.

The knowledge of all these metabolic reactions which may convert an inert chemical agent into a potent electrophylic reactive agent (f i. vinyl chloride) has made possible the understanding of the

correlation between carcinogenic and mutagenic activities (both
activities depend for some class of chemicals on these metabolic
reactions) and moreover the development of suitable in vitro or
in vivo methodological procedures for evaluating the potential mu
tagenic activity of those chemicals which are subjected to a metabolic conversion by mammalian enzymatic reaction. The resutls of
these studies have indicated how many possible mutagenic agents
are present in our environment.

5. DIFFERENT METHODOLOGICAL PROCEDURES FOR IDENTIFYING CHEMICAL
MUTAGENS.

As it has been stateg earlier, there are two ways of altering
the genetic material, namely the production of gene mutation and
the alteration in the structural organization of a chromosome or
in the numerical organization of a genome's structure; other types of genetic effects, such as recombination and gene-conversion
may moreover represent partly a genetic risk, as these processes
could allow the expression of recessive harmful mutations present
in a heterozygous individual. For the above reasons, a comprehensive approach cf evaluating the potential mutagenic activity of a
chemical should be based on biological systems which include: (a)
a variety of biological organization; (b) a variety of ultimate
genetic effects, including all types of genetic alterations; (c)
a variety of initial events at the DNA level.

Results of mutagenicity studies developed with different mutational assays have gemonstrated to some extent the presence of
specificity of the mutagenic activity: Natulan, Bleomycin, Uretha-
ne, Auramine, o-Toluidine, Ethionine, Dimethylhydrazine, Stilbestrol, Chloroform are mutagenic in some genetic assays only: the
reascns might be due to the existence of a peculiar kinetics of
the metabolic conversion of the compound, or to a need for a particular error-prone repair process, or to the existence cf a cell-
stage specificity.

Since the aim of a mutagenicity study is the assessment whether a chemical compound induces a mutagenic effect which can be transmitted to the next generation, or the type of the induced mutagenic change (gene or chromosome mutation) and the frequency of the induced mutagenic events, genetic research has developed extensive studies on various genetic systems in different organisms which make possible the definitions of all possible genetic effects produced by chemicals.

Tables 6 and 7 report the most validated assays which have been defined during recent years: they represent different organisms and genetic systems which might allow the evaluation of all possible types of mutation inducible by chemical agents.

6. PREDICTIVE VALUE FOR CARCINOGENICITY OF MUTAGENICITY TESTS.

Molecular biology researches have developed several information which demonstrate that some mutational events might cause the stage of initiation of a cell transformation process: both mutational and cancerogenic processess are associated with a phenotypic change of hereditary type. Mutations are by definitions the results of a permanent change in the DNA structure; a cancer cell is by definition the result of different functions and gene-expressions which have occurred in the basic structure of the cell.

It is well known at the present that the final form of a precarcinogenic chemical is an electrophylic agent which is able to react with nucleophylic centers of cellular macromolecules including the DNA: all metabolic reactions which occur in the cell are common to both carcinogens, as well to mutagens (fig. 3), and the effects that the two classes of compounds may produce in the DNA molecule are all correlated with steps on which it depends the evaluation of a mutational event (fig. 4). A valid support to the hypothesis that carcinogenic compounds are also mutagens has been produced by the data collected by McCANN et al. during 1975-76 with chemical mutagens/carcinogens tested on the bacterium S.typhi-

TABLE 6

ORGANISMS AND GENETIC TEST SYSTEMS FOR THE ASSESSMENT OF GENE MU-
TATIONS INDUCED BY CHEMICAL COMFOUNDS

ORGANISM	GENETIC SYSTEM	GENETIC END POINT
A. BACTERIAL TESTS		
1. Salmonella typhimurium	a. Reverse Mutation	Base-pair changes Base Insertions & Deletions.
2. Escherichia coli	a. Reverse Mutation	Base-pair changes
B. YEAST TESTS		
1. Schizosaccharomyces pombe	a. Forward Mutation	Base-pair changes
	b. Reverse Mutation	Base Insertions & Deletions
2. Saccharomyces cerevisiae	a. Forward Mutation	
	b. Reverse Mutation	Base Insertions & Deletions
C. FUNGAL TESTS		
1. Neurospora crassa	a. Forward Mutation	Base-pair changes Base Insertions & Deletions Small Deletions
2. Aspergillus nidulans	a. Forward Mutation	Base-pair changes
	b. Reverse Mutation	

D. MAMMALIAN CELLS

    1. AZA-Resistance V-79   a. Forward   Intragenic mutations
                                  Mutation

    2. TK Mutation L5178Y   a. Forward   Intragenic mutations
                                    Mutation
                                  b. Reverse
                                  Mutation

E. INSECTS

    1. Drosophila   a. X-linked   Intragenic mutations
       melanogaster   Recessive   & small deletions
                                  Mutation
                                  (Forward
                                  Mutation)

F. MAMMALS

    1. Mouse specific   a. Recessive
       Locus Test   Mutation
                                  (Forward
                                  Mutation)   Intragenic mutation

    2. Mouse spot test*   a. Recessive
                                  Mutation
                                  (Forward
                                  Mutation)   &

    3. Sperm abnormality* a. Recessive
                                  Mutation   Small Deletions
                                  (Forward
                                  Mutation)

G. HOST MEDIATED ASSAY   Forward   The same as in A,B,C,D
                                  Mutation
                                  Reverse
                                  Mutation

---

* Tests not well validated, difficult to perform, or organism requires additional genetic characterization.

TABLE 7

ORGANISMS AND GENETIC TEST SYSTEMS FOR THE ASSESSMENT OF CHROMOSO-
ME MUTATIONS INDUCED BY CHEMICAL COMPOUNDS

A. MAMMALS (in vitro)	a. Peripheral blood lymphocyte	Chromosome aberrations
	b. Somatic cell line	Chromosome aberrations
		Sister Chromatid Exchange (SCE)
B. MAMMALS (in vivo)	a. Micronucleus	Somatic chromosome aberrations
	b. Bone marrow cells	Somatic chromosome aberrations
	c. Germ cell cytogenet	Germ cell chromosome aberrations
	d. Dominant lethal	Heritable chromosome aberrations
	e. Heritable translocation	Heritable chromosome aberrations
	f. Somatic cell	Sister Chromatid Exchange (SCE)
C. Drosophila	a. Dominanth lethal	Germ cell chromosome aberrations
	b. Translocation	Heritable chromosome aberrations
D. YEASTS & FUNGI	a. Mitotic recombination	Chromosome rearrangements
	b. Gene conversion	Gene rearrangements
	c. Non-Disjunctions	Genome mutations

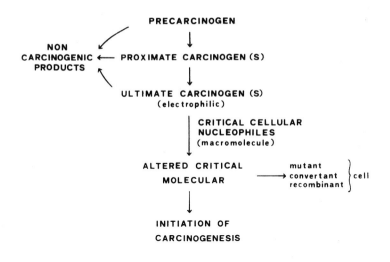

SCHEME FOR ACTIVATION AND DETOXIFICATION OF CHEMICAL
CARCINOGEN

Fig. 3

A) REPAIR OF MODIFIED DNA'S

B) STRUCTURAL DEFECTS IN DNA

C) EFFECTS ON TEMPLATE FUNCTIONS

D) CHROMOSOMAL ABERRATION

E) PRODUCTION OF GENETIC INFORMATION CHANGE

F) POLYPLOIDIZATION SEGREGATION

G) CHANGE IN GENE DOSAGE

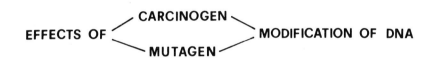

Fig. 4

murium (Ames test): according to these results the Ames test can identify about the 90% of carcinogens (sensitivity of the test) and can reject on the base of negative results about the 87% of non carcinogens (specificity of the test) (fig. 5): although the validity of this assumption resides in the percentage of carcino-gens present in the sample of chemicals analyzed, on the chemical nature of the analyzed chemicals, and on the metabolic reactions, several other studies have demonstrated that these results are ge-nerally valid (table 8).

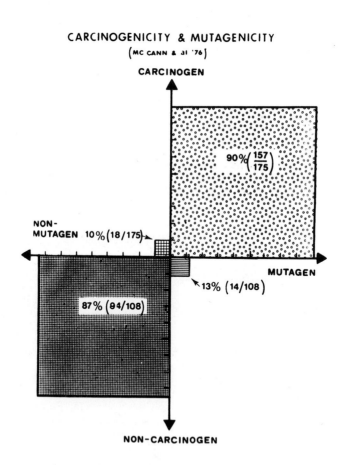

Fig. 5

TABLE 8

RESULTS OF MUTAGENICITY ASSAYS OF SEVERAL GROUPS OF CARCINOGENS/
NON CARCINOGENS ON SALMONELLA

AUTHOR	TOTAL Nº OF CHEMICALS ANALYZED	PERCENTAGES OF MUTAGENIC COMPOUNDS	
		CARCINOGENS	NON CARCINOGENS
J. McCANN et al. (1975)	300	89.7	13.0
T. SUGIMURA et al. (1976)	240	92.8	22.9
B. COMMONER (1976)	100	82.0	18.0
T. SUGIMURA et al. (1977)	241	85.0	26.0
M.M. BROWN et al. (1979)	52	84.0	25.0
H.S. ROSENKRANZ and L.A. POIRIER (1979)	87	51.7	16.6
V.F. SIMMON (1979)	87	63.7	36.3
H. BARTSCH (1979)	180	76.0	43.0

(*) false positives.

The best present estimate of the ability of <u>Salmonella</u> test to
identify chemical carcinogens as mutagens indicates a value in the
range of 70-80%.

Other short-term mutagenicity assays may, however, be combined
with the Ames test to improve the identification of carcinogens.
A recent programme developed by different institutions has shown

how feasible is the possibility of identifying the carcinogenic chemical compounds by several different mutagenic assays.

Although there are limitations to the use of short-term mutagenicity tests _in vitro_ assays in the assessment of carcinogenic compounds which depends on several factors, as f.i. those indicated in Table 9, the use of mutagenicity tests has resulted as the only practical possibility for the evaluation of thousands chemicals present in the human environment as a prescreening method for carcinogenic compounds.

Short-term tests for chemical carcinogens presently do not constitute a definitive evidence as to whether a substance does represent a carcinogenic hazard to humans, but positive results indicate a suggestive evidence for a carcinogenic hazard.

7. CONCLUSIONS

"Having been at last successfully alerted to the genetic dangers of ionizing radiation, civilized man did not need much persuasion to accept the geneticists warning against the dangers of potential mutagens among the countless new substances that are used in medicine, industry pest control, food preservation, etc. In fact, there is a risk that geneticists, by stressing these dangers, may make the public over-anxious. Yet, it is quite possible and even probable that the overall effects of all these chemicals, acting separately or in combination, may be a far greater genetic hazard than that posed by ionizing radiation. It is the inescapable duty of geneticist to assess this hazard as accurately as possible, of governments to lay down guidelines for the clearance of substances and collaborate in the testing" (C. AUERBACH, 1976).

TABLE 9

FACTORS THAT DETERMINE THE PROCESSES OF CANCER DEVELOPMENT IN VI
VO AND ARE NOT DUPLICATED BY MUTAGENICITY SYSTEMS

---

1. BIOLOGICAL ABSORPTION AND DISTRIBUTION
2. THE CONCENTRATION OF ULTIMATE REACTIVE METABOLITES AVAILABLE
   FOR REACTIONS IN ORGANS AND ANIMAL SPECIES WITH CELLULAR MA-
   CROMOELCULES
3. THE BIOLOGICAL HALF-LIFE OF METABOLITES
4. DNA REPAIR MECHANISMS BETWEEN THE TEST SYSTEM AND THE WHOLE
   ANIMAL
5. IMMUNO SURVEILLANCE
6. ORGAN-SPECIFIC RELEASE OF PROXIMATE OR ULTIMATE CARCINOGENS
   BY ENZYMATIC DECONJUGATION
7. DEACTIVATION REACTIONS WHICH CAN LEAD TO COMPOUNDS POSSESSING
   EITHER NO CARCINOGENIC ACTIVITY OR LESS CARCINOGENIC POTENTIAL
   THAN THE PARENT COMPOUND

This sentence summarizes the aim of genetic toxicology and the
importance of the metodologies developed for assessing the mutagenic risk as a possible preventive measure to be useg to reduce the
burden of those human diseases due to mutations produced by environmental chemicals.

8. GENERAL BIBLIOGRAPHY

1. AUERBACH, C.: Mutation Research. Problems, results and perspectives. Chapman & Hall, London, 1976.
2. BOWERS, J.Z. and G.P. VELO: Drug Assessment: Criteria and Metho
   ds. Elsevier, Amsterdam, 1979.
3. GALLI, C.L. et al.: Chemical Toxicology of food. Elsevier, Amsterdam, 1978.
4. HIATT, H.H. et al.: Origins of human cancer. Cold Spring Harbor
   Laboratory, 1977.

124

5. HOLLAENDER, A. and F.J. DE SERRES: Chemical Mutagens. Principles and methods for their detections. voll. 1-5, Plenum Press, New York, 1971-1978.

6. KILBEY, B. et al.: Handbook of mutagenicity test procedures, Elsevier, Amsterdam, 1977.

7. LOPRIENO, N.: Mutagenicity tests for evaluating chemical substances, ETS, Pisa, 1978.

8. SCOTT, D. et al.: Progress in Genetic Toxicology, Elsevier, Amsterdam, 1977.

© 1980 Elsevier/North-Holland Biomedical Press
The Principles and Methods in Modern Toxicology
C.L. Galli, S.D. Murphy and R. Paoletti, editors.

REPRODUCTIVE TOXICITY

IAN C. MUNRO

Director, Bureau of Chemical Safety, Food Directorate, Health Protection Branch, Health & Welfare Canada, Tunney's Pasture, Ottawa, Ontario, K1A 0L2, Canada.

The study of reproductive toxicology affords the opportunity to examine the effects of chemical substances on the reproductive cycle. Reproductive toxicity testing is a mandatory requirement of most government authorities for premarket clearance of drugs, food additives, pesticides and in some instances, environmental chemicals. In this connection, guidelines for conducting these laboratory tests have been developed by most national authorities concerned with controlling human exposure to chemical substances. Reference to published guidelines is given in the reference list.

Evidence that has accrued to date demonstrates the importance of undertaking these tests prior to premarket clearance of chemicals. For example, the demonstration of fetotoxicity and teratogenicity following exposure of pregnant rats to the ethylenebis-dithiocarbamate herbicides clearly demonstrates the need for carefully conducted tests to assess reproductive toxicity[1]. Studies in monkeys by Allen et al.,[2] demonstrate the unique susceptibility of the rhesus monkey to PCB's and dioxins and further underscores the value of these tests in assessing the toxicity of chemicals to which man may be exposed.

In evaluating the reproductive toxicity of chemical substances, it is important to keep in mind the unique opportunity this affords to obtain information on metabolism and pharmacokinetics in both the mother and fetus under repeated dose conditions. These data are extremely valuable in interpreting reproductive tests and in extrapolating the results to man. Up to the present, too little attention has been given to obtaining this information, with the consequence that the results of many tests are difficult to interpret in terms of human health. It also can be safely stated that in the past, reproductive studies have tended to focus on gross effects such as decreased litter size or pup weight and little attention has been given to detailed pathological examination or to postnatal development of major organ systems such as the brain.

So let us begin by examining the objectives of reproductive toxicity tests from the perspective of modern toxicology. Reproductive tests should be designed so as to detect adverse effects on any segment of the reproductive cycle. During this period of development several processes related to the reproductive cycle, listed in Table 1, are vulnerable to toxic insult by chemicals. The classical approach to screening chemicals for

TABLE 1

TOXICOLOGICALLY VULNERABLE STAGES OF THE REPRODUCTIVE CYCLE

Gametogenesis

Copulation

Fertilization

Preimplantation Period

Implantation

Embryonic Period

Fetal Period

Maternal-Placental-Fetal Relationships

Parturition

Suckling

Postnatal Development to Puberty

potential effects on reproduction involves exposure of both sexes of the selected species, usually rats and mice, to the test chemical for a minimum of one gametogenic cycle prior to mating. A broad range of parameters is assessed during the reproductive test and include those used in standard toxicity tests such as food consumption and weight gain as well as special parameters including normality of the estrus cycle, mating behavior, conception rates, fertility, embryotoxicity, fetotoxicity, weight of the newborn, sex distribution and the presence of malformations. During the postnatal period, observations are recorded on growth and survival of the offspring, suckling habits, toxicity which may develop during lactation (since some chemicals are excreted in the milk), and finally the reproductive ability of the offspring.

Although normally, such studies are confined to rodents, recent experience with some of the halogenated hydrocarbons demonstrates the need of careful evaluation in the selection of species to ensure an appropriate species is selected for the chemical class under investigation.

Usually, treatment is continued for one or more generations as shown in Figure 1. The three-generation protocol implies that adverse effects may be magnified, and hence more easily detected as they are passed from one generation to the next. At present, the only

REPRODUCTIVE TOXICITY TESTING SCHEME:

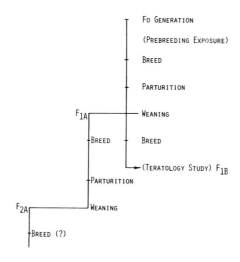

plausible mechanism by which this could occur is through mutation. Since few tests for reproductive performance are conducted as genetic tests and since mutational effects are not likely to be observed following only three generations of exposure, the wisdom of conducting reproduction tests beyond two generations has been questioned. Indeed, there have been very few reports of effects on reproduction observed in three-generation tests that were not observed in one- or two-generation tests. However, the need for the two-generation test may be substantiated on the basis that animals exposed in utero should be allowed to mature and mate, thus permitting an evaluation of the total reproductive cycle. Generally, it can be concluded that in most cases a two-generation test would suffice for hazard evaluation of environmental chemicals, provided no adverse effects are noted such as would lead to the continuation of the test for subsequent generations.

Because of the important role played by reproductive toxicity in safety evaluation of food chemicals, there is a growing need to develop a more complete understanding of mechanisms involved in the genesis of toxic events induced in utero. In this connection, postnatal toxicology, metabolism and pharmacokinetics and perinatal carcinogenesis are the areas of toxicology where gaps in present knowledge are greatest. The remainder of this paper will concentrate on these issues.

POSTNATAL TOXICOLOGY

It is becoming increasingly obvious that subtle postnatal effects warrant more detailed consideration than that which they have received in the past. In this regard, detailed assessment of the anatomical and functional integrity of the neonate is of paramount importance. The prime concern is not with readily detectable overt toxicity but with subtle forms of toxicity which may be manifest as behavioral alterations such as learning deficits and hyperactivity. This is recognized now by some as the logical extension of teratology studies yet it needs to be pursued in more depth in reproduction studies. Data taken from the work of Khera and Tryphonas[1] demonstrate the advantages of careful assessment of postnatal effects.

Ethylenethiourea (ETU), a major degradation product of the ethylenebisdithio-carbamates, is a potent teratogen in the rat. Single maternal doses in the range of 60-480 mg/kg induced a wide range of fetal anomalies such as hydrocephalus, anophthalmia, cleft lip and anomalies of the fore and hind limbs. Encephalocele, or extrusion of part of the brain from the skull is commonly seen as well. At lower doses of 30 mg/kg no anomalies or other signs of toxicity were noted at birth but after 9-10 weeks several of the offspring from mothers given 30 mg/kg developed an anomalous hopping-type gait. Most of these animals displayed learning difficulties and alterations in scheduled-controlled behavior. The focus of interest was in determining whether the behavioral changes were a result of anatomical alterations in the nervous system or were due to more subtle effects of ETU on the higher brain centers associated with learning and behavior. When the pups were sacrificed at 64 weeks of age, mild hydrocephalus with dimpling of the cerebral hemispheres was seen along with histological lesions in the brain. These findings demonstrated that the behavioral effects were probably due to structural changes in the nervous system induced by ETU. There are few, if any, examples of irreversible behavioral alterations induced by food chemicals that are not associated with gross or microscopic pathological changes. From a public point of view, it is of paramount importance to determine if irreversible behavioral changes do occur in the absence of overt pathological alterations in nervous tissue. Thus, when functional defects are observed in motor or sensory systems histological investigations should be undertaken to determine whether or not the observed effects are due to visible pathological or biochemical changes in various areas of the peripheral and central nervous systems. In the past, it has not been common practice in safety evaluation to examine tissues histologically during the neonatal period and indeed the study of normal tissue histology or neonates has been somewhat neglected. A need exists to develop a better understanding of neonatal pathology particularly as it relates to the pathogenesis of lesions induced in utero or during suckling. Nowhere is this need more evident than in the evaluation of studies undertaken to assess the potential carcinogenicity of chemicals using the in utero exposure model, particularly as it relates to the possible mechanisms involved.

PHARMACOKINETICS AND METABOLISM

Preliminary pharmacokinetic studies that are designed to assess the rate of uptake, tissue distribution and rate of elimination of the test substance are of critical importance in the assessment of toxic events and provide information that is essential to the design and interpretation of reproduction studies. Since humans are likely to be exposed to uniform doses of food chemicals, it is desirable that the animal studies reflect this exposure pattern. Thus, it is important to achieve steady-state tissue concentrations prior to mating of the animals. This will ensure a uniform exposure of the developing fetus to the test compound during gestation. Data on the pharmacokinetics of saccharin and methylmercury exemplify these points (Figure 2). The half-life for the elimination of

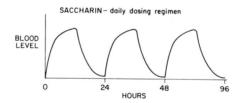

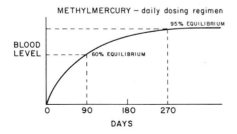

saccharin is less than 24 hours. Thus, steady-state blood levels, so far as they can be achieved, are reached rather quickly. This indicates that even if mating commenced one week following initial exposure of the dams, the fetuses would be exposed to a uniform dose of saccharin. On the other hand, methylmercury slowly accumulates in the maternal tissues and reaches equilibrium concentrations only after prolonged exposure. Since methylmercury readily crosses the placenta, commencement of mating prior to achieving steady-state maternal blood levels would result in the fetus being exposed to increasing doses of methylmercury over the gestation period even though the maternal dose was constant. Obviously, this would preclude the establishment of any valid relationships between exposure level, body burden and adverse effects induced in utero.

Data on the red food color, amaranth, serve as another example of the usefulness of conducting pharmacokinetic and tissue distribution studies prior to designing reproduction studies. Amaranth is an "azo dye" which is metabolized to naphthionic acid and amino-R-acid by azo reductase enzymes found in the gut microflora and the liver[3, 4]. Subsequent metabolism can produce several additional metabolites[5, 6]. Metabolic studies in the rat have demonstrated that only about 3% of the amaranth is absorbed intact from the gut[7] while the metabolites are absorbed to a somewhat greater extent (Table 2). Studies in

TABLE 2

RETENTION OF RADIOLABELLED AMARANTH IN THE RAT

Percent of Dose Excreted	
Urine	7.4 ± 1.0
Feces	78.3 ± 4.1
Percent of Dose Retained	14.2 ± 3.3

which Wistar rats were dosed orally with (^{14}C) (U)-amaranth demonstrate that about 14% of the radioactivity was retained in the body over 24 hours. An additional 7% of the radioactivity was excreted in urine over the 24 hour period giving a total absorption of amaranth plus all metabolites of about 21%. These data are in agreement with those of Pritchard et al.[8] and Radomsky and Millinger[6], indicating that about 20% of the naphthionic acid produced in the gut was absorbed. The radioactivity was quickly excreted from the body via the kidney, the elimination half-period for blood being about 6

131

hours[6, 8].

Studies were undertaken to determine whether amaranth and its metabolites would cross the placenta. Because insufficient radiolabelled amaranth could be given orally to assess placental transfer, pregnant rats were dosed intravenously with either 0.74 or 7.91 mg amaranth/kg body wt. containing (^{14}C) (U)-amaranth (specific activity - 26.7 uC/mg). A substantial portion of the amaranth given iv was quickly metabolized by liver azo reductase enzymes to naphthionic acid and other metabolites. The pregnant rats were necropsied 1 1/2 hours post-dosing and maternal blood and organs and entire fetuses were analyzed for total radioactivity by liquid scintillation counting techniques. Using the iv route would undoubtedly present a "worth case" situation with respect to placental transfer. Table 3 shows the absolute dpm of radioactivity in maternal blood and fetal tissues and the fetal/maternal ratio from these experiments. The levels of radioactivity in maternal blood were 28 to 30 times higher than in the fetuses. The eleven fold increase in maternal dose resulted in a nine and eight fold increase in radioactivity in maternal blood and fetal tissues respectively. Even so, the placental transfer was so low that the levels of radioactivity in the fetuses were not significantly above background at either dose level. These preliminary data indicate that only a small amount of amaranth or its

TABLE 3
PLACENTAL TRANSFER OF ^{14}C-RADIOACTIVITY
FOLLOWING INTRAVENOUS ADMINISTRATION OF ^{14}C(U)-AMARANTH

Amaranth Dose I.V. mg/kg body wt.	Maternal Blood dpm/ml	Fetus dpm/g	Fetal/Maternal Ratio
0.74	4785	171	0.06
7.91	41973	1381	0.03

metabolites can traverse the placenta to the fetus. From these data the conclusion can be drawn that amaranth would not likely produce any direct teratogenic or reproductive effects particularly at doses humans are likely to obtain from foods and this has indeed been shown to be the case[9, 10, 11, 12].

These data on the pharmacokinetics and distribution of amaranth raise questions regarding the need for detailed multigeneration reproduction studies for substances that are poorly absorbed from the gut and do not readily cross the placenta. The only justification for such studies on these types of chemicals would be the potential for adverse reproductive effects mediated through alterations in the physiological functions of the dam that may indirectly affect the fetus. For chemicals that do not readily cross the placenta yet produce adverse effects on reproduction, pharmacokinetic and tissue distribution studies will assist in the evaluation of adverse maternal effects that may lead to fetotoxicity.

Moving to the use of pharmacokinetic studies in postnatal studies, attention is drawn to some recent studies we have conducted in infant mokeys. In these studies, a group of infant Cynomalogus monkeys was fed a human infant formula milk diet and was dosed with lead acetate at the rate of 2 mg Pb per kg body weight per day. A control group received the same diet but were not treated with lead. After approximately 12 months of treatment both the control and treated monkeys were transferred to an adult primate diet. Throughout the period of treatment, the blood lead and free erythrocyte porphyrin levels were measured. As can be seen in Figure 3, the blood lead levels rose quickly following treatment and tended to stabilize at about 80-90 ug per 100 ml. Following

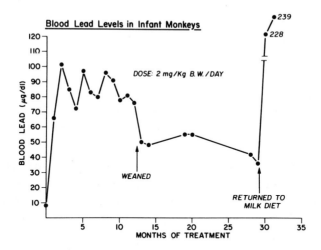

weaning, however, the blood lead levels abruptly declined. This decline was attributed to the change to the adult diet. When the animals were placed back on a milk diet the blood lead levels rapidly increased and in fact exceeded previous values. At this stage, one of the animals displayed epileptiform seizures, a condition not noted prior to weaning. Although not shown here, the blood lead levels declined abruptly when the animals were once again placed on the adult ration.

The effect of the diet on blood levels was reflected in the results of the free erthrocyte porphyrin (FEP) analysis. In Figure 4 it will be noted that the increase in FEP in treated animals roughly paralleled the blood lead levels and fell dramatically to control values once the diet was changed to the adult primate diet.

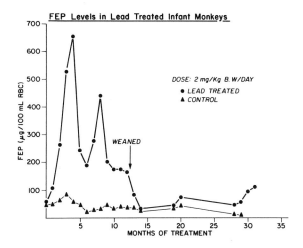

The results of these investigations clearly demonstrated the value of pharmacokinetic studies in interpreting toxic effects. If, for example, no data were available regarding blood lead levels in these monkeys one would be hard pressed indeed to interpret the FEP data.

Data on the uptake and elimination rates of the test compound and its metabolites in blood and critical organs permit a realistic assignment of dose levels and assist in selecting the duration of exposure required for the establishment of steady-state blood levels of the test chemical during the studies. Data on tissue distribution of the compound and its metabolites allow an assessment of the potential for accumulation in various fetal and maternal organ systems. Finally, these data greatly assist in the comparison and extrapolation of toxicity data between species.

IN UTERO EXPOSURE CANCER STUDIES

Recently, the in utero exposure model for evaluation of chemical carcinogenesis has received increased attention by oncologists and its application in regulatory toxicology has been the subject of much heated discussion. In such studies the parent or Fo generation is dosed with the test chemical for some time prior to impregnation as well as during pregnancy and lactation. The offspring in the F1 generation are then dosed with the chemcial for the remainder of their lifetime or for a period thereof. The second generation is thus exposed to the chemical in utero and through the mother's milk (if the chemical gains entrance to the fetal or newborn animal via these compartments) as well as through the diet after weaning.

The Need For In Utero Exposure Studies

In the practical sense, the in utero exposure model mimics the human situation, particularly in the case of food additives and certain environmental contaminants. These chemicals are often consumed unknowingly and may be ingested by humans throughout their lifetime, including the pregnancy and lactation periods. Thus, there is the potential for the perinatal human to receive the chemical or its metabolites via the placenta or from mother's milk.

In addition, the use of this model is based on the expectation that in utero exposure may Increase the sensitivity of cancer bioassays. This increased sensitivity may be expressed in terms of an increased incidence or reduced latent period of tumors seen in the offspring or in the induction of unique tumors not frequently seen in the parents. However, this assertion is based on somewhat limited published data. The incidence of tumors in animals exposed in utero to aflatoxin, saccharin or the ethyl derivatives of the nitrosamides is somewhat greater than that in animals treated only from weaning[13, 14, 15]. However, substances such as methylnitrosourea, 1,2-dimethyl-hydrazine, 1,phenyl-3,-3-dimethyltriazine and azoxylethane appear to be more carcino-genic in the adult[16].

The hypothesis of increased sensitivity is supported by the observation that diethyl-stilbestrol induces tumors of the vagina in young women whose mothers were given this drug for pregnancy maintenance[17, 18]. Although this appears to be a unique carcinogenic event not yet observed in the parents, there is some suggestion[19, 20, 21] that DES may increase the incidence and decrease the latent period of breast cancer in the mothers. Thus, it cannot be concluded on the basis of these data that DES is carcinogenic only in the offspring. A somewhat analogous situation has been reported by Druckery[22] who observed that rats exposed in utero to certain nitroso compounds developed mainly neurogenic tumors whereas tumors at other sites predominated in animals treated post weaning.

These apparent differences in sensitivity may be due to a variety of factors including the pharmacokinetics and metabolism of the test compound and the immunologic competence of the host. In addition, the rapidly dividing cells of the fetus may be more or less susceptible to carcinogenic substances, depending upon their metabolic capability and stage of development.

Regulatory Considerations

From the regulatory point of view the in utero exposure model would appear to be most useful as an instrument for detecting those compounds which may be carcinogenic only in the offspring. If the test compound is found to be carcinogenic only in the offspring. If the test compound is found to be carcinogenic in the parent as well as the progeny, regulatory action will be based primarily on the fact that it is a carcinogen, not because it induced tumors at different doses or with a different latent period or even at different sites in the F0 and F1 generations. While, in principle, these arguments are valid, the decision to proceed with the two-generation cancer study can be taken only after careful consideration of a variety of factors. There has been little experience with this model for assessing the carcinogenic potential of chemicals, therefore, its validation as an acceptable procedure for safety evaluation must be considered in an orderly and systematic fashion.

Our limited experience with the in utero exposure model has identified a number of deficiencies in current knowledge that must be evaluated prior to general acceptance of this system for carcinogenicity testing. First there is the question of dose selection. Many have criticized the use of high doses in cancer testing not only in relation to the F1 cancer studies but also in relation to the more traditional test procedures. Since the acquirement of dose-response information is critical to an adequate safety evaluation of a chemical, it is necessary to employ large enough doses to produce undesirable effects. The problem is most difficult in the interpretation of data generated as a result of using only one or two very high doses that greatly exceed human exposure levels. This problem is not unique to carcinogenesis but spans the gamut of toxicity testing procedures, even including the in vitro systems.

The data presented on amaranth suggest that the in utero model may not be applicable in all cases. The results of pharmacokinetic studies with amaranth demonstrate that the material does not reach the fetus in any significant concentration. Since the fetus would be exposed to very low levels of amaranth even at high maternal doses, positive effects on the F1 generation would have to be interpreted with great caution were they observed. Thus, it is apparent that the pharmacokinetic studies will provide information critical to the decision to proceed with in utero testing and will assist in the selection of a range of adequate doses. Further pharmacokinetic data of this type are required in order to determine if other compounds are handled in the same way as saccharin and amaranth.

Another factor that must be taken into consideration in the selection of doses for in utero testing, is the potential for adverse effects on reproduction. Obviously, a compound that is fetotoxic cannot be administered in the in utero exposure model at doses as high as can be achieved in conventional tests. Studies we have done with hexachlorobenzene demonstrated reproductive toxicity at 80 ppm in the diet, while in subacute studies 200 ppm were required to produce a discernible toxic effect[23]. In the in utero cancer test, however, 40 ppm was the maximum dose of hexachlorobenzene that could be given in order to achieve an acceptable level of survival in the offspring. This is an instance where the in utero exposure model was not as rigorous a test as conventional cancer studies due to limitations in dosage. Probably this would be the case with most of the aromatic chlorinated hydrocarbons that accumulate in tissues and readily traverse the placenta. Based on these data, it is apparent that involvement of in utero exposure in cancer testing may in some cases decrease the possibility of obtaining information on potential carcinogenic effects of chemicals.

Another point that requires consideration is the selection of pups of the F1 generation. Statisticians claim that the maximum sensitivity of the test will result when one male and one female are selected from each litter of the F0 generation. A problem in this selection relates to the intra-litter variation in transplacental exposure to chemicals, so a study was undertaken in which pregnant Wistar rats were administered a single oral dose of ^{14}C-saccharin after twenty days gestation. At thirty minutes post-dosing, the amount of saccharin in each fetus was measured by scintillation counting.

As is noted in Table 4, the inter-litter variation in saccharin concentration exceeded the intra-litter variation by a factor of 2.6. The variation between litters in the exposure via the placenta was highly significant (P <.001) whereas the variation within litters was not.

TABLE 4

MEASURE OF VARIANCE FOR INTRA AND INTER LITTER DISTRIBUTION OF SACCHARIN (DPM/G)^2

SOURCE OF VARIANCE	VARIANCE
intra-litter	33447
inter-litter	85175
ratio of variances	2.6

These data demonstrate that the selection of the F1 generation animals should be done at random. One procedure involves culling to a maximum of eight per litter at four or five days of age in order to balance the burden placed on the dams and to ensure an equitable food supply and distribution of test chemical among littermates. Culling should be done at random but so as to leave four males and four females whenever possible. Finally, one male and one female should be randomly selected at weaning to continue on test in the F1 generation.

The saccharin data demonstrated a remarkably consistent distribution between fetuses within litters which suggests that intra-litter variation in the concentration of chemical may not be as difficult a problem as originally anticipated. Nevertheless, there are insufficient data to make any firm conclusions regarding the intra-litter distribution of chemicals, which is required to establish the validity of the in utero exposure protocol. In addition, actual bioassay data are needed in order to establish whether or not the litter effects noted above are also characteristic of the toxic endpoints of interest in a chronic study.

138

SUMMARY

This paper has forward on current thinking regarding reproductive toxicity tests. It is important to bear in mind that these tests, when properly designed and executed, provide a great deal of information regarding potential adverse effects of chemical substances. In the past too little attention has been given to assessing postnatal effects of chemical substances and few investigators have incorporated pharmacokinetic studies into their protocols. These important aspects of reproductive toxicology should not be overlooked.

REFERENCES

1. Khera, K.S. and Tryphonas, L. (1977) Toxicol. Appl. Pharmacol. 42:85-97.

2. Allen, J.R., et al. (1979) Annals of New York Academy of Sciences, Part VI, Reproductive Effects, pp. 419-425.

3. Roxon, J.J., et al. (1967) Fd. Cosmet. Toxicol. 5:367.

4. Walker, R. (1970) Fd. Cosmet. Toxicol. 8:659.

5. Singh, M. (1970) J. Assoc. Agric. Chem. 53:23.

6. Radomsky, J.L. and Millinger, T.J. (1962) J. Pharmacol. Exp. Ther. 136:259.

7. Ruddick, J., et al. (1978) Unpublished data.

8. Pritchard, A.B., et al. (1976) Toxicol. Appl. Pharmacol. 35:1.

9. Collins, T.F.X., et al. (1975) Toxicol. 3:115.

10 Collins, T.F.X., et al. (1976) J. Toxicol. Environ. Health 18:851.

11. Khera, K.S., et al. (1974) Fd. Cosmet. Toxicol. 12:507.

12. Khera, K.S., et al. (1976) Toxicol. Appl. Pharmacol. 38:389.

13. Grice, H.C., et al. (1973) Can. Res. 33:262-268.

14. Arnold, D.L., et al. (1979) Toxicol. Appl. Pharmacol. (in press).

15. Druckrey, H., et al. (1970) Z. Krebsforsch 74:141-161.

16. Ivankovic, S. (19) IARC Scientific Publication, No. 4:90-99.

17. Herbst, A.L., et al. (1971) New England J. of Medicine 284:878-881.

18. Herbst, A.L., et al. (1974) Am. J. Obstet. Gynecol. pp. 713-724.

19. Bibbo, M., et al. (1978) New England J. of Medicine 298:763-767.

20. Ryan, K.J. (1978) New England J. of Medicine 298:794-795.

21. U.S. Department of Health, Education and Welfare (1978) DES Task Force, Summary Report, DHEW publication number (NIH) 79-1688.

22. Druckery, H., et al. (1966) Naturwissenschaften 53:410-411.

23. Kuiper-Goodman, T., et al. (1977) Toxicol. Appl. Pharmacol. 40:529-549.

© 1980 Elsevier/North-Holland Biomedical Press
The Principles and Methods in Modern Toxicology
C.L. Galli, S.D. Murphy and R. Paoletti, editors.

TERATOLOGY AND SAFETY EVALUATION

AK PALMER

Huntingdon Research Centre, Huntingdon, Cambridgeshire PE18 6ES

Teratology studies for safety evaluation of new drugs are a composite drawn from the two multidisciplinary sciences of toxicology and teratology. From each of these we must take those compatible factors that can be amalgamated to create a consistent, balanced system that will

<blockquote>a) prevent the uncontrolled use of dangerous materials in man</blockquote>

without   b) inadvertently preventing the use of beneficial materials in man.

As such, in aims and interpretation, safety evaluation studies should be considered in a different manner to those more academic studies that occupy the bulk of published literature on teratology. Screening tests in general, and those with positive results in particular are rarely published.

Understandably therefore, attainment of the correct balance is not easy and resultant misconceptions at times have generated a low opinion of the value of screening tests. (4) Among the misconceptions consider the use of the term 'false' positive to explain away the apparent discrepancy when drugs with long established use in man are found to be positive in animal tests. Can any terminology be more ridiculous considering the ever increasing list of materials (which include common salt and inert sand grains) that consistently can cause adverse effects in animals ? Use of the term 'false' positive is based on the misconception that materials can be categorised absolutely as teratogens or non-teratogens, a belief that is contrary to one of the basic principles of teratology, namely, that <u>any material may be teratogenic if given to the right species at the right time at the right dosage</u>.

In respect of the latter, consider aspirin, originally dubbed as a 'false' positive because initially it was suggested that only rats were susceptible; later studies however showed embryotoxicity and teratogenicity in primates. Consider corticosteroids originally considered to be 'false' positives because cortisone affected only mice; later, however, the more powerful fluorinated corticosteroids were shown to be capable of inducing malformations in a host of species including primates.[3] Faced with such examples, who would dare assume that these and other materials would remain 'false' positives were we to experiment in man with the same vigour employed in animal tests. However, we do not need to go to such extremes as the examples already exist. Consider oxygen, which can cause cataracts in premature infants and which may be implicated in some cases of patent ductus arteriosus; without oxygen we would die and a 'reduced dosage' would lead to hypoxia which in itself can cause teratogenic effects in a variety of species, including man. As less extreme examples consider that certain antidiabetic, antiepileptic and anticancer agents have been implicated in human teratogenesis yet their use will continue as their removal from the medical armoury could be even more damaging.

It seems obvious therefore that for safety evaluation determination of whether or not a material is teratogenic is not enough. What we also need to know is whether teratogenic or other adverse effects will be encountered in human use. To answer one question without the other is to eat eggs without bacon or to eat Italian food without pasta; the results may be interesting but never complete.

To answer both questions it is important that teratology studies are conducted and interpreted in concert with all other pre clinical tests of pharmacology, pharmacokinetics and general toxicity. In particular, as almost all countries now require a fertility (or general reproductive) study and a peri and post-natal study in addition to teratology tests in two species, it is important that the three segments are planned and executed as a single co-ordinated unit.

In the broader framework it is no longer surprising that anti tumour agents designed to interfere with cell multiplication will also interfere with embryogenesis, or that drugs affecting blood flow and pressure in the adult may also exert the same action in the embryo thereby affecting development of the ventricular septum. Nor should it be surprising that drugs designed to affect cholinergic or adrenergic nerve impulses to smooth muscles of heart or intestines may similarly affect smooth muscle of reproductive organs such as the uterus thereby disturbing the proximate environment of the embryos and affecting their development.

In such cases (and there are many) where adverse effects would be natural extension of the intended pharmacological activity, interpretation becomes a quantitative exercise, in which one has to determine the margin between dosages eliciting the desired effect and those eliciting an undesired effect : for this purpose the more reference points there are to other studies, the better. Even with apparently qualitative differences between species references to other studies are important for how could we accept the use of materials such as imipramine or meclozine were it not for the fact that metabolic studies show that the metabolites inducing the adverse effects in test species are not normally found in man.

Performance of teratology studies in isolation can leave loose ends that will be siezed upon by the bureaucratically inclined who unfortunately tend to emphasise the superficial differences between national requirements and ignore the more important similarities in concept. In turn this can lead to an unnecessary duplication of studies and a waste of valuable resources.

If this last hint of political and economic aspects of teratology studies in safety evaluation seems out of place it would be as well to remember that experience shows that failure to understand or apply basic philosophical aspects causes far more problems than the mechanistics of study performance. This latter point is also reflected in the remaining commentary on the performance of teratology studies per se since more attention has been given to problem areas than to attaining a correct balance of factors.

Teratology studies

A basic requirement for all national agencies is that studies should be performed in at least two species, one preferably being a non-rodent. Pregnant females are dosed with the test compound during the period of organogenesis (embryonic differentiation) usually with three test dosages. A negative group must be included and the addition of a positive control group is sometimes recommended - unfortunately.

Females are killed one or two days prior to parturition, numbers of live and dead young are counted, foetuses are weighed and examined for external, internal, soft tissue and skeletal abnormalities. Some national agencies recommend that a proportion of litters are allowed to be born and the offspring reared to maturity to determine latent physiological or behavioural deficits : others require this step to be taken in either the reproductive or peri and post-natal studies.

It is in the further expansion and interpretation of these requirements that inter-agency divergence becomes apparent and can even extend to intra-agency divergence both chronologically and for different spokesmen at the same time. These differences can be all the more frustrating and irritating when pseudo-scientific logic masks an underlying political or bureaucratic motivation. Some further comments on the details of the basic study design are as follows :

Choice of material(s)

Even before the advent of GLP legislation, it was important to characterise and ensure the quality, consistency and stability in dosing formulations of the test material. For example, many of the negative results obtained with thalidomide may be attributed to its hydrolysis when dissolved in sodium hydroxide,[7] whilst the herbicide 2,4,5-T was labelled as a teratogen when more probably the real cause was a highly toxic dioxin contaminant.[2] A range of subtle to profound differences in results can accrue from differences in the vehicle, the dose volume and the concentration employed; particle size can be particularly important in suspensions.

Choice of species

First and foremost one must counteract the fairy story that there is an 'ideal species' for the performance of general purpose studies such as those of teratology in safety evaluation.

In reality, test species are chosen because they are available, economical and easy to manage.[1] These practical considerations often legitimately outweigh more theoretical considerations (eg. exact similarity in metabolism), and because of the greater use of these animals we have accumulated a wealth of information on basic physiology, embryology, rates of malformations, response to drug types etc. all of which is extremely important for the performance and interpretation of studies. From this accumulation of knowledge 'scientific' explanations for the choice of species may be given but it should be remembered that these are post hoc rationalisations to disguise the fact that we use the 'devil we know'.[5]

No species reflect this situation more than the rat and all agencies require teratology studies in this species. Among the many practical assets of the rat, which make it widely used in other pre-clinical safety tests, the short regular oestrous cycle and gestation period, the relative ease and accuracy of determination of mating are extremely advantageous to the teratologist.

For the interpretation of results the rats shows a low rate of spontaneous malformations so that 'negative' or 'positive' results are fairly readily identified as such. As a corollary in some quarters this low background is considered to indicate that the rat may not be sensitive to a wide range of teratogenic actions, eg. its lack of response to thalidomide. This belief is not necessarily altered by the fact that the rat can be especially sensitive to specific compounds, for example in its teratogenic response to salicylates and parabendazole type antihelminthics ; the toxic effects of anti inflammatory agents at parturition or during late pregnancy can be problematical if offspring are to be reared.

For regulatory tests the rabbit is the most widely used second species and in the UK reasons have to be given if it is not used. For most countries, the rabbit is considered as a non-rodent for reproductive studies but not for general toxicity studies thereby providing a further illustration that species are chosen for practical rather than 'scientific' reasons. Of course it sounds better to suggest that the rabbit was used because its susceptibility to thalidomide guarantees that it will be susceptible to other teratogens. This belief is of course erroneous as not all teratogens work in the same way.

More relevant are the practical factors that led to the rabbit being used to test thalidomide in the first place. These include the ease with which mating can be achieved and the precision with which pregnancy can be determined, factors which had led to pre-existing background information on embryological development and physiology of reproduction and with its use in screening tests further knowledge has accumulated.

Of the common species used the rabbit shows the highest rate of more varied abnormalities[6] perhaps partly as a consequence of its use for purposes other than as a laboratory animal. Another factor is the convenient size of the foetuses which allows more detailed examination for abnormalities in both soft and skeletal tissues.   For example, whilst studies in mice might suggest that corticosteroids only cause cleft palate, studies in rabbits reveal cleft palate and a variety of other deformations not so readily seen in the small mouse foetus.

For interpretation the higher incidence of more varied abnormalities suggests that the rabbit may be more sensitive to a variety of teratogenic actions than the rat. Unfortunately, this advantage must be set against the inevitable disadvantage that because of the greater background 'noise' more effort, thought and judgement is required to distinguish 'negative' and 'positive' responses.

One disadvantage of the rabbit is that being herbivorous both general or specific stress can readily result in enteric disorder making it extremely difficult to distinguish between induced and coincidental effects on the parent animal, and also difficult to maintain stocks of animals in prime condition. Such maternal changes must be monitored as in all species embryonic malformations can arise secondarily to impaired maternal economy.

It is now widely known that the rabbit is unduly sensitive to antibiotics specifically affecting gram positive bacteria which are a necessary component of the rabbits' gastro intestinal tract. Less readily recognised is the fact that the rabbit can also be very sensitive to anti cholinergic or β adrenergic blocking agents since these can affect the motility of the all important sensitive gastro intestinal tract.

The third most widely used species in regulatory teratology is the mouse and various real and imagined reasons have been given as to why it has not retained the higher position it holds in non regulatory teratology. Comparison of the differing responses of mice and rats to cortisone or tricyclic antidepressants shows that they cannot be considered to be merely little and large versions of the same species and perhaps there is greater truth in the view that whilst rats and mice show many of the same practical advantages, on an overall basis the rat shows them to a greater degree. For example, mice tend to be less docile than rats making them less easy to handle and dose; they are also smaller making examination of foetuses more difficult. Also in comparison with the rat the more rapid late foetal development leads to greater individual variation in the degree of maturity eg. skeletal ossification; there is also a higher background incidence of spontaneous malformations often occurring in a clonic pattern. Both of the latter can cause difficulties in interpretation of results.

As the mouse cannot effectively compete with the rat it is mostly used as an additional species or as a replacement for the rabbit when the latter species can be shown to be unsuitable.

From time to time   other species have been suggested and used but even with the most likely contenders such as the ferret (because it is a small carnivore) and the hamster, they lack the all round balance of practical assets necessary for general purpose use. For example, how does one dose a hamster intravenously ?

Generally, it is best to use unconventional species for the sole purpose of confirming positive responses with a strong teratogen, for example using primates to demonstrate the potential of thalidomide. Using an unconventional species to demonstrate negative responses is a form of Russian roulette and investigators get away with it solely because the odds are in their favour. In other words as malformations are low frequency phenomena the laws of

probability would decree that a negative result would be the most likely outcome even with a moderate teratogen. Conversely if one is unlikely enough to find a malformation or two in the test group the numbers used would usually be too low to objectively determine whether the malformations were coincidental or treatment related.

Dosages   (8)

Currently most authorities recommend the use of three test groups as follows :-

        a) a high dosage causing minimal maternal toxicity or being the
           maximum tolerated.

        b) a low dosage causing the clinically intended effect in the test
           species or being a low multiple of the intended human dosage.

        c) an intermediate dosage logarithmically spaced between high and
           low doses.

Given such simple rules it is surprising how many mistakes are made usually through lack of attention to detail or attempts to take short cuts. For example, using single dose LD_{50} values to determine the high dosage for a repeated dose study is frequently fatal, even within the same species; it is even more likely to be disastrous if one uses an LD_{50} value in rats to choose a high dosage for a rabbit teratology study. Quite frequently such short cuts lead to loss of the entire study through maternal death, or if not that, through the occurrence of marked embryonic effects secondary to maternal toxicity.

At the other end of the scale one can end up choosing too low a high dosage if selection is based on the end results of toxicity studies of 6 months or longer. For choosing a high dosage with accuracy, there is no real substitute for a specifically designed range finding study in which the test material is administered to female animals of the intended species, by the intended route of administration, at the intended concentrations and for the intended dosing period (ie. 10 days to 2 weeks usually). Regarding the question as to whether pregnant or non-pregnant females should be used for such studies the answer is so simple that it is often unrecognised. Thus, if one has prior knowledge that the test material is likely to be teratogenic, embryotoxic, an abortifacient, or will be considerably more toxic to pregnant than non-pregnant animals, then it is more appropriate to use pregnant animals.

If there is no prior evidence of such selective or specific effects, which is the case for most new materials, then it is cheaper, quicker and more convenient to use non-pregnant animals. In particular, bearing in mind that teratology studies are still subject to emotive, rather than objective assessment it avoids the occurrence of adverse effects on embryos in uninterpretable circumstances.

On occasions use of non-pregnant animals in preliminary studies will lead to loss of embryonic material in the main study due to the occurrence of a greater toxic effect in the pregnant female. To the academic teratologist this may seem to be wasteful but in terms of safety evaluation it represents the acquisition of important information obtained in reliable circumstances.

From these preliminary studies some thought must be given as to what constitutes a minimally toxic effect. For material inducing a dosage related retardation in weight gain it is relatively simple to select a dosage that will cause a minimal reduction in weight gain, ie. not more than 10%. In some cases however, whilst a marginal reduction in weight gain may be achievable it is not desirable, because of alternative effects occurring at lower dosages. Such cases may include materials causing an extended pharmacological reaction that will interfere with maternal economy; prolonged sedation or interference with hormonal balance are obvious examples.

Conversely, for some materials such as anti-inflammatory agents, and hypoglycaemics where the end response may be sudden death a 'minimally toxic' dosage is pointless and it is better to choose a maximum tolerated dosage than can be shown to be meaningful by reference to range finding studies, ie. it can be clearly demonstrated from dose response that the next logical higher dosage would cause lethal effects.

There are of course occasions when it is impossible to provoke any response of a pharmacological or toxicological nature at the maximum practical dosage. For routes of administration such as ocular, nasal and vaginal installation, intramuscular injection of small species; inhalation or in dermal application in any species, dosage may be severely limited by physical factors. All that can be done is to permutate combinations of vehicle, concentration of material, dosage volumes and frequency of administration to obtain the highest practical dosage possible.

However, with more convenient routes of administration such as gavage or subcutaneous injection allowing administration of much higher dosages, the absence of a biological response should be followed by questions as to whether the test material is of any value and as to whether the right species has been chosen for the studies before resorting to the use of the highest practical dosage.

Having established the highest dosage the most practical means of selecting the two lower dosages is to follow a descending sequence using relatively small intervals such as $\frac{1}{2}$ to $\frac{1}{4}$ according to the slope of the dosage response. If the results are negative there is no point in investigating lower dosages; if the results are positive or equivocal there is usually sufficient margin above clinical dosage (human or animal) to continue in a logical pattern.

The more theoretical approach of establishing a low dosage on clinical response in the test species is rarely realisable and even when it is possible it may necessitate the use of several intermediate dosages which will be expensive, or necessitate the use of large intervals between dosages. The latter can form an inconvenient basis for further investigation.

On one last point, having selected the three test dosages it is often possible to make slight adjustments so that at least the low and intermediate dosages match those employed in other toxicity studies : this matching can prove extremely useful in the interpretation of equivocal or positive results.

Control groups

For all studies a negative control group should be included and should be treated in an identical manner to the test groups, except for omission of the active principle. Where the vehicle itself is likely to induce effects, eg. syrups and alcohol bases for rabbits, or when the dosing procedure may be traumatic, eg. insertion of medical devices, inhalation, it is also advisable to include an untreated control group. Well recorded, consistent, historical control values are also of value.[6] It is sometimes recommended that positive control groups be included proving that 'you can fool some of the people all of the time'. In the vast majority of cases the time, money and effort spent on positive control groups would have been better spent on adding a further test group of more negative controls.

The only time 'positive' controls are of any value for the interpretation of results is when they relate closely to the new test material and can then be called comparative controls. For example, aspirin can be a useful comparative control in rats when testing another salicylate and dexa- or beta-methasone can be useful comparative controls in any species when testing a new fluorinated corticosteroid. However, to include these or any other teratogen that is unrelated to the test material in no way guarantees that the test system is suitable for the test material. This should be patently obvious from the fact that aspirin is a potent teratogen in rats but not other species, cortisone is a potent teratogen in some strains of mice but not rats, and thalidomide is a potent teratogen in rabbits but not rats and mice.

The less fallacial view that inclusion of a 'positive' control group will assure assessors of the capabilities of the investigators, is still naive since it requires no great skill to be able to detect malformations such as exencephaly, gastroschisis or cranioschisis. By far the best guide of an investigators capability is provided by the consistency with which he can detect a range of minor changes in the foetuses of 'negative' control groups.

Route of administration

Most authorities recommend that the test material be administered by the route or routes intended for man, an eminently sensible suggestion since it does not always follow that the route allowing the higher rate of administration will always provide the greatest effect. Hexachlorophene is a good example since it causes little effect orally, due to its break-down by intestinal bacteria, but it will induce maternal toxicity and teratogenic effects when applied topically or by the vaginal route. We have also encountered greater effects following dermal application than by subcutaneous administration.

Conversely to these examples it is extremely infuriating to have to perform a series of time consuming investigations in teratology and pharmacokinetics to counteract adverse results obtained by injection of materials which when applied by intended topical or oral routes are never absorbed to any meaningful extent in either animals or man.

In occasional instances and particularly with unusual routes of administration such as inhalation or installation into body orifices or intra muscular injections in small animals it is necessary to compromise in order to attain either a sufficient margin above the clinical dosage or to avoid unnecessary repetitive testing as would be the case for the different routes of parenteral administration.

Such compromises should be made carefully and preferably be supported by the performance of comparative pharmacokinetic and/or toxicity tests to ensure correct interpretation of results.

Frequency of dosing

All authorities require that the test material be administered once daily during the critical period or organ differentiation. For most countries this means days 6 to 15 inclusive of pregnancy for rats and mice and days 6 to 18 for rabbits. Japan is an exception requiring dosing on days 7 to 17 of pregnancy for rats.

Observation of spermatozoa in vaginal smears of rats and mice and observation of coitus (or artificial insemination) is considered to represent day 0 of pregnancy.

It is in respect of the frequency of dosing that teratology for safety evaluation diverges from academic teratology and thereby causes confusion. This confusion could perhaps be reduced if people would realise that the aims are different. In simplistic terms the academic teratologist tries to establish an optimal dosage regime which will maximise the occurrence of malformations relative to the occurrence of other adverse effects : this objective is more usually obtained by dosing on one or at the most two days of pregnancy following the basic principle that malformations are induced by the application of a precise dosage, at a precise time of organ differentiation.

For safety evaluation, however, the primary objective is to determine the lowest dosage that will provoke any adverse effect, be this malformations, embryotoxicity, growth retardation or maternal toxicity; moreover, one must allow for the fact drugs are rarely administered as single doses, must allow for the occurrence of cumulative effects, or accumulation of metabolites and must accept that the whole period of organogenesis be covered, since there is no prior indication of which stage (ie. day of pregnancy) will show the greatest susceptibility. All of these aspects would not necessarily be examined by dosing animals on only one or two days and then covering the entire organic period by the expensive and time consuming process of performing 5 to 10 studies instead of one.

Whilst it would be ridiculous to go to this extreme it is also equally ridiculous for investigators to rigidly follow governmental guidelines when they have the information to perform a better study. Examples would include the use of more than one daily dose, when physical limitations of the dosing technique preclude administration of a daily dosage of reasonable magnitude, or when investigating highly active compounds with a short half life. Conversely, for long acting materials or depot preparations intervals of 2 to 3 days between doses may be more appropriate. In the case of drugs with pronounced cumulative toxicity, or with pronounced enzyme inducing properties, it would be more appropriate in many cases to reduce the total dosing period to a few days and perform 2 or 3 studies. For example, in rats one study may be dosed during days 6 to 10 and the other during days 10 to 15.

Numbers of animals

Different national agencies vary only slightly in their specification for the number of pregnant animals per group, usual values being about 20 for rats and mice and 10 to 15 for rabbits. For Japan an extra 10 rats per group must be added to form a rearing phase. Whether these values represent the numbers that should be present at the beginning of the study or at termination is not always clearly stated.

The numbers suggested have been arrived at empirically, or on practical or economic grounds, there being no scientific basis for allowing the use of smaller numbers of rabbits than rats or even smaller numbers of species such as pigs or primates. Phrases such as 'there must be sufficient to permit statistical analysis' are frequently meaningless as until one knows the parameters that will be affected, the way they will be affected, or whether the response occurs as a discrete, semi-discrete or a continuous variable, one cannot determine the most suitable method of analysis.

On empirical grounds experience suggests that for the generally negative responses of screening tests consistency within and between studies tends to decrease rapidly below 10

to 12 animals per group. Reasonable consistency occurs between 12 to 20 per group.
Above 20 to 25 per group theoretical gains in statistical terms are usually negated by added
difficulties of chronological dispersion of the total experiment and by diminishing global
control. To provide numbers sufficient for valid statistical analysis of low frequency events
such as malformations would usually require a marked jump from 20 animals per group to
above a minimum of 60, whatever the species.

Examination

The different aims of safety evaluation compared with academic teratology that necessitate
use of repeated dosing techniques also influence the methods of examination in several
respects.

One of these is that greater attention must be paid to maternal parameters, eg. weight gain,
as these provide the all important links with other toxicity studies and allow the results of
the teratology study to be put in perspective. In particular this enables us to determine
whether a selective effect has been encountered and whether previous estimates of safety
margins have been altered.

The academic teratologist on the other hand often does his utmost to avoid these perspectives
in order to maximise his harvest of abnormal foetuses and in so doing may forget that the
dosages he has used to obtain malformations may be far in excess of dosages that because of
other toxic effects would never be contemplated in human use.

For a number of reasons not the least being the facts that most materials examined will be
of low teratogenic potency and that the priority aims of providing a broad cover and
establishing perspectives reduce the chances of attaining an optimum regime for inducing
malformations, high rates of obvious malformations are rarely encountered in screening
tests. Indeed values are usually so low that in isolation distinction between treatment
induced and coincidental abnormalities cannot be made objectively.

In consequence, the teratologist in safety evaluation must broaden the scope of his
examination in order to be able to utilise the more frequent and therefore most analysable
and reliable events that inevitably accompany teratogenic activity. To this end it would
be a considerable help if we stopped referring to 'Teratology Studies' and used more
appropriate terminology such as calling them 'Tests for selective embryopathy'. For example

even under optimum conditions rarely if ever, are increased rates of malformations observed without being accompanied by increased embryonic death, or reduced foetal weight or increased incidences of minor structural changes occurring at or below the optimum dosage for induction of malformations.

To this end the numbers of live and dead implantations must be recorded, for dead implants (ie. resorptions) it may be useful to distinguish between early embryonic deaths (resorptions) and late embryonic deaths as, more frequently than not, teratogens increase the number of early deaths relative to the number of late deaths. If primiparous rats or mice are used the uteri of apparently non pregnant females should be examined for early total resorptions by the Salewski technique. (The technique does not work in rabbits and can be confusing for animals that have undergone a previous pregnancy). For viable foetuses it is important to stimulate respiration to facilitate future examination and it helps to kill dams by exposure to CO_2 in the case of rats or cervical dislocation in the case of rabbits and mice. Sacrifice of dams with barbiturates can depress respiration in foetuses if they are not removed from the dam extremely rapidly.

The almost universal practice of recording the position of live, malformed and dead embryos in the uterine horns leads almost invariably to the collection of useless data. If a test compound induces an increased incidence of affected foetuses a government assessor is not going to alter his decision on the basis of their uterine position. Information on individual foetal weights is also rarely used and the main value is to be able to link foetal weight with immaturity or malformation. A more convenient less time consuming practice is to weigh the entire litter to obtain litter weight and then calculate foetal weight from this. Occasional individual foetuses with external abnormalities or which obviously differ in size from the norm can be weighed as individuals and tagged to ensure that there is a link with subsequent examinations. Pregnancy rate should also be recorded since the timing of initial treatment is such that it would be possible for a highly active compound to kill embryos at or just after implantation so that at termination the animal merely appears to be non-pregnant. This event has been recorded in our laboratories.

For rats and rabbits or other polytocous species, it is advisable to record corpora lutea counts their value being to ensure that differences in numbers of live and dead young are not attributed to treatment when they are due to earlier coincidental factors. It must be remembered, however, that the facility to count corpora lutea decreases with decreasing body size hence for rats and rabbits counts must be regarded as estimates which can be reliable for a group of animals but not for specific individuals. For mice and hamsters accurate estimates can only be made by recourse to time consuming methods (eg. histopathological examination) and their insurance value may not be worth the effort.

Following determination of litter values and examination of live foetuses for external malformations, foetuses must be further examined for more subtle skeletal and visceral changes. Some people will also examine dead foetuses but this usually results in confusion because of artefacts and also seems pointless as there can be no greater insult than death.

There are various methods available for further examination of foetuses and irrespective of what a government regulation may say, the most important factor is that the investigator chooses methods with which he is comfortable. For example, the two main methods of visceral examination of rats and mice are the Wilson sectioning technique and micro-dissection. At its very best the hand sectioning technique is probably slightly better than microdissection as one is able to detect slightly higher incidences of minor cardiovascular changes and can detect as many as can be recorded by histopathological serial sectioning techniques. The best however, is very difficult to achieve requiring not only an innate ability to translate from two dimensions into three but also the opportunity to constantly examine relatively large numbers of foetuses.

In the absence of this combination of factors microdissection may be the better technique as adequate levels of examination can be attained and retained more readily. Micro-dissection has the added advantage that if the number of litters examined per day is low it is feasible to perform microdissection on fresh specimens which allows examination for both soft tissue and skeletal abnormalities in the same foetus.

Indeed for larger foetuses from the size of a rabbit or above, the fresh microdissection is often more effective, than hand sectioning (or even microdissection of fixed foetuses) and it makes more sense to examine individual foetuses for both skeletal and soft tissue defects.

In respect of skeletal examinations for rat, rabbit and mouse foetuses the alizarin staining technique is far superior to X ray methods as indicated by the certainty and consistency with which minor skeletal changes can be observed; moreover, one can always re-examine the foetus or turn it round slightly to be certain that one is not looking at an artefact.

X ray examinations are preferred for very large foetuses such as pigs for reasons of convenience, but for smaller foetuses they only begin to approach the accuracy of alizarin staining if one is prepared to go through the time consuming process of disarticulating the skeleton to layout the various parts in a single plane.

There are several variations to these techniques all of which can be employed and the key to determining whether the correct methods are being employed is the ability to consistently observe and record the minor structural anomalies that are always present in the normal population. Failure to observe these minor changes in soft and skeletal tissues of <u>negative</u> control animals indicates inadequate examination.

Categorisation of abnormalities

Efficient examination inevitably leads to higher background incidences of structural changes and it is important to ensure that this does not lead to confusion. To this end results should always be presented so that the overall picture of the number of foetuses and number of litters affected is accurately portrayed and not artifically magnified by counting foetuses with more than one change several times.

Bearing in mind that results are usually negative and that frank malformations will occur in low frequency it is important not to mask important irreversible changes with trivial ones. To this end it is useful to adopt a categorisation system and the semi-quantitative one used in our laboratories is as follows [6] :

<u>Major malformations</u> : include those irreversible changes that are obviously detrimental to survival or are extremely rare, examples are cyclopia, gastroschisis, exencephaly.

<u>Minor anomalies</u> : are not obviously detrimental and, probably because of this, occur with greater frequency than major malformations. They can be obviously irreversible, for example agenesis of the gall bladder in rabbits or persistent right sided azygos vein in rats or short tail or hemi vertebrae in any species, or they can be obviously reversible as in the case of unossified occipital bones in mice, unossified phalangeal bones in rats or incompletely descended testes in rats and mice.

Common variants : can also be constituted of a mixture of irreversible changes such as extra ribs or obviously reversible changes such as unossified sternebrae. They differ from minor anomalies in that they can be consistently recorded in more than 5% of the population. Categorisations of this nature are not easy since structural changes can readily fall on the borderline between categories. Nor is it logical to expect all investigators to work to exactly the same system since a difference in strain of animals, day of sacrifice or recognition level can markedly alter the incidence of some of the more subtle changes. Despite these difficulties if the investigator follows a system he can apply consistently, organisation and interpretation of essentially negative results is greatly facilitated. Moreover, one of the prime indications of teratogenic activity is disruption of the category system as increasing incidences of similar anomalies merge imperceptibly from one category to another. Thus with increasing dosages of a salicylate not only does the incidence of extra ribbed pups increase but the extra ribs get longer and there can often be two or more extra pairs. We have also recorded progressively increasing incidences and degrees of change in the cardiovascular system and in another example there was a continuous reduction in the digits ranging from a degree of change that was almost indistinguishable from controls through degrees of obvious minor reductions through to frank oligo- and ectrodactyly.

In all cases small but recognisable increase in the incidence of frank abnormalities was preceded at lower dosages by significant increases in the incidence of more subtle changes.
Assessment of results
Detailed analysis over several hundreds of studies shows that for polytocous species the litter rather than the foetus represents the only valid sample unit and that litter values generally show non-normal distributions (Poisson or beta binomial are the most common). Failure to recognise these factors can result in meaningless and troublesome statistically significant differences and make authoritarian requests for 'standard deviations' laughable. Non parametric methods of analysis are the most useful for general purpose use but like all statistical methods should not be used as a substitute for biological judgement. Indeed in this respect meaningful differences in incidences of major malformations usually fulfil Berksons Intra ocular Traumatic Test (ie. they hit you between the eyes) long before they can be shown to be 'statistically' significant by valid methods of analysis.

For example, on statistical grounds to detect marked increases, say from a basic 0.1% to a 10% incidence, group sizes ranging from 60 per group to several hundreds of litters would be required. In one study where a particular abnormality was the only criterion of effect we had to use between 1000 to 1500 rats to be certain that statistical analysis was valid. These statistical criteria particularly apply to monotocous species such as primates where there is little chance of using altnerative parameters to detect effects.

It is fortunate therefore that the primary aim in screening tests is to determine the lowest dosage at which any adverse effect may occur and a relief to know that on currently available information malformations will only occur at higher dosages. As previously stated to date there is no known teratogen that will induce malformations at dosages lower than those that will cause other more detectable adverse effects. Particularly in standard screening tests, other effects such as increased numbers of embryonic deaths, lower foetal weights, increased incidences of variants and/or minor anomalies will be recorded at dosages below those inducing major malformations.

For most real or possible teratogens adverse effects will be obtained at dosages close to those causing maternal toxicity, thereby, not materially altering previous estimations of safety margins. If on valid extrapolation the existence of a wide and real safety margin above the human dosage can be demonstrated it will probably be unnecessary to perform more precise studies ti distinguish between teratogenic and other effects or to determine whether these are primary direct effects or secondary consequences of maternal toxicity.

In rare cases the investigator may record adverse effects at dosages markedly lower than those causing maternal toxicity and thereby materially reduce previous estimates of the safety margin. Again it may not be necessary to make fine distinctions between terato-genicity, embryotoxicity or growth retardation since none would be considered acceptable in the human case. Only in very special cases will it be necessary to determine precisely whether the adverse effects recorded are independent, or linked to real teratogenic potential. This will usually be when the drug appears to afford such therapeutic advantages that its use at or close to dosages causing adverse effect must be considered. Anti cancer drugs are the most obvious examples. In such circumstances secondary stage studies may need to be performed but since these will be on an individual basis and intended to answer specific questions their design and interpretation must be approached in a different way and this must not be confused with the approach required for general screening.

References

1. Brown, A.M. (1963) In : Animals for Research : 261-285, Ed. W. Lane-Petter, Publ. Academic Press.

2. Courtney, K.D. et al (1970) : Science 168 : 864-866

3. Hendrickx, A.G. et al (1975) : Fed. Proc. 34 : 1661

4. Palmer, A.K. (1976) : Environ. Health Prespectives 18 : 97-104.

5. Ibid   (1978) : In Handbook of Teratology 4 : 215-253. Ed. J.G. Wilson and F. Clarke Frazer. Publ. Plenum.

6. Ibid   (1977) : In Methods in Prenatal Toxicology : 57-71. Ed. D Neubert et al Publ. George Thieme

7. Schumaker, H. et al (1968) : J. Pharmacol. Exp. Therap. 10 (i) : 189-197.

8. WHO (1967) : Principles for testing drugs for teratogenicity : WHO Tech. Report Series No. 364

TESTING FOR CARCINOGENICITY

GIUSEPPE DELLA PORTA and TOMMASO A. DRAGANI
Division of Experimental Oncology A, Istituto Nazionale per lo
Studio e la Cura dei Tumori, Via G. Venezian 1, 20133 Milan, Italy

It is difficult, and perhaps unwise particularly in this moment,
to give precise instructions on how to perform an assay for
carcinogenesis. There are large differences in requirements among
countries, and even in the same country most often in relation to
the use of the material to be tested and to the extent of exposure
of the human population. However, an effort is underway in the
attempt to harmonize legislation on toxicology within the European
Community and, hopefully, with the USA. Perhaps this attempt is
somewhat easier for long-term assays, where many national and
international committees have prepared guide-lines over the last
10 years, and no great differences in the general approach have
emerged, although considerable improvements in the design and
conduct of the experiments have been made. Clearly, harmonization
of minimun standards required by the various governmental agencies
will prove to be useful in dealing with various environmental
situations, but a good degree of scientific freedom, and uncertainty, in testing procedures will eventually prove benificial in the
sense that more research will be undertaken in an effort to make
the results more reliable and perhaps the assay simpler. Not enough
research is being done in this specific field, and many assumptions,
which are generally accepted, need to be more scientifically
substantiated.

Rather than going into details, which can be found in many
publications, we shall try to indicate some of the major
difficulties involved in a long-term bioassay for carcinogenesis,
referring in particular to the problems which are specifically
connected with this type of study. It should be understood that
most of the problems involved in the design and conduct of the
study and in the reporting of the results are covered by good
laboratory practice regulations, are common to various types of

toxicology assays, and will be discussed elsewhere during this
course. We would like, however, to mention that in a long-term
bioassay more than in others, it is necessary to assign specific
responsibilities to each component of the team that follows the
experiment, but there must be also a close contact between the
professional and technical staff, because over a long period of
time errors are more likely to occur. In addition, it is important
to recognize that at least ideally the same pathologist who reads
the slides at the microscope should follow the autopsy procedures
and be informed of the development of the experiment.

The diet is an issue of the greatest importance in a long-term
experiment. An open-formula diet composed of natural ingredients
is preferred, should be prepared in small batches and not stored
for extended periods of time. Periodic controls should be made
not only for the quality and quantity of the essential nutrients
but also for contaminants, particularly for pesticides,nitrosamines
and mycotoxins.

The design of the experiment

The design of the experiment is strictly related to the available information on the test material, which must include the
chemical and physical properties of the compound, its stability,
method of analysis and types and level of impurities. The problem
of impurities is of great importance, particularly in a long-term
experiment where the administration over a long period of time
even of minute amounts may profoundly alter the results and may
be entirely responsible for the observed toxic effects. Connected
with the problem of impurities is that of the selection of the
technical grade versus the highly purified compound. Practically,
a step-by-step approach may be suggested, where the technical
grade material is tested first, followed, in the case of positive
results, by the pure compound and then by the impurities.

Another aspect of great importance is the comparative metabolism
and pharmacokinetics of the compound. Obviously, this may dictate
the choice of the species to be tested, when differences are
apparent and the metabolism in humans is known. The results of the
acute and subchronic toxicity tests must also be available.
Finally, it is necessary to be informed about the major ways human

exposure may occur, both in qualitative and quantitative terms.

In the past, certain types of medium-term experiments have been suggested as a means of screening carcinogens. Two types deserve mention. The first is the lung adenoma assay, which uses strain A mice with a large incidence of spontaneous lung adenomas, and has as the end point the increase and acceleration of their occurrence. The second type is the subcutaneous test, usually performed in the rat with the end point of observing chiefly, if not only, local tumors. Both types of assay, although they have some merits, should not be considered in formal testing for carcinogenesis, particularly because now the so-called short-term tests may provide more meaningful information that can be used in a prescreening program.

Another point that should be discussed is the straight carcinogenesis experiment versus the combined chronic toxicity and carcinogenesis study, the aim of the latter approach being a decreased cost. However, several confounding effects may be introduced in the carcinogenesis test. In any case, since the chronic toxicity is done in the rat, the issue concerns only the rat and not the mouse. If a combined experiment is designed, most workers are in favor of satellite groups, which are treated separately and used for interim killing and biochemical observations. The multigenerational approach will be discussed elsewhere during this course.

At least two species of rodents should be included in the study, usually the mouse and the rat, less frequently the hamster particularly for respiratory tract carcinogenesis. A non-rodent species is no longer required, partially because of practical reasons but also because not enough data are available to prove that a non-rodent animal will give more valid information than the rodents. On the other hand, the two rodent species are requested again on practical grounds. Two are better than one, three or four are too expensive.

Not enough attention is given to the selection of the strains. Animals from well-controlled and well-known outbred closed colonies are adequate. Inbred strains are often preferred because their spontaneous incidence of tumors is more stable. Hybrids between two inbred strains are also highly recommended because they are strong animals. It is important to select a strain or a hybrid with a low incidence of spontaneous tumors. On logical grounds, two strains with a different pattern of spontaneous tumors should be the best choice, but we do not have enough information to say that a combination of two strains of the same species, e.g. the mouse, could validly substitute the two species.

Dose selection is another very important issue, and, again, although certain rules are now generally accepted, not enough research and thought are given to the problem. In most instances two or three levels plus the O level are used. The high dose, in most cases,is the equivalent of the maximum tolerated dose, defined as the highest dose that produces a minimal toxicity, such as a 10% decrease or delay in body growth, or some enzyme alteration, without impairing well-being and survival. This level should be determined by an accurate 90-day subchronic test. When the compound does not produce toxicity at all, the dose should not go up to unreasonable levels, and, for example, should not exceed 5% if given in the diet or in the drinking water. Why use such a high dose? The rationale is that if a level is used that is comparable to that of the human exposure, the small number of animals that can be used in the experimental situation will not allow the detection of the induction of a low percentage of a given type of tumor, let us say 1%. This percentage, however, would be of considerable relevance in the human situation. It is believed that the sensitivity of the system can be increased by increasing the dose. This concept is open to criticism, because it does not take into account the possibility that a non-specific toxicity, which may indeed be present, may interfere,in both directions, with the mechanisms of tumor induction.

One high and one low dose, e.g., one-half or one-fourth of the high dose, are believed to be sufficient to discover whether or not the chemical is carcinogenic. However, a third lower dose should be added when the 90-day study indicates major differences in pharmacokinetics according to the dosage level. At least 3 dose levels should be used, if the experiment is carried out for risk assessment. It should also be noted that the high dose could produce an unpredicted toxicity with a poor survival rate.

As for the controls, each study must have its concurrent
control group, which must be identical in every aspect to the
treated group except for the exposure to the test material. When
a vehicle is used, a control group treated with the vehicle is
necessary. In theory, the vehicle control group should be an
adequate control, but it is better to have an untreated control
group as well. It must be emphasized that it is of great
importance that the investigator knows very well the animals he
uses and has precise information on their spontaneous incidence
of tumors. If this is not the case, a larger control group or
perhaps two control groups, should be concurrently kept under
observation. It is also important that each laboratory collects
and keeps historical data on previous control groups, to be used
in the final evaluation of the experiment.

It is now generally accepted that 50 animals per sex should be
included in each treated and control group. It is also recognized
that some increase in the group size, e.g., 80 animals, will
decrease so slightly the probability of false negatives that it
does not justify the increase in work and cost. If, for any
purpose, interim killing or special observations, such as blood
chemistry, are required,then satellite groups should be added and
treated as completely independent sets.

The oral, dermal and respiratory routes are the most frequently
used routes of administration. The choice depends upon the way
human exposure occurs and upon the physical and chemical
characteristics of the compound to assure a proper absorption.
There is a general consensus that the experimental route of
exposure should be as close as possible to the human exposure.
However, quite often, particularly with industrial chemicals,
human exposure could be by more than one route, e.g., inhalation
and dermal absorption. The oral route certainly has many advantages,
provided that the chemical is absorbed and can be mixed in the
diet or in the drinking water, since it is technically simple and
can assure a continuous exposure. Cutaneous exposure may be useful
as a model system for induction of skin tumors, particularly in
initiation and promotion experiments, but has limitations for the
induction of internal tumors, since the quantitative absorption
is difficult to ascertain. The respiratory route is certainly

important, particularly when gaseous or powdered materials have to be tested. However, the inhalation system poses many serious technical problems, which can be dealt with only by highly specialized laboratories equipped with chambers for exposure to aerosols. An alternative to inhalation is intratracheal instillation for particulate material.

The administration of the compound should be continuous through-out the experiment. In the case the material is given by stomach tube or by dermal application, the frequency should be at daily intervals unless pharmacokinetic data suggest differently.

The animals should be introduce into the experiment as soon as possible after weaning, and treatment should start preferably at 6 weeks of age. It has been suggested that pre- and perinatal treatment may enhance susceptibility to tumor induction, particularly in specific tissue. However, there is little evidence that a carcinogenic action would not have been demonstrated if the treatment had been started in the post-weaning age.

The treatment should last for the greatest part of life, but the often suggested procedure of continuing treatment until the last animal has died spontaneously should not be followed, because it may postpone the end of the experiment unnecessarily only because a few animals are surviving to a much older age than the others. This practice may greatly complicate the evaluation, even in statistical terms, of the experiment. Actually, we need some large experimentations to prove whether a treatment lasting about half of the mean survival of the animal used, when followed by a suitable time of observation, is adequate for the induction of tumors. At present, it is recommended that the treatment is continued for 24 months for mice and hamsters and 30 months for rats. However, the study can be terminated earlier, when mortality reaches 75% in the control or in the lowest dose group. The study should obviously continue if a high mortality is present only in the highest dose. The two sexes should be considered as two separate experiments. On the other hand, a negative experiment should be taken as valid only if at least 50% of the animals in any group are surviving at 18 months for mice and hamsters and at 24 months for rats. The duration of exposure, usually coincides with the observation period, that is the animals are killed soon after termination of treatment. However, in certain situations where treatment is causing some toxic effect, a further period of observation without treatment may, on the one hand, favor the development of the already induced tumors and, on the other hand, facilitate the pathologic assessment of tumors after recovery from a nonspecific toxic pathology.

The conduct of the experiment

The methods of randomization are relatively simple, and is necessary to have a good source of random numbers either computerized or in tabular form. However, it has to be decided if one wants to take into consideration the position of the cages in the room. In this case, it is possible to first assign the animals to groups and then give a random ordering of the sequentially numbered cages, using a random permutation of a series of numbers. More important than the position of the cages is to ascertain with careful observation made by a competent person that all the animals are in good condition and to discharge, e.g. on a body weight basis, all abnormal animals before starting any type of randomization.

During the entire course of the experiment, animals must be checked daily, and preferably twice a day, to monitor animals likely to die soon. Cannibalized or decomposed animals are a great loss in this type of experiment, and, in principle, they could be assumed to be bearers of an unknown tumor. If the percentage of lost animals reaches 10% in any of the groups, the entire experiment can be invalidated.

Body weights must be recorded on an individual basis once a week for the first 13 weeks of the experiment, then every 4 weeks. Animals loosing weight, in poor condition, or presenting superficial or internal masses should be followed carefully and, if necessary, sacrificed. In my opinion, clinical chemistry should not be included in carcinogenicity studies, since it must be already programmed for the chronic toxicity test. The only procedure which may be useful is a blood smear from an animal which has an enlarged spleen or lymph node. Food and water intake should be recorded periodically.

Pathology

Pathologic examination is the most important and difficult
moment in a carcinogenicity study. A blood smear should be made
from all killed animals. A complete and accurate necropsy of all
animals, dying or killed during or at the end of the experiment,
should be performed under the supervision of an experienced
pathologist, and all lesions should be properly described.
Necropsy should be done soon after death, but it must be kept in
mind that even a decomposed and partially cannibalized animal
should not be abandoned without a complete as possible gross
examination. After careful examination of all organs by appropriate
sectioning, representative specimens of all tissues and gross
lesions should be fixed for histology and preserved until
completion of the pathology report.

Considerable controversy exists over the number of tissues to
be examined microscopically and whether or not all animals of all
groups should be treated alike. Practical reasons together with a
scientific rationale can suggest a satisfactory compromise between
the various positions. All organs of all animals of the high dose
group and control group and all grossly seen or suspected tumorous
lesions of all animals of all groups must be examined microscopically. If a different tumor incidence in a given organ is observed
among groups, then that target organ should be examined
microscopically in all animals of all groups. It must be recognized
however, that, even though in most instances tumors can be
discovered at gross examination, it is unlikely that a random
histologic section and even multiple sections of large organs
can demonstrate a minute lesion overlooked at necropsy.Conversely,
minute lesions in small organs (such as pituitary, thyroid,
adrenals, testes, and harderian glands) are seldom seen grossly,
whereas they can be easily detected by microscopic examination.
It can, therefore, be suggested that these organs should be
examined in all animals.

Analysis and interpretation of the results

Provided that the study has been correctly designed and
conducted and that no invalidating events have occurred, in
particular no high loss of animals without pathologic examination,

the results can be examined by statistical methods. Analysis of the growth curves and survival are of a great importance, on the one hand, because a slight weight depression in the high-dose groups will prove that the highest possible dose level has been used, and, on the other hand, because significant differences in survival curves for causes other than tumors may greatly reduce the validity of the test.

Analysis of tumor incidence requires a proper recording of data for each individual animal, with a consistent terminology to describe lesions. The analysis of the overall incidence of tumor-bearing animals has little meaning, because tumors are often multiple and each may arise through a different pathogenetic process. Each type of tumor in each organ should, therefore, be treated separately, although it is the duty of the pathologist to group various tumors according to a similar histogenesis and pathogenesis. It is also important to separately report benign and malignant tumors, although they may be grouped for statistical analysis, particularly when distinction between a benign and malignant tumor may be difficult and ambiguous and progression from benign to malignant status is known to occur frequently. Extreme care and competence is necessary, however, to distinguish hyperplastic, reversible lesions from tumors.

Tumor incidence can be statistically examined with various unadjusted and time-adjusted analyses. A final interpretation of the results should also take into consideration historical controls, i.e., groups of untreated animals of the same species and strain, kept under the same experimental conditions. In fact, it has recently become evident that large variations of spontaneous tumors may occur among control groups without any known reason. A comparison of the tumor incidence in the experimental and matched control groups with that seen in historical controls may be useful to give more or less strength to the observed differences, particularly in the case of rare tumors.

Evidence of carcinogenicity

The evaluation of evidence of carcinogenicity of a compound is a complex process which must take into account the results of all available long-term studies, as well as of mutagenicity and other

short-term tests. An increased incidence of malignant tumors may
be sufficient evidence of carcinogenicity if observed in multiple
species, strains or experiments, or when a high incidence or
various types of tumors is observed. Conversly, limited evidence
of carcinogenicity may derive from a single experiment, from
partially inadequate experiments, or from an increased incidence
of neoplasms which often occur spontaneously or are difficult to
classify as malignant. Several criteria can be listed to arrive
at a score of evidence. However, they always need a good
scientific judgment, which must cope with the multiple variations
observed in each experiment and the many unknown factors involved
in carcinogenesis. It should always be kept in mind that the most
commonly observed tumors of the mouse either can be induced by
viruses (lymphomas and mammary carcinomas) or are under genetic
control (lung adenomas and hepatomas), whereas those of the rat
are often under endocrine control. Therefore, the best evidence of
a direct carcinogenic action, which can dissipate the doubt of an
indirect mechanism which may not be equally operational in
different species, comes from an experiment where multiple types
of tumors, including rare ones, are produced, even though not with
a high incidence.

© 1980 Elsevier/North-Holland Biomedical ...
The Principles and Methods in Modern Toxicology
C.L. Galli, S.D. Murphy and R. Paoletti, editors.

SUBCHRONIC TOXICITY STUDIES: METHODOLOGY, INTERPRETATIONS AND PROBLEMS

P.S. ELIAS, MD, MFCM, B.Sc., MRIC, C.Chem.

International Food Irradiation Project
Federal Research Centre for Nutrition
Postfach 3640, D-7500 Karlsruhe
Federal Republic of Germany

OBJECTIVES

The primary objective of a subchronic study as part of the toxicological appraisal of a xenobiotic is the characterisation of its physiological impact following repeated administration over a significant fraction of the life span of the test species. Subchronic studies also permit a judgement on the need for additional or more extended studies to delineate more clearly the toxicological profile of the substance under test. They are invaluable for determining the appropriate dosage levels for conducting chronic toxicity studies, because they provide information on the major toxic effects of the test compound, on dose-response relationships and on the reversibility of any phenomena observed. Apart from giving an indication of the minimum dose causing any toxic effect, such studies point to the existence of species differences in the nature of the response and to the effects of environmental variables on the characteristics of the observed toxicity.

A major objective of subchronic studies is the establishment of the spectrum of toxicological effects of a compound, their nature and severity, in an animal species in which the metabolic pathways of the same or analogous substances are as similar as possible to those in man.

In many instances it has been possible to make a judgement with respect to the suitability of a substance as a component of the human environment on the basis of the results of subchronic studies. The extent to which subchronic tests can be relied upon to evaluate the safety of a substance depends on a number of factors such as chemical structure, the nature and extent of human exposure, and the character of the biological responses of animals to exaggerated dosage with the compound.

EXPERIMENTAL DESIGNS

Conventional subchronic toxicity studies are usually limited to dietary or other appropriate exposure of two laboratory species for a period varying from 90 days to 1 year, generally representing 10% of the life span of the species selected. In the common laboratory rodents e.g. the rat, mouse and hamster, this period extends conventionally over 90 days. In the longer lived species, such as the dog, pig and subhuman primates, it may be extending over 1-2 years. One rodent and one non-rodent species are frequently employed. Traditionally the rat and the dog are used, but a second rodent species, the mouse, is frequently resorted to because of its availability. In order to benefit from the existing data base and background information it is preferable to use conventional strains of rodents unless know-ledge of the comparative metabolism and toxic effects in man and other species dictates otherwise. Both sexes should be studied in order to detect differences due to sex hormone effects.

The methodology of subchronic studies has been standardised over many years. The minimum recommended group size is 20 rodents of each sex per group but other authorities suggest 10 to 30 animals per group. With the larger non-rodent species (dog, cat, monkey, pig etc.) groups larger than 4 per sex are unusual. With such small numbers statistical evaluation is often not warranted, the data from these species being largely regarded as qualitative rather than quantitative. Suitable numbers of animals of the same age, body weight and sex as the test animals, randomly selected, should be used as controls. These animals are handled and subjected to the same measurements as the test groups. They are given the dosing vehicle or the basic diet without the test material in equivalent amounts to the test groups. The same observations are made with the same precision and frequency and are then compared with the responses obtained in the test groups.

On the basis of acute toxicity data and on estimated or predicted intake levels under conditions of use, at least five dose levels are selected in the hope of bracketing the "no observed adverse effect" level for the species under the specific conditions. Studies in which all dosage levels reveal no observable toxic effects are regarded as inconclusive. It may be expedient to initiate the study with larger numbers of test levels and to discontinue those which prove too toxic after the first few weeks. During this period, significant deviations from control data in any observed parameters are considered "effects". The degree of significance depends, of course, on the size of groups employed, the number of animals exhibiting adverse signs, and their severity. The number and extent of the examinations made in such studies vary somewhat with the known properties of the compound and the purpose of the test but it is useful to establish a routine of careful clinical assessment.

In general, these observations include daily observations for overt signs of toxicity (quality of hair and coat, general condition of eyes, mouth, teeth, nose and ears, posture, gait, behaviour or activity, character of excreta) by competent animal laboratory technicians under the supervision of a veterinarian expert in laboratory animal medicine. Weekly examinations include records of body weight and food consumption, assessment of cardiac and respiratory functions by simple auscultation. Periodic haematological and biochemical examinations of the bood and urine, hepatic, renal and gastro-intestinal functional tests are also carried out. When indicated, other parameters are examined such as blood pressure, rectal temperature, neurological reflexes and other more detailed neurological examinations, if nervous system effects are expected, ophthalmological examinations by ophthalmoscopy and slit lamp techniques, if ocular toxicity is suspected. External and internal structures are palpated and any tissue masses recorded.

Electrocardiographic and electroencephalographic studies (the latter performed on dogs or primates) can be included although their significance may become questionable where it is necessary to anesthetize the animal. In the usual 90-day protocol, such observations are made after 6 and 12 weeks (termination) on test.

In the larger mammals, pretest or "day 0" data are also obtained.

All animals are routinely sacrificed and examined at autopsy for gross pathologic changes including the weights of the major organs and glands. Representative specimens of all major tissues and organs are preserved for histopathological examination. At a minimum, histopathological examinations are made in the highest dosage groups and control groups to discover target organs or systems. Depending on the type and severity of the pathological lesions, organs should be examined from either representative animals, or in some instances, all animals at lower dosage levels. Detailed records of all clinical observations must be maintained.

The need for greater emphasis on the reproductive performance of test animals has become apparent in recent years. Concern has increased over placental transfer mechanisms and how this may influence development of the embryo and the survival of the fetus to term. It is therefore desirable to incorporate at least preliminary observations on any teratologic effects into the subchronic phase of toxicologic investigations. While this is not feasible with larger species such as dogs, it can be done in small rodents by expanding the protocol to include a minimum of one reproductive cycle carried through parturition and lactation, followed by a second with delivery by Caesarian section and examination of the uterine contents for evidence of nidation failure or the occurrence of terata. This scheme fits well with protocols calling for the use of test animals exposed in utero (i.e. F_1 weanlings), and also provides young males which can be used at maturity in a dominant lethal assay, if that assay is required.

SELECTION OF TEST SPECIES

The selection of the rat and the dog as test species for subchronic studies has been based primarily on convenience and cost rather than on a consideration of physiological fit between the animal and man which would render the tests more predictive in terms of safety for humans. This is not to say that these two laboratory animals were physiologically or metabolically in-appropriate or that the data so obtained are not relevant except in rare cases. However, it is now a generally accepted principle that the subchronic phase of any investigation is best considered in at least two steps. In the first of these, relatively short range finding studies in more than one species of rodent and in perhaps two or more non-rodents should be conducted with emphasis placed on the pharmacokinetic aspects of the compound; i.e., its rates of absorption, distribution in blood and organs, route and rate of excretion either unchanged or as a metabolite and the relationships of blood and tissue levels of the test compound to the development of toxic lesions. To the extent they are known, data on human toxic effects should be compared with those of the test animal, using information in analogous compounds where direct evidence is not available. Because subchronic studies usually involve exaggerated dose levels, it is important to determine the effect of the dose on the route of metabolism and on normal detoxication mechanisms. Differences in metabolizing enzyme systems exist among various species which may profoundly affect the qualitative or quantitative manifestations of toxicity and may lead to erroneous judgements as to safety in use. Hence care must be exercised in selecting appropriate animal species for metabolism and pharmacokinetic studies. If metabolic information were available, it would serve as guidance in the selection of the test species. In any case, cost or convenience should not determine the choice in cases where the metabolism or pharmaco-kinetics of a substance in any species are known to differ significantly from that in man.

ROUTE OF ADMINISTRATION

The main route of administration should mimic human exposure. Food additives, pesticides and most environmental chemicals are likely to enter the food supply or drinking water. For these substances the main route of administration of the test substance should be by incorporation in the diet. Drinking water may be used where physical incompatibility or chemical reactions may make the animal diet unsuitable as the vehicle. The inhalational, percutaneous or parenteral route may be appropriate in other instances.

'here are certain basic considerations which govern the dosage

of test substance absorbed within a given time interval. Administration by gavage has been employed where for some reason
(e.g. high volatility) it is not feasible to measure accurately
the daily food or water intake, hence the dosage. Local irritation of gastric or duodenal mucosa may be a factor in addition to
the trauma associated with the introduction of the dosing tube or
needle into the esophagus. It is obvious that gavage must be
limited to the administration of relatively small amounts of
material and, hence, is useful only with substances of high toxic
potential. If gavage is employed then control animals should be
treated with the suspending vehicle in equivalent amounts. This
route, however, is least representative of the normal route of
ingestion of food components inasmuch as it results in relatively
high peaks of blood and tissue levels over a short period
compared with absorption via the diet. The aqueous or oily
vehicle used for direct intragastric dosage may influence absorption at a rate and to a degree significantly different from that
resulting from consumption when incorporated in the diet. Moreover the latter permits greater opportunity for chemical or
microbial action to take place in the gut, which also is more
characteristic of normal ingestion.

Parenteral administration, inhalation or percutaneous administration bypasses the gastrointestinal tract with its ab-
sorptive mechanisms, which latter may modify the toxicity of a
substance.

SELECTION OF DOSAGE LEVELS

The requirement that the range of test levels must extend from
one producing some adverse but non-lethal effect to a level of
no-observable effect may lead to unrealistic attempts at dietary
incorporation when the test substance is relatively innocuous
(e.g., a food, per se). When this requirement is coupled with a
desire to achieve the highest possible "safety factor" between
the no-effect level for the animal and the expected human intake,
care must be taken that the resulting ration is not nutritionally
inadequate or unbalanced particularly with respect to vitamins or
minerals. In the extreme situation where a diet contains 5 per
cent or more of the test material, it should be checked for

acceptability and nutritional adequacy.

The range of doses selected for subchronic toxicity tests should ideally include at least one evoking a clearly toxic but not lethal response, one showing no demonstrable effect, and three or more intermediate dosages, usually at semilogarithmic intervals, so that at least two more positive response levels will be found. Various approaches have been employed with this purpose in mind. Assuming that the LD_{50} of the substance has been established, some fraction of that dose may be predicted to be sub-lethal but toxic over the subchronic test period. This dose has often been found to fall between 10 and 25 per cent of the LD_{50}, depending largely on the slope of the acute dose-response curve, i.e., the steeper the slope the smaller the fraction of the LD_{50}.

A better procedure for choosing dosages involves preliminary range-finding tests in five or more groups of rodents (perhaps as few as 2 or 3 animals per group) for a period of 3 to 4 weeks, with doses at 3- to 5-fold (but in any case not greater than 10-fold) intervals. Too few dose levels, or spacing them too closely together, run the risk that none, or only one, falls within the positive range. Ideally, the lowest dose in subchronic studies should induce no observable adverse effect and be a reasonably large multiple of the estimated human daily intake. The zero dose level represents the control reference point. Dosages are difficult to select for compounds which bioaccumulate. Selection here depends on kinetic studies of the half-time of elimination.

When test materials are incorporated in animal diets, it becomes imperative to obtain accurate food consumption data. From these the actual intake of the compound is derived, expressed in terms of mg/kg body weight per day.

Thus, diet composition without corresponding food intake data may be meaningless since the latter is affected by various factors, including caloric density and palatability, and by the diminishing rate of food consumption on a body weight basis with growth. One aspect of toxicity may be true appetite depression leading to reduction of test dosage intake as well as of nutritionally essential dietary components thus confounding the observed effects. Paired feeding experiments, in which the daily intake of each animal in a control group is limited to that of its "mate" in a test group, have been proposed in the attempt to differentiate between nutritional and toxic effects. However, this presents obvious difficulties in multiple dose level studies.

Of particular significance in the subchronic studies using immature rodents is the initial high metabolic activity which causes the weanling animal normally to eat several times as much food per unit of body weight as the adult.

In order to maintain approximately uniform dosage on a body weight basis, it is therefore essential in studies commencing with weanling rats to adjust the dietary concentration of the test substance at weekly, or at least biweekly periods to compensate for the changing rate of food consumption. Immediately post-weaning, rats on normal diets consume about 2.5 times the adult level, which they generally attain at about 15-16 weeks of age. Post-weaning animals would be markedly overdosed until the anticipated adult dose level is attained. If the concentration of the test compound in the diet is held constant from weaning to maturity, the actual dose received may affect the toxic response. In dogs it is preferable to choose the dietary route and to employ capsule administration for unpalatable compounds.

DIET PREPARATION

Of prime importance in toxicological feeding studies is knowledge of the composition of the basal diet. Most suppliers of commercial laboratory feeds are willing to state the qualitative composition, but have been reluctant to reveal quantitative formulas, which may vary depending on the supply and cost of ingredients. There is a growing demand not only for detailed "open formula" information but for guarantees of the freedom of commercial diets from pesticide residues or other contaminants which, even though present in miniscule amounts, may affect the toxic response to the test substance, either synergistically or antagonistically. Monitoring batches of commercial diets for contaminants presents a major problem, the list of potential pesticide residues, mycotoxins, and heavy metal contaminants being almost unlimited, and there is generally no a priori basis for suspecting which are likely to be present. At the least, screening tests should be performed for common contaminants, such as organo-chlorine compounds, aflatoxin and nitrosamines.

The alternative of preparing one's own basal ration does not appeal to most toxicologists in part because of the time and expense involved and in part because it does not entirely avoid the difficulties mentioned above.

To avoid uncertainties associated with natural-type diets some investigators have recommended the use of "semi-synthetic" or "purified" diets composed of casein or lactalbumin as the source of protein, starch, dextrin, dextrose and/or sucrose as the carbohydrate source, with partially hydrogenated vegetable fat, mineral salts, and synthetic vitamins, making up the balance. Practical experience with these diets has not been uniformly satisfactory, especially in longer studies or where reproduction is involved. However, their use may be justified by special circumstances for subchronic tests, bearing in mind that they deviate radically in composition from typical natural diets for either animals or man.

ANIMAL HUSBANDRY

If no own rodent breeding colonies are maintained, it is necessary to have access to reliable supplies of animals of known genetic origin, bred under uniform conditions, delivered in healthy conditions, and checked for freedom from parasites. Knowledge of litter origin is of advantage for assigning animals to test and control groups. To minimize inter-litter differences in initial body weight, breeders should cull large litters at the fourth day to eight or ten per litter, discarding runts and balancing the sex distribution to the extent possible.

The choice between barrier maintained (SPP) and conventionally reared strains of rodents will depend on the requirements of the protocol and the type of facilities available. In either case, all animals exposed to the rigors of shipment should be quarantined on arrival until their status has been evaluated and risk of contamination with an infectious agent is past. Without exception, the established rules of good laboratory practice with respect to animal care should be adhered to. Individual caging and the use of scatter-resistant feeders are essential in any study in which food consumption is to be measured. Cognizance should be taken of the fact that rodents practice coprophagy (mice even more than rats), the effect of which is partially mitigated by the use of wire-bottom cages. While housing in basket type cages reduces the chance of intercurrent respiratory infection, it increases the possibility of ingesting feces which may contain toxic metabolites of the test material. Larger mammals require particular attention since they are less standard-ized than rodents and more susceptible to infection.

OBSERVATIONS

The kind and frequency of interim observations made during the course of subchronic tests may vary widely depending on the objectives of the investigation. In the classic case, however, certain basic parameters constitute a minimum if the data are to have significant predictive value in terms of safety evaluation or the design of subsequent chronic studies. The frequency with which observations are made will also be determined by circum-stances. Shorter intervals will be specified when the toxic potential of the compounds are unknown or unpredictable as com-pared with confirmatory studies on analogues or substances for which a large data base already exists. Obviously, the earlier in a study that deviations from normal or expected values are recognized, the more latitude accrues for the modification of the protocol.

Physical observations include twice daily check for appear-ance, morbidity and mortality, daily examination for toxic signs, weekly records of body weight and food consumption, periodic neurological, ophthalmological and organ function tests. Special physiological measurements, where indicated, would be ECG changes for cardiotoxic compounds since these changes may precede the development or give an indication of the existence of myocardial necrosis. Routine methods exist for recording ECGs in dogs and rats and these may be supplemented by recording heart rate and respiratory rate.

Haematological examinations should be performed on randomly selected subgroups of rodents prior to the start of the test, at

30 day intervals and terminally on all animals. It should include red, white and differential cell counts, haemoglobin level, haematocrit, cell morphology, reticulocyte count, platelet count and determination of standard clotting parameters e.g. prothrombin time, clot retraction, fibrinolysis and factor assays. Bone marrow examinations should also be done terminally on all animals. In the case of non-rodents all animals need to be examined at regular intervals.

Biomedical evaluations of serum and plasma parameters as well as determinations of serum enzyme levels should be performed. Urine analysis should cover the semiquantitative tests as well as microscopic examination of centrifuged sediment. Any of these examinations may be omitted, or others possibly added where justified by the known properties of the test material. Usually, a full set of observations is recorded after 6 and 12 weeks and once again prior to terminal sacrifice, if the test period exceeds 3 months. Studies with rodents started at weaning preclude an initial blood drawing and reliance is usually placed on historic colony data or on analyses of blood from litter-mates sacrificed at the time the animals are assigned to groups. The terminal set of observations is the most significant. At autopsy, a sample of bladder urine should be drawn by syringe where possible since cage-collected urine samples are often contaminated.

In addition to these routine observations, a modern protocol will also include special studies designed to yield information on the pharmacokinetics of the compound, particularly as almost all biochemical mechanisms are rate limiting in one or more steps of a multistep process. As discussed earlier, elucidation of the metabolic fate of a substance and the enzyme systems involved in its passage through the body, as well as its ability to induce drug metabolizing enzymes, have become increasingly important in assessing the potential hazard to man as well as the appropriateness of the animal species. Hence, where special techniques are required to obtain suitable samples of blood or tissues (e.g., liver) at the time of sacrifice, the protocol should so indicate. The nature of the metabolites and the rates of metabolic transformations should be studied in blood, urine and faeces. For determining the kinetics of any possible accumulation in various body compartments serial sacrifices at 3 week intervals may be necessary. It may be preferable to include an extra group of animals from the start, in which the kinetics of elimination of the test compound and its metabolites could be studied after completion of the dosing period.

PATHOLOGY

Among the observations included in any subchronic study, those designed to detect alterations in morphology of cellular structures within the organs and tissues of the animal require emphasis. As a rule range-finding trials do not justify extensive pathologic evaluation since significant pathological changes usually do not occur until after longer exposure. The exceptions would be highly toxic compounds where it is desired to determine the immediate tissue response. Pathological alterations which are more subtle, and which develop only after repeated and cumulative dosage, especially at low levels, are of greater significance.

While it is imperative that every animal that dies or is sacrificed be subjected to gross pathologic examination at autopsy, the extent to which the tissues and organs should be examined for histological aberrations can vary widely. In the absence of overt signs of toxicity at any dosage, including gross examination of the viscera, histopathologic evaluation may be limited to all the main tissues from all animals in the highest treatment and control groups. The identification of treatment-related lesions at the highest dose should be followed by the detailed examination of the same organs or tissues in the lower dose groups until the "no observed adverse effect level" is found. All major organs should be weighed and the organ/body weight ratios calculated.

ORGAN FUNCTION TESTS

The use of non-rodents permits the application of a wide range of organ function tests because large samples of blood or urine can be collected on a routine basis. If rodents are used, only a few tests can be selected. Organ function studies should be

carried out prior to starting the test, repeated at 3 and 10 days
after initiation of dosing, and subsequently performed at 30 day
intervals throughout the test including a terminal examination.

For hepatotoxic effects various clearance tests (BSP) or serum
enzyme (sorbitol dehydrogenase, glutamic oxaloacetic transminase,
glutamic-pyruvic transaminase, alkaline phosphatase) activity
estimations or serum bilirubin levels are useful for diagnosis.
Cardiac function may be related to serum creatine phosphokinase
activity. Useful indices of renal function are serum creatinine
and blood urea nitrogen levels.

RESULTS AND INTERPRETATIONS

The results of subchronic studies require careful interpretation, particularly if they are to be used for deciding on the
need for further chronic toxicity testing. The nature of the
toxicity, the target organs involved and the dose-response relationships observed are important parameters in the toxicological
evaluation of a substance. The full complement of clinical,
biochemical, metabolic and pathological observations has to be
assessed by comparing data from groups fed several graded dosage
levels of the substance under study with those data from control
groups.

The weight gain or body weight change for each group should be
plotted against time to check for differences between test groups
and between test and control groups. If any differences are
found these should be subjected to trend analysis. Food and
water consumption should also be plotted and analysed in a
similar fashion. The finding of reduced weight gain or body
weight in otherwise healthy animals may be due to toxic appetite
depression or mere inappetance and unpalatability of the diet.
Paired feeding experiments may help to distinguish between these
effects. Organ weight, biochemical and haematological data
should be compared with those obtained on the contemporary
controls. Any findings, whether positive or negative, should be
correlated with the pathological observations. Reversible shifts
in the homeostasis are obviously not important in the absence of
other evidence of toxicity. Similarly, organ function changes
should be correlated with histopathological data to enable judge-

ment of the toxicological significance of any observed changes.

Subchronic studies are only of limited value for predicting the toxic effect of life span exposure for several reasons. The nature and degree of the toxic response is known to vary when test animals are dosed repeatedly over varying periods. The process of ageing alters the sensitivity and metabolic capability of tissues and is accompanied by spontaneous occurrence of disease. In man the effects of chronic exposure may be modified by the intervention of intercurrent degenerative diseases e.g. heart disease, chronic renal failure or neoplasia. Moreover no prediction can be made from subchronic tests regarding the carcinogenic, mutagenic or teratogenic potential of a substance or about its effects on reproduction except for primary effects on the gonads.

If a "no observed adverse effect" level of dosage can be determined, this may be used in certain circumstances for establishing acceptable daily intakes (ADIs) for intentional food additives, for setting tolerances and residue levels for unintentional additives and contaminants, or for establishing acceptable levels of exposure, such as threshold limit values and maximum acceptable concentrations, for industrial chemicals at the work place.

Emphasis must be placed on the uncertainties in toxicological interpretation which arise from qualitative and quantitative differences in the reactions of animals and man to chemical substances. The similarities must also not be overlooked. Toxicology relies heavily on the similarities in the anatomy, biochemistry, physiology and reactions to biologically active substances of different species. There are numerous examples of parallelism of qualitative and quantitative response to chemicals in animals and man; nevertheless, differences frequently occur. Similarity between species must never be assumed but evidence must always be sought to establish its existence for each chemical studied.

A few examples of qualitative differences between animal species and man in their reactions to chemicals will illustrate the problem of interpreting the results of a toxicological study. Morphine causes a marked central nervous stimulation in cats but has a depressive effect in man. Prolonged treatment of rats with cyclacillin causes chronic proliferative and degenerative nephropathy in male rats but not in female rats, beagle dogs, rhesus monkeys or man. In the mouse, hamster, dog, monkey and man, 2-naphthylamine induces cancers but it has little effect in the rat and rabbit. Caecal ulceration in guinea pigs and rabbits develops on administration of degraded carrageenan, while experience in the rat and man suggests that no such abnormality occurs.

It must also be recognised that the ability of animals to predict human reactions to chemicals is limited and some types cannot be reproduced at all in animals. Subjective symptoms such as nausea, headache or depression cannot be predicted from animal experiments and their detection requires human exposure. The guinea pig is the only experimental animal of value in demonstrating the capability of a chemical to cause allergic sensitisation. Blood dyscrasias, e.g. agranulocytosis, arising from the toxic action of a chemical such as benzene or chloramphenicol, or via an immunological reaction as with amidopyrine were found only when humans were exposed to them.

There are many examples of animal species reacting in a qualitatively similar but quantitatively different way to chemicals. The data on methyl mercury toxicity, for example, suggest that mice were the least sensitive species, followed, in order of increasing sensitivity, by rats, monkeys, ferrets and cats. Miniature pigs were much more sensitive than beagle dogs.

The amounts and type of food as well as its composition and vitamin content may influence the reaction of animals to chemical substances. Caecal ulceration developed within 2 weeks in guinea pigs given 2% degraded carrageenan in drinking water but no lesions appeared when the same concentration was administered in milk even after 18 weeks. Dehydration and calorie restriction have been demonstrated to affect the susceptibility of animals to the toxic effects of chemicals and the same may apply to man. Synergistic and antagonistic effects of other chemicals have to be borne in mind because man seldom comes into contact with one chemical substance at a time. For example, the administration of carbon tetrachloride reduced the lethal effects of fenitrothion,

but not of some other organophosphorus compounds. The tumoroge-
nicity of diethylnitrosamine is increased by the enzyme-inducing
activity of phenobarbitone but the induction of intestinal
tumours with azoxymethane is inhibited by BHT, another powerful
inducer of hepatic microsomal enzymes.

Age, state of health, the nature of the gastrointestinal
microbial flora, cyclic variations in function, the existence of
stress and the development of tolerance are all factors which may
affect the experimental outcome. They must be allowed for when
evaluating the results and making extrapolations to man.
Technical factors associated with the design of the experiment
must be taken into account when interpreting the results. The
practice of administering concentrations of substances to animals
which are considerable exaggerated compared to those experienced
by man may cause adverse effects over and above those due to
direct toxicity. Substances may be very irritant or produce some
other irrelevant abnormality at the concentrations needed to
provide a high margin between animal and human exposure, but may
not produce these effects at the concentrations to which man is
likely to be exposed. The physiology of some animals makes the
interpretation of results of toxicological experiments particularly prone to error. For example, while the dog and cat can
vomit and are thus species of value in examining substances which
may induce vomiting in man through their local irritant action or
through a central nervous effect, the rat is unable to vomit nor
does it appear to have a cough reflex. This rodent is therefore
without two protective mechanisms available to man.

Enlargement of the large intestine is uncommon in man and
believed to be related to a neuromuscular deficiency. In the rats
however, caecal enlargements is relatively common in germ free
animals, when receiving antibiotics, when fed modified starches,
lactose, magnesium sulphate etc. It has been postulated that the
size of the rat caecum is controlled by the bulk of the caecal
contents and is an adaptation to their retention. In man the
normal response to bulk in the large intestine is expulsion.
Hence the toxicological significance of the finding of caecal
enlargement may be none if it is a physiological adaptation or
may be highly relevant if due to some pathological process.

REVERSIBILITY STUDIES

One problem in the evaluation of observations during the terminal stages of a subchronic study is the degree of importance to be attached to reversible clinical and biochemical findings. It has been argued that reversible changes often represent normal physiologic response to stress. The stress in such cases being the adaptation to an unusual load on some metabolic pathway through which the animal attempts to mitigate the effects of the substance by accelerating an existing enzyme reaction, initiating a new one (enzyme induction), or overtaxing an excretory process. An example of a commonly seen reversible effect is the mild liver enlargement frequently observed after feeding certain compounds without any detectable alteration in the histological architecture of the organ. It is felt by some authorities that complete return of the organ (or function) to normal upon removal of the stress is evidence of "no toxicity" and simply indicates the capacity of the animal to adapt to external stresses in a physiological manner. Thus it has been recommended that some proportion of the survivors of a subchronic study be continued on the basal control diet for up to 3 months after cessation of exposure and then examined for reversal of adverse effects as seen in those sacrificed earlier. Kinetic studies may assist in determining the appropriate exposure and reversibility periods.

The obvious difficulty with this concept is that no sharp line separates the reversible from the irreversible change, which, like most physiological phenomena, may well be time-dose dependent. The point at which the change becomes irreversible will obviously determine an adverse response.

The practical problem of demonstrating reversibility in any instance of this type depends for its solution on the early recognition of the change, whatever the parameter involved. It is also dependent on the availability of a sufficient number of animals in the affected group to permit a significant number to be returned to the control (non-treatment) regime and on the ability to follow them long enough for the reversal effect to become manifest. Since the likelihood of a reversible effect is not usually predictable, the investigator must start a sufficient number of animals per group to allow for such a contingency or be prepared to repeat the study once the need has been demonstrated. This recognition often occurs only at the end of the predeter- mined time-span, after all or some of the animals have been sacrificed. The result is the need to repeat the experiment, perhaps with a modified protocol, in order to be able to verify the assumption that the effect was actually reversible, and if so, at what dosage level and after what length of exposure.

EXTENDED SUBCHRONIC STUDIES

Extended protocols for subchronic studies have been developed in response to the need for early indication of the potential effects of a new compound on reproductive performance. Such information was not obtained in the conventional 90-day rat feeding study. However, a significant time and cost saving benefit can be gained by combining these two phases into one experiment rather than conducting separate reproduction and tera- tologic tests.

Thus, weanling animals are reared to maturity on the test diets, mated, and the F_{1a} progeny carried through one complete maturation and reproductive cycle in the course of which all the conventional behavioural and clinical observations can be made. Data for reproductive efficiency and performance are recorded and indices calculated for conception and gestation, the number and size of litters, the weight of pups at birth and their viability, survival and growth through lactation. Under special circum- stances, for example when mutagenicity is suspected, reproduction studies extending into several generations may be required.

Following the weaning of the first (F_{1a}) litters, the F_0 females are mated for the second time with males from the same treatment group. Half the number of gravid does are sacrificed 24-48 hours prior to the expected onset of parturition (cal- culated from the appearance of sperm in the vagina after mating) and the usual observations made according to protocols accepted for teratological studies. These include for each sacrificed doe the number of mature corpora lutea, and the number, sex, and weight of mature fetuses, identified according to position in each horn of the uterus. The presence of early resorption sites and of dead or partially resorbed fetuses is also noted.

After weighing, all fetuses are examined for the presence of abnormalities grossly observed (terata). Half of the fetuses (including those with gross terata) are fixed in Bouin's solution and subsequently sectioned by the Wilson free-hand procedure to detect aberrations of the internal soft tissue structures. The other half of the pups are cleared in alkali, stained with alizarin red and examined for skeletal malformations.

The other half number of pregnant does is allowed to deliver the F_{1b} generation of pups. The latter are carried through to weaning, during which time data for growth, viability and post-natal development are recorded. At weaning both the F_0 and the F_{1b} generation are sacrificed and subjected to gross and histo-pathological post-mortem examination. If desired, the F_{1a} generation may be used to produce an F_{2a} generation for investigation of transplacental mechanisms or subsequent dominant lethality studies.

The additional data supplied by this modified reproduction and teratologic phase of the subchronic study, while quite adequate in terms of the numbers and types of observations, differs from most published procedures in that exposure of the dam is con-tinuous from the moment of insemination to the end of the pregnancy. In cases where the number of implantations is re-duced, an increased incidence of abnormalities is observed, the relationship between dose and severity or frequency of effect appears significant, or it is desired to establish the embryonic stage at which the conceptus is most sensitive, appropriate teratologic testing in greater depth may be required. It should be remembered, however, that a dose-response relationship may not be obvious in teratologic studies since the intervention of maternal metabolism and the protection afforded by the placental barrier are important factors.

The disadvantages of extended subchronic studies are the con-siderable increase in the length and cost of the study and the larger requirements for the test substance and experimental animals.

REFERENCES

Casarett, L.J. and Doull, J. (Eds.) (1975) Toxicology - The Basic Science of Poisons. Macmillan Publishing Co., Inc., New York.

Commission of the European Communities (1978) General Guidelines for the Toxicological Evaluation of Chemical Substances. Document No. V/F/1/78/26, Luxembourg, April 1978.

Dixon, R.L. (1976) Problems in extrapolating toxicity data for laboratory animals to man. Environm. Health Perspect., 13, 43.

Food and Drug Administration Advisory Committee on Protocols for Safety Evaluation (1970) Panel on Reproduction Report on Reproduction Studies in the Safety Evaluation of Food Additives and Pesticide Residues. Toxic. Appl. Pharmac., 16, 264.

Food Safety Council (1978) Proposed System for Food Safety Assessment prepared by the Scientific Committee. Food Cosm. Tox., 16 (12) Supplement 2, pp. 83-92.

Golberg, L. (1975) Safety evaluation concepts. J. Assoc. Offic. Agric. Chemists, 58, 635.

Joint FAO/WHO Expert Committee on Food Additives - Second Report (1958) Procedures for the Testing of Intentional Food Additives to Establish Their Safety for Use. Tech. Rep. Ser. Wld Hlth Org. 144.

Joint FAO/WHO Expert Committee on Food Additives - 17th Report (1974) Toxicological Evaluation of Certain Food Additives with a Review of General Principles and of Specifications. Tech. Rep. Ser. Wld Hlth Org. 539.

Loomis, T.V. (1968) Essentials of Toxicology, Lea & Febiger, Philadelphia.

McNamara, B.P. (1976) Concepts in health evaluation of commercial and industrial chemicals. In Advances in Modern Toxicology, I, Part 1: New Concepts in Safety Evaluation. Edited by M.A. Mehlman, R.E. Shapiro and H. Blumenthal. John Wiley & Sons, New York.

National Academy of Sciences - National Research Council (1970) Evaluating the Safety of Food Chemicals. NAS-NRC, Washington, D.C. p. 49.

National Academy of Sciences - National Research Council. Committee on Food Protection (1972) Subcommittee on Review of GRAS List (Phase II). A Comprehensive Survey of Industry on the Use of Food Chemicals Generally Recognized as Safe (GRAS). Washington, D.C.

National Academy of Sciences - National Research Council (1975) Principles for Evaluating Chemicals in the Environment. NAS-NRC, Washington, D.C. p. 97.

New Concepts in Safety Evaluation, I, part 1: Advances in Modern Toxicology (1976) Edited by M.A. Mehlman, R.E. Shapiro and H. Blumenthal. John Wiley & Sons, New York.

Oser, B.L. and Hall, R.L. (1978) Criteria employed by the expert panel of FEMA for the GRAS evaluation of flavouring substances. Food Cosm. Toxicol. 15, 457.

Weil, C.S. (1972) Guidelines for experiments to predict the degree of safety of a material for man. Toxic. Appl. Pharmac., 21, 194.

Weil, C.S. (1972) Statistics vs safety factors and scientific judgement in the evaluation of safety for man. Toxic. Appl. Pharmac. 21, 454.

Weil, C.S. (1975) Toxicology experimental design and conduct measured by interlaboratory collaborative studies. J. Assoc. Offic. Agric. Chemists, 88, 683.

World Health Organization, Tech. Rep. Ser. 348 (1967) Procedures for Investigating Intentional and Unintentional Food Additives. Report of a WHO Scientific Group, Geneva.

World Health Organization (1978) Environmental Health Criteria No. 6. Principles and Methods for Evaluating the Toxicity of Chemicals, Part I, Geneva.

Zbinden, G. (1973 and 1976) Progress in Toxicology. Special Topics, Vols 1 & 2. Springer-Verlag, New York.

© 1980 Elsevier/North-Holland Biomedical Press
The Principles and Methods in Modern Toxicology
C.L. Galli, S.D. Murphy and R. Paoletti, editors.

CHRONIC STUDIES

R. L. BARON
Health Effects Research Laboratory
U.S. Environmental Protection Agency
Research Triangle Park, North Carolina 27711

In principle as in practice, chronic toxicity studies have not changed dramatically over the past 25 years, nor has the need changed for the data from such studies. "Chronic oral toxicity tests are designed to provide data adequate to evaluate the safety of substances which might be ingested by man." These sentiments were expressed by Fitzhugh in one of the first modern day essays relating to such studies.[4] In more recent times, with the widespread directed introduction of chemicals into the environment for such uses as agricultural plant protection or in food processing, the inadvertent environmental contamination through industrial processes and the industrial and non-industrial exposure of humans to a variety of chemical agents, the need for such tests has been expanded to include more than ingestion or dietary considerations. However, the basic premise is the same--the need for chronic studies exists because it can be readily realized that target organs and tissues found to be affected in short-term acute studies are not always the same as those following repeated exposures for long periods of time. The ultimate use of data from highly structured chronic studies in animals and less sophisticated, generally retrospective, epidemiological experiences is the determination of dosage levels which can be used to estimate an acceptable exposure level from which the inherent safety of proposed use patterns can be evaluated.

The classical approaches to the study of toxicity have been described in a variety of publications.[6,10,11] These generally involve studies in one or more species of animals for periods of time ranging from several weeks to several years with appropriate dosages and routes of administration. A variety of specific tests, conducted at prescribed intervals during each study, allows assessment of anatomical and functional changes measured by the use of biochemical, physiological, pathological, and more recently, behavioral methodology.

There are no specific routine animal investigations which can be universally applied to define the toxicological significance of exposure to all
materials. The consequences of such studies and the realization that an
assessment of safety must always be subject to continuous review and the
data to subsequent reevaluation is important in consideration of planning
studies designed to evaluate the toxicological hazard to man. For example,
the criteria for a "no effect level" or "no observable effect level" has
changed (1) as the methods for detecting abnormalities have increased in
sensitivity, (2) as the mechanisms underlying toxic responses have been
elucidated and (3) as the significance of certain abnormalities has been
evaluated. A variety of effects of questioned significance in previous
years have been reevaluated under the present state of knowledge. For
example, the significance of liver hypertrophy following stimulation of
inductive processes has been a focal point of extensive investigations over
the past few years and takes on more significance as biochemical interactions are further described.

The basic toxicity studies that are conducted today have not changed with
respect to fundamental concepts. They have been enlarged in scope, refined
in measurement and greatly increased in cost. They are more comprehensive
and precise and there is little doubt of their value in identifying those
chemical agents that induce profound organotropic events, especially if they
do so in more than one species. However, with consideration of such factors
as genetic homogeneity in the test animals, a controlled environment
(including diet) in the testing program, and restrictive insults (i.e.,
neurological, neurotoxicological and behavioral) versus the heterogeneity of
such conditions in man, the potential for relevant extrapolation to man of
animal data from chronic studies is limited.

In consideration of the relationship of man to experimental animal models,
a mathematical approach to safety (or risk assessments) must take into
account differences in the responses of experimental animals from those of
man. Until such time as the data base for human response is adequate for
use and until mathematical considerations directly use data from man as part
of the equation, safety factors must be used. The value most commonly used
in connection with food additives and pesticides as dietary constituents was
brought to the scientific community about 25 years ago by Lehman and Fitzhugh
of the U. S. Food and Drug Administration.[8] Because of inter- and intra-
species variations, the factor of 100 was used, reflecting that man is about
10 times more sensitive to poisoning than the rat and that some persons may

be as much as 10 times more susceptible than others. This concept was and continues to be commonly recognized as a relative yardstick of safety, high enough to reduce the hazard of intentional food additives to a minimum and at the same time low enough to permit the use of some chemicals, particularly those necessary in food production. In most instances, the safety factor of 100 is used in conjunction with a no-effect level in chronic studies using laboratory animals to estimate an Acceptable Daily Intake (ADI) for man. The Joint Meeting on Pesticide Residues (JMPR) has defined an Acceptable Daily Intake as that daily dosage of a chemical which, during an entire lifetime, appears to be without appreciable risk on the basis of all the facts known at that time. The ADI for man is an empirical figure. It is derived by a simple mathematical operation from the experimentally observed no-effect level of a chemical administered to a sensitive and appropriate laboratory species generally throughout its lifetime. The no-effect level is adjusted by an appropriate safety factor to arrive at the ADI for man, expressed in milligrams of the chemical per kilogram body weight. In less than chronic studies, that is, where the duration of exposure is for less than one half the expected lifetime, an additional margin of safety has been recommended varying from 10 to 20 fold. While this puts an added burden on the quantity of chemical additive allowable in food, it allows for greater assurances of safety to man.

That a safety factor can be used to evaluate the safety of all chemically induced toxic effects has been a subject of extensive debate. This has been principally true with respect to potential human carcinogens. Except for the legal mandates of the 1958 Delaney amendment to the U.S. Food, Drug and Cosmetic Act[1] prohibiting the intentional addition of a carcinogen to food, there is no clearcut answer to the problem of potential human carcinogens as food additives. The World Health Organization and the Food and Agriculture Organization, through the JMPR, have shown some indifference to the U. S. considerations of the presence of certain carcinogens as residues in food. Through an extensive review of the toxicological data and recognizing the need for low levels, including unintentional residues, of specific pesticides in food, the JMPR, using more exaggerated safety margins, has accepted the consideration that certain potential human carcinogens may be tolerated as contaminants in the diet (amitrole, DDT, and several other chlorinated hydrocarbon pesticides).

Over the past 16 years, the JMPR has considered a large number of food additives and pesticides with respect to estimating an ADI for man.[5] An

ADI has been allocated to those chemicals which have been considered not to present a toxicological hazard to man under the conditions specified for their use. The JMPR has published a series of reports containing summary reviews of the available toxicological information and use patterns of pesticides and food additives, dealing not only with those materials specific to a single country or region, but with all materials proposed to enter world trade and impacting large populations. Because of practical considerations of world trade in food and because it has become well accepted that the intentional additives (either pesticide or non-pesticide chemicals) have rarely attained such a level in the actual diet as to approach the ADI, the JMPR has tended to give decreasing attention to the ADI as an absolute figure and increasing attention to those use patterns which result in the need for pesticide tolerances or maximum residue limits in food. With respect to certain basic toxicological concepts, it has been reasonable to assume that there is an amount of chemical which can be ingested every day in the diet for a lifetime without causing any appreciable harm to health and with the practical certainty that no injury to health will result from this exposure. The uncertainties in these considerations have been in part offset by such concepts as the use of safety factors and the heterogeneity of diet which preclude that a chemical will be present in the diet to which man will be exposed every day for his lifetime. In the sixteen years of its existence, the presence of only two chemical agents (DDT and Dieldrin) in food consumed by humans has been shown to approach the ADI as established by the JMPR.

While the ADI has been useful in the evaluation of safety in use of food additives or pesticides and has provided a scientific approach to the setting of intentional and unintentional maximum limits of these materials in food, the ADI is probably the most misrepresented concept in toxicology. The ADI is not an inherent fundamental property of the chemical in question and as such must remain solely a guide with respect to the intentional and unintentional addition of materials to food.

CHRONIC STUDIES

The biological experimentation employed, while inherently imprecise, inconsistent and unpredictable with respect to extrapolating the data to man, is invariably the chronic study in appropriate animal species. While it is evident that such studies require individual consideration, there are some general considerations that can be appreciated and it is to these that this discussion is addressed.

On August 28, 1978[3] and May 9, 1979,[2] the EPA proposed test standards for chronic toxicity studies and requested comments on the standards under the Federal Insecticide Fungicide Rodenticide Act (FIFRA) and the Toxic Substances Control Act of 1976 (TSCA). In these test standards, both carcinogenic and non-carcinogenic responses are to be evaluated. The test standards proposed under both programs are very similar. There are some differences in TSCA and FIFRA test standards which will be resolved before the U.S. Environmental Protection Agency proposes one uniform testing standard for chronic studies.

The major objectives of both programs to evaluate chronic effects are: to determine whether and to what extent the chemical in question produces specific damage to tissues and organs such as kidney damage, liver damage or the induction of tumors in test animals; to develop data that will permit an estimate of the probable magnitude of harm to exposed animals; and to provide data that can be used in an assessment of the nature and extent of risk of exposure. The importance and utility of long term animal bioassay for development of test data on chronic health effects cannot be overemphasized. In many instances, studies cannot be conducted in man for ethical or legal reasons. Data from retrospective and prospective epidemiological studies in man are, in many instances, impractical to relate to a direct exposure to a specific chemical and are difficult to use in a risk assessment. In the absence of direct information, long-term animal bioassays provide data that can be used for identification and quantitation of risk of exposure.

Several definitions may be helpful within the reference of this discussion. Chronic effects refer to the endpoints noted from those disease processes which have a long latency period for development, result from long-term exposure, are long-term illnesses or combinations of these factors. Certain chronic effects such as tumors are life-shortening and generally become apparent later in life, regardless of exposure. Other chronic effects such as liver or kidney damage may be similar to acute or subchronic effects noted in short-term exposure. These appear as chronic effects under conditions of less intense but longer-term exposure which might result in a gradual accumulation of tissue damage to the point of ultimate organ dysfunction. Oncogenicity relates to one specific type of chronic effect requiring special consideration. The term oncogenic has been used rather than carcinogenic as this best reflects tumor induction or neoplasia. By strict definition, carcinogenicity pertains to invasive (or malignant) neoplasia resulting from epithelial cells. The term oncogenicity includes those disease processes that result in benign and/or malignant neoplasms of any cell type. Thus, the term oncogenic may be more appropriate than carcinogenic. Benign neo-plasms are significant for several reasons, the primary one being that benign tumors may have serious consequences with respect to tissue crowding and transformation to malignancy. Thus, the term oncogen is defined as a chemical agent that either initiates, promotes or causes biological changes that result in benign and/or malignant neoplasms.

There are several basic requirements in the chronic studies as suggested by the EPA. These include: personnel, chemical analyses, dietary con-siderations, reporting requirements and the actual test standards to be employed.

One of the most critical elements in any studies, but especially chronic studies, is having a knowledgeable and motivated scientific staff to manage and conduct the studies. To this end, pathologists have been recognized having a key role.

In addition to pathologists, a veterinarian must meet rigid standards to be in charge of animal care and welfare. With the exception of these two categories, there are no other specific personnel criteria. It is recognized that there are no simple solutions to some situations, such as the possible shortage of experimental pathologists and adequately trained veterinarians and toxicologists to perform these studies.

Analytical chemical tests are to be performed to provide reasonable assurance that the test mixture contains the level of test substance required and that the material is equally dispersed in the administering medium. Chronic toxicity test standards propose a specific diet for use in long-term studies as well as chemical analyses for nutrients and dietary contaminants. The diet is a significant source of variance in all studies. The longevity of animal species, including humans, has been shown to be influenced by the quality and quantity of the diet. It is essential that a nutritionally adequate diet meets the needs for long-term health.

TABLE 1

PROPOSED TSCA CHRONIC STUDY STANDARDS

SPECIES	MOUSE (Combined and Oncogenic) RAT (All Studies) DOG (Combined and Non-Oncogenic)
STRAINS	ALL ESTABLISHED STRAINS
SEX	BOTH MALES AND FEMALES
NUMBER	50 of each sex--Rodents 6 of each sex--Dog 8 of each sex--each clinical trial
AGE	6 weeks for Rodents 10 weeks for Dogs
CONTROLS	MATCHED WITH TEST GROUPS
ROUTES AND FREQUENCY OF EXPOSURE	Gavage--daily for study duration Dietary--ad libitum Inhalation--5 days/week, 6 hours/day

For oncogenic test standards, rats and mice have been found to be reliable models for human oncogenicity. Similar results in both species markedly increases the degree of confidence when extrapolations to humans must be made. Both sexes of both species are proposed because of the obvious differences demonstrated in previous testing regimes with respect to the response of females and males to various chemicals. With the exception of arsenic, virtually all human oncogens have been confirmed in animal studies using rats and mice. The choice of rodents has been based on a number of parameters including economic and the time necessary to produce meaningful data. With rodents, the normal lifespan is 2-3 years, while with dogs or monkeys, the species must be maintained for 7-10 years. This would greatly increase the cost but would not assure that the data available would be more meaningful.

For non-oncogenic chronic studies, rats and a non-rodent species (usually a dog) are recommended under the TSCA standards while only rats are recommended under the FIFRA guidelines (short-term dog studies are, however, recommended in the FIFRA standards). The basis for the TSCA recommendation is that non-oncogenic chronic effects are sometimes detectable in non-rodents but not in rodents. Another reason for the use of a non-rodent species is the enhanced capability to conduct more precise clinical evaluations using larger animals. While there has been considerable discussion on the practicality of proposing a non-rodent species, dose-related effects obtained with larger animals have, in some instances, more nearly approximated those

expected to occur in humans. Dogs have been extensively used as the usual
non-rodent species, whose lifespan duration is between that expected for
humans and laboratory rodents. Non-human primates have also been recommended
as surrogates for humans based primarily on the phylogenetic relationship
and similarity in physiologic function. However, non-human primates are
expensive and difficult to obtain, with many countries having restricted
exportation quotas. For routine testing, the advantages of non-human primates
over dogs does not offset the procurement costs, management costs and problems
found in the maintenance and use of primates.

For combined chronic test studies, three species have been proposed
under TSCA while two rodent species have been proposed under FIFRA. Under
the conditions of this combined test, as both oncogenic and non-oncogenic
chronic effects must be evaluated, it has been suggested that the mouse and
rat (and dog for TSCA) be used in the study. The use of inbred, hybrid or
outbred strains of animals is known to be a controversial point. While
inbred strains are more predictable in response, outbred strains are more
resistant to diseases.

An area of controversy is the use of both negative and positive controls
in monitoring the technical procedures in the study. The validity of the
data, of course, depends on the results of comparisons of the data with
negative control groups. One way to determine sensitivity of the animals is
to employ positive control groups which have advantages in monitoring technical
procedures and controls such as diet mixture and environmental conditions.
However, it is questionable whether positive controls will be a major factor
in many chronic studies.

It is proposed that animals be started on test at the earliest practical
age, preferably immediately after weaning and acclimatization. This will be
no later than six weeks of age for rodents and ten weeks of age for dogs.
Initiation of the study in utero would, of course, provide for greater
sensitivity, especially with respect to evaluating oncogenic effects.
However, the extent of the enhanced sensitivity is difficult to evaluate.
Too few chemicals have been tested using in utero exposure followed by a
chronic testing program. Considerably greater costs and difficulties of
adjusting exposure, randomization and maintenance of animals preclude the
serious consideration of this type of exposure on a routine basis.

In general, the route of exposure of individual chemicals should simulate
as nearly as possible the expected or known human exposure. Such experimental
design would provide greater confidence in extrapolating the data to predict

the human hazard. The chemical to be tested should be administered by the same route and in the same frequency for the duration of the study; for gavage, the test substances should be administered daily; for feeding, ad libitum; for inhalation exposure, a minimum of five days per week six hours per day. A key factor is to insure that the chemical substance to be tested reaches the target site (if it is known) in the appropriate metabolic stage of degradation as is expected to occur in humans. The route of administration bears heavily on subsequent metabolic and pharmacokinetic factors.

TABLE 2

PROPOSED TSCA CHRONIC STUDY STANDARDS

	Oncogenic	Non-Oncogenic and Combined
DURATION	24-30 months	24 months for dogs 30 months for rodents
DOSE LEVELS	3 + control	4-5 + control for rat 3 + control for mouse and dog
DOSE SELECTION	MTD and FRACTIONS	NOEL to TOXICOLOGIC EFFECT
CLINICAL PARAMETERS	Daily 12 hour observations for behavior, mortality, etc.	
	Weekly and biweekly growth and food and water consumption	
	Hematology - Animal	Hematology, urinalysis, blood chemistry, organ function,* residue analysis at 3, 6, 12, 18 and 24 months (* - also at onset)
PATHOLOGY	Gross examination only	Gross examination and tissue weights
	Microscopic examination of specified prepared tissues and organs from all animals on study.	

Under the TSCA chronic study standards, the material should be tested for a minimum of 24 months for rodent species but no longer than 30 months. In non-rodent species, the tests should be 24 months in length. For non-oncogenic and combined chronic effects exposure to mice and dogs should be for 24 months with 30 months proposed for the rat. The dose level will presumably be adjusted weekly for the first six months of the study during which active growth of rodents is noted. The dose levels may be modified throughout the course of the study depending upon the species involved.

Chronic studies in animals are complex procedures requiring control of many variables for several years. Professional experience and knowledge of the relevant parameters is needed for adequate control. The primary purpose of these studies is to provide maximum opportunity for the detection of an adverse biologic effect. Obviously, the longer the period of observation, the better the chance of detecting such effects. However, a point of diminishing returns can be reached when intercurrent disease and/or survival of the animals make the observation or evaluation difficult. The most optimal study is that which includes exposure and observation through all or nearly all the expected lifespan of the animal under study. Exposure from conception to old-age death provides the maximal data upon which a hazard assessment can be made. Negative results decrease in value as the exposure and observation periods are shortened. They become practically meaningless if these periods are shorter than one-half the lifespan of the animals under test.

Chronic studies should be performed at doses likely to yield effects whose impact can be extrapolated to humans. Animal bioassays with the use of a few dozen (or even a few hundred) animals have relatively low sensitivity for the detection of adverse biological effects. In the human population, individuals and groups of individuals exist which have varying degrees of sensitivity and exposure. The test animal must in many ways be regarded as a surrogate of a large number of humans. This is a gross oversimplification of the situation but one that has no alternative under the current hazard evaluation programs. A practical approach for a routine test for oncogenic properties, for example, is to use high dose level exposure. While it has been recognized that most oncogenic effects show a positive dose response relationship, maximum tumor incidents may not occur at the highest dose level, especially when additional toxicity factors interact. Thus, it has been suggested to use multiple dose levels in these studies, especially where potential oncogenic effects are to be evaluated. Chronic bioassays, done at doses and under conditions permitting maximum expression of the potential adverse effects, provide the soundest bases for the assessment of hazard to humans.

The proposed TSCA and FIFRA oncogenic test standards recommend three dose levels; under TSCA the highest dose level should be "slightly toxic," the second a multiple of the first, usually one-half to one-quarter, and the third to be no more than one-half of the second dose and no less than 10% of the high dose. The high dose level does not necessarily refer to "the maximum tolerated dose" (MTD) so often seen in the literature and recommended under FIFRA. The high dose level should be that which would be "slightly toxic" (a term that is not fully defined but one above which survival of the population is impaired). For non-oncogenic tests, the dose level must be selected to provide data that would allow a "no-observable effect level" (NOEL) to be estimated. It is widely believed that threshold levels exist with most toxic responses and a dose response estimation can be used in subsequent risk assessments. It is expected that from three to five dose levels may be necessary to provide data appropriate to meeting all of the requirements of these non-oncogenic studies. Under FIFRA oncogenicity standards, the MTD concept has been recommended.

Subchronic short term tests will, in many instances, provide sufficient data to choose appropriate dose levels for chronic studies. In most instances, a ninety-day study should be used to provide such preliminary data. Pharmaco-kinetic and metabolic data may be of some value in defining dose levels for chronic studies.

It must be pointed out that many noted scientists have stated that except for oncogenic (and perhaps mutagenic) events, any toxic signs that will be produced at a given dose will occur in 90 days. McNamara[9] has suggested that long-term, no-effect doses may be predicted from short term studies. In many instances, especially for drug toxicity and safety evaluations, this concept may hold. However, for long-term events to be predictive of potential human hazards, there is little to suggest that appropriate risk or hazard assessments can be made on the basis of shorter term studies.

Appropriate clinical procedures are necessary to assure high standards in chronic studies. In an attempt to assure that no more than five percent of the animals under study are lost due to autolysis, cannibalism, loss, etc., it is expected that frequent, clinical procedures will be followed. Routine clinical examinations will include daily observations and body weights and food and water consumption data taken weekly for the first thirteen weeks and biweekly thereafter. Changes in behavior and pharmacologic effects are included in the clinical examinations. In the oncogenic chronic studies, routine hematology has been recommended. In the non-oncogenic studies, in addition to hematology, blood chemistry, urinalysis and organ function studies have been proposed. Hematology studies are to be performed at the one-year interval and at the termination of the study. Table 3 is a listing of the suggested clinical tests.

TABLE 3

CLINICAL PROCEDURES

<u>Hematology</u>

    Hematocrit
    Hemoglobin (reticulocyte count if RBC is low)
    Erythrocyte count
    Total and differential leukocyte
    Platelet count
    Clotting time
    Prothrombin time

<u>Chemistry</u>

    Lactic dehydrogenase
    Glutamic-pyruvic transaminase
    Alkaline phosphatase
    Creatinine kinase
    Blood Urea Nitrogen
    Creatinine
    Direct and total bilirubin
    Cholesterol
    Triglycerides
    Electrolytes--calcium, sodium, potassium and chloride
    Gamma glutamyl transpeptidase
    Ornithine carbamoyl transferase
    Uric acid
    Albumin
    Globulin
    Protein

<u>Urinalysis</u>

    Specific gravity or osmolarity
    pH
    Protein
    Glucose
    Sediments (by microscopic examination)
    Ketone
    Bilirubin
    Urobilinogen

<u>Functional Tests</u>

    Renal - Water dilution
           Water concentration
    Hepatic - BSP excretion
    Pulmonary - Total lung capacity
             Residual volume
    Cardiovascular - EEG
                blood pressure
                exercise recovery

The key to an adequate chronic study rests on the extent and accuracy
with which tissues and organs of both treated and control animals are examined
for morphologic changes. Quality and extent of pathologic documentation are
major factors in establishing the validity of bioassays in animals. Inadequate
pathologic examinations can significantly reduce the value of an otherwise
well-conducted chronic study. Carcinogenic and other chronic toxic effects
of a chemical develop through a series of stages from minimal changes to
those that are more advanced and possibly fatal. With carcinogenesis, the
process may go through early stages including a typical hyperplasia, carcinoma
in situ and/or historically benign tumor before progressing to a clearly
malignant stage. Although the stage of development is important in clinical
treatment, it is not relevant in deciding whether a chemical is a carcinogen.
Induction of pre-neoplastic lesions in the process of oncogenic development
is an indication that the test substance is capable of inducing an oncogenic
response given sufficient exposure and time.

As histopathology represents such a significant portion of a chronic
study, significant attention should be paid to this aspect. Routine gross
examinations must either be carried out with "qualified" pathologists, or
technicians under the direct supervision of such personnel. Microscopic
examinations can only be carried out by a qualified pathologist. Fixation
and treatment of tissues and organs and slide preparations with appropriate
H&E staining procedures are routine in this program. Table 4 is a listing
of tissues to be examined (in addition to any tissues that show gross evidence
of neoplasm or an unusual lesion).

Additionally, microscopic examination of ten randomly selected animals
from long-term rodent survivors and all non-rodent animals of each test
should be performed.

Metabolic and pharmacokinetic studies should be performed in conjunction
with chronic bioassays. These studies may give some indication of the toxic
potential of a chemical under examination.

TABLE 4

TISSUES TO BE EXAMINED UNDER PATHOLOGY PROCEDURES

Gross Pathology

1. Physical Examination

2. Tissue Weights and Visible Condition

Heart	Testes	Brain
Liver	Spleen	Adrenal Glands
Kidney	Lung	Thyroid Glands (with parathyroid)

Microscopic Pathology

Brain
  (Fore, mid and hindbrain)
Spinal Cord
  (cervical, lumbar and thoracic sections)
Eyes (with continuous Harderian gland)
Heart and Aorta (3 sections)
Trachea and Lungs (with bronchi)
Esophagus
Stomach
Intestines (small and 3 sections of large)
Pancreas
Liver (2 lobes)
Vagina, corpus and cervis uteri, ovaries
  and fallopian tubes

Gall Bladder
Spleen
Kidney
Urinary Bladder
Lymph Nodes
Bone (with marrow)
Skin
Skeletal Muscle
Oral Mucous Membrane (tongue,
buccal mucosa, alveolar
mucosa, pharynx and
nasopharynx)
Testes, Prostate and all male
accessory organs

Glands:

Pituitary	Thyroid (with parathyroid)
Salivary	Mammary
Thymus	Zymbals
Adrenal	

SHORT-TERM TEST FOR ONCOGENESIS

Oncogenic tests have been traditionally based on the experimental
induction of tumors in laboratory animals. Such tests usually involve the
observation of treated animals for the majority of their lifespan. Recently,
short-term methodologies have been developed to provide more rapid markers
for the tentative identification of oncogenic effects. These methods are
directed towards the study of mechanisms underlying neoplastic transformation
as well as towards providing rapid, reproducible and inexpensive bioassay
methods for testing chemicals and physical agents for potential carcinogenic
activity.

At the present time, no one of the short-term tests can be used to establish whether a compound will or will not be carcinogenic in humans or experimental animals. Positive results obtained in these bioassay screening systems suggest further extensive testing of the agent is needed in the long-term animal bioassays. Negative results in the short-term test, however, do not establish the safety of the compound.

Testing for mutagenic events has been developed to assess the ability of a substance to induce genetic alteration. The resulting information can be used for considering the genetic hazard of chemical agents to man. Because of the similarities of basic molecular mechanisms by which chemical mutagens and most chemical carcinogens appear to induce genetic effects, it has been postulated that mutagenic effects can be used to predict carcinogenicity. The use of a battery or variety of short-term genetic tests has been recommended in order to minimize false negative and false positive results. Data from these bioassays are being used to select and prioritize compounds for further long-term investigation. Several bioassay systems are now available at the mammalian cell level for the identification and study of substances that represent a possible oncogenic hazard. In tests for neoplastic transformation, the cells derived from transformed colonies when innoculated into immunosuppressed animals grow as malignant tumors. Although the most definitive evidence for neoplastic transformations of cells in culture is the ability to increase tumors on innoculation into animals, a number of phenotypic changes in the treated cultured cells are commonly used as bioindicators.

The study of carcinogenesis at the cellular level presently offers an effective means to identify potential carcinogenic effects and to examine mechanisms of action. Short-term tests for chemical carcinogens presently do not, in the absence of confirming long-term bioassays and epidemiological data, constitute definitive evidence that a substance does or does not pose a carcinogenic hazard to humans. However, positive responses in these tests are considered suggestive evidence of a carcinogenic hazard. In some instances, results from short-term tests may conflict with animal bioassay data. Positive responses to short-term tests are sufficient to provide suggestive evidence of carcinogenicity even if the substance has shown only negative responses in some animal bioassays. Short-term test results also provide supporting evidence for prospective epidemiological studies. As the degree of certainty attached to negative responses in animal bioassays increases, because the observation is reproduced in other animal species, strains, or

under more rigorous test conditions, the suspicion about the oncogenic
potential test chemical noted as a result of short-term tests may be reduced
and eventually eliminated.

Under TSCA, the cost per chemical for a chronic bioassay is estimated to
be approximately $400,000 for the oncogenicity studies and $550,000 for the
non-oncogenic chronic studies. Where combined oncogenic and non-oncogenic
studies are performed, it is estimated the total cost will be approximately
$800,000. The cost of pre-chronic range finding studies ranges from $50,000
for an oncogenic study to $100,000 for non-oncogenic study, and to $130,000
for combined studies. The actual cost estimates will, of course, vary. The
question of whether the ultimate cost will inhibit industrial development
and growth in such areas as pharmaceuticals, agricultural, chemical or food
additives has yet to be fully answered. The proposed regulatory programs
will bear heavily on the safety of man and his environment. The ultimate
costs and the impact on chemical developments, however, have yet to be
calculated.

REFERENCES

1.   Delaney Amendment - 21 U. S. Code of Federal Regulations Section 409(c)
     (3)(A); Section 512(d)(1)(H) animal growth promoters as food additives;
     and Section 706(b)(5)(B) food colors, 1958.

2.   Environmental Protection Agency. (1979) Proposed Health Effects Test
     Standards for Toxic Substances Control Act Test Rules. Fed. Register,
     44(91), 27334-27362.

3.   Environmental Protection Agency. (1978) Proposed Guidelines for Regis-
     tering Pesticides in the U.S.; Hazard Evaluation: Human and Domestic
     Animals. Fed. Register, 43(163), 37336-403.

4.   Fitzhugh, O. G. (1959) Chronic Oral Toxicity. In Appraisal of the
     Safety of Chemicals in Foods, Drugs and Cosmetics. Association of Food
     and Drug Officials of the U. S.

5.   Food and Agriculture Organization. (1978) Pesticide Residues in Food,
     AGP: 1978/m/5.

6.   Food Safety Council. (1978) Proposed System for Food Safety Assessment.
     Report of the Scientific Committee.

7.   Food and Drug Administration. (1978) Nonclinical Laboratory Studies.
     Good Laboratory Practice Regulations. Fed. Register, 43 (247), 59986-
     60025.

8.   Lehman, A. J. and Fitzhugh, O. G. (1954) 100 Fold Margin of Safety.
     Food and Drug Officials Quart. Bulletin.

9.   McNamara, B. P. (1976) Concepts in Health Evaluation of Commercial and
     Industrial Chemicals. In Advances in Modern Toxicology, Vol. 1, Part 1,
     edited by Mehlman, M. A., Shapiro, R. E. and Blumenthal, H.

10. National Academy of Sciences. (1975) Principles for Evaluating Chemicals
     in the Environment. A report for the Working Conference on Principles of
     Protocols for Evaluating Chemicals in the Environment.

11. Sontag, J. M., Page, N. P. and Saffiotti, U. (1976) Guidelines for
     carcinogen bioassays in small rodents. Natl. Cancer Inst. Carcinogenesis
     Tech. Rep. Ser. No. 1. National Institutes of Health. DHEW Publ. No.
     (NIH) 76-801. Washington, D. C.

© 1980 Elsevier/North-Holland Biomedical Press
The Principles and Methods in Modern Toxicology
C.L. Galli, S.D. Murphy and R. Paoletti, editors.

SHORT-TERM TESTS FOR CARCINOGENICITY

CHRISTIAN SCHLATTER and WERNER K. LUTZ

Institute of Toxicology, Swiss Federal Institute of Technology and University of Zürich, Schorenstrasse 16, CH-8603 Schwerzenbach (Switzerland)

There is no doubt that long-term carcinogenicity studies show many disadvantages. First, they last a long time, at least two to three years, only rodents are suitable for such tests due to their relatively short lifespan, and the studies have to be carried out with a large number of animals. Another point which causes some concern and problems in interpretation, is the need of high dose levels to guarantee a sufficiently high safety factor. Consequently one has to extrapolate by orders of magnitude to the dose levels to which man is exposed, but a high dose level may induce toxicity, and toxicity by itself could modify the tumour response. High dose levels also can overwhelm the metabolic capacity of the animal.   In such a case a mathematical extrapolation to man's exposure would not be justified. Also, there are only a few laboratories in the world where long-term studies can be performed in a sufficiently controlled and competent manner. Other important factors influencing the tumour incidence are the strain of animals and mostly unknown environmental and dietary components which leads to problems in standardization of the tests.

Therefore, there is a great need for finding other methods of carcinogenicity testing. The current concept of tumour induction is shown in Figure 1.

In the following we will focus on the importance of chemical structure, interaction with DNA and induction of mutations and cell transformation.

CHEMICAL STRUCTURE

The majority of carcinogenic chemicals enter the organism as biologically inactive compounds. Once in the body they are converted to reactive metabolites by enzymatic action, only a small group of chemicals are reactive without enzymatic activation. Unfortunately there are no short-term tests giving information on interferences in the events occurring between cell transformation and tumour induction. The main chemical property of a reactive compound is its electrophilicity[1]. For example the reaction of an activated nitrosamine with nucleophilic centers of bases of a nucleic acid, e.g. N-7 of guanine or 0(6) is shown in Figure 2.

208

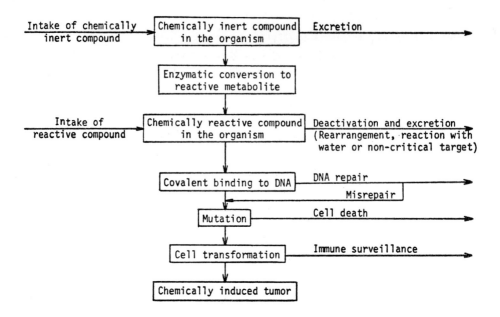

Fig. 1.   Sequence of events in the chemical induction of a tumour.

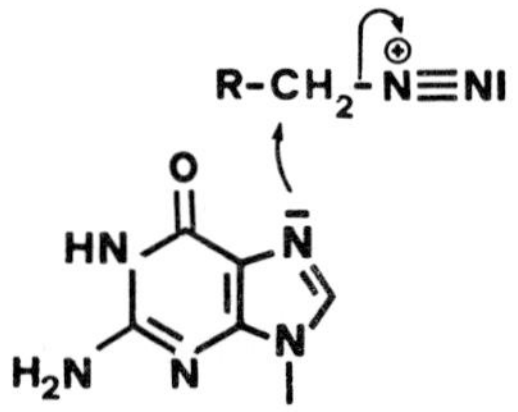

Fig. 2.   Nucleophilic attack of nitrogen-7 of guanine on a diazonium ion.

The main prerequisite for reaching the microsomal enzymes and the cell
nucleus is a considerable lipophilicity of the compound. The organic chemist
can deduce from his knowledge of the chemical properties of chemicals that
methyl methanesulphonate, e.g., is lipophilic as well as electrophilic and
therefore,a reaction with DNA leading eventually to tumours is likely. Other
compounds which can react without enzymatic activation are listed in Figure 3.

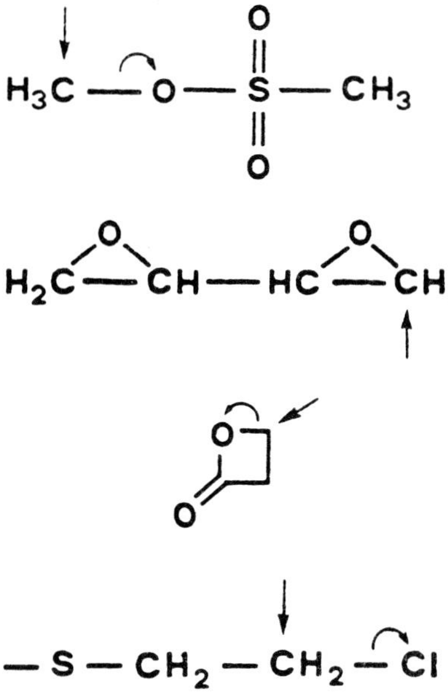

Fig. 3. Selection of directly acting carcinogens. From the top: methyl methanesulphonate; 1,2,3,4-diepoxybutane; β-propiolactone; a sulphur mustard.

However, no simple prediction of their biological properties is possible for the large class of compounds which must be activated in the body. Sites and ways of activation are not easily predictable. Examples for activation are given in Figure 4.

Without having done extensive biological and metabolic studies it would not have been possible to recognize the r-7,t-8-dihydroxy-t-9,10-epoxy-7,8,9,10-tetrahydro-benzo(a)pyrene as the most active carcinogenic metabolite of benzo(a)pyrene.

The case of saccharin shall be used as an illustration of the general features discussed above (Figure 5).

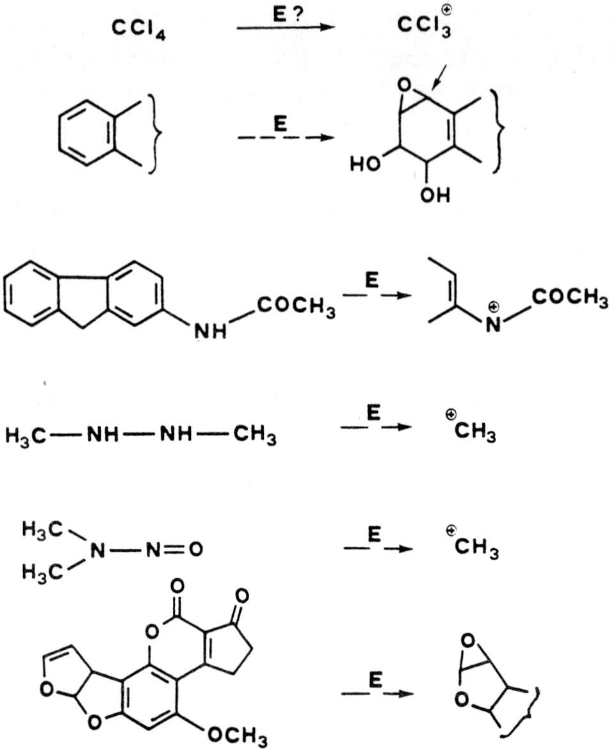

Fig. 4. Selection of carcinogens which need enzymatic activation. From the top: carbon tetrachloride; a polycyclic aromatic hydrocarbon (the reactive metabolite shown is known from benzo(a)pyrene); 2-acetylaminofluorene; 1,2-dimethylhydrazine; N,N-dimethylnitrosamine; aflatoxin B_1.

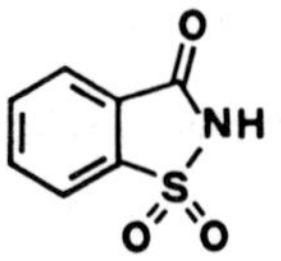

Fig. 5. Chemical structure of saccharin.

The main characteristic of this compound is nucleophilic, and there are no structures of which an electrophilic cation could be formed. Also, saccharin is very polar, it lacks the essential lipophilicity to penetrate the different cell membranes. Therefore, after consideration of the structure of saccharin one can conclude that it is unlikely it will ever act as a direct carcinogen able to interact with DNA. This presumption was recently confirmed experimentally[2].

Another example relates to aromatic amines. It was shown mainly with the model compound 2-acetylaminofluorene that for the activation to an electro-philic intermediate a free ortho-position is important. Thus by blocking the ortho-positions the carcinogenicity of an aromatic amine should disappear. This was shown to be true for the tetramethyl derivative of the carcinogen benzidine[3] (Figure 6).

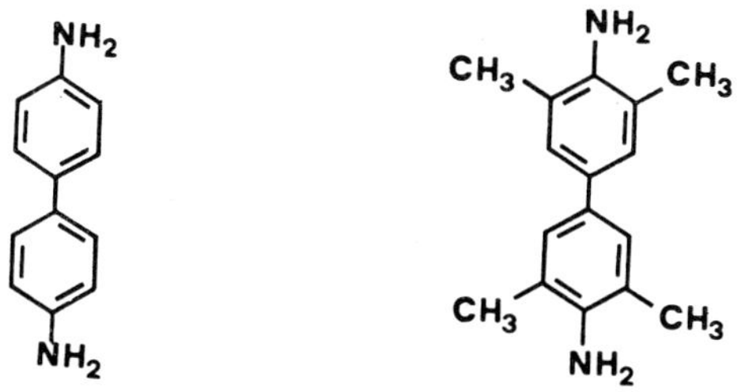

Fig. 6. Chemical structures of benzidine and its 3,5,3',5'-tetramethyl derivative.

Another example is shown by the carcinogenicity of substituted ethylenes. Once the carcinogenicity of vinyl chloride was detected the suspicion was raised that the other related compounds (Figure 7) are most probably also carcinogenic.

Long-term bioassays confirmed this suspicion, except for styrene[4]. Like the other compounds, styrene is metabolised to the intermediate expoxide which was shown to be carcinogenic[5]. Most probably styrene itself is not carcinogenic because any intermediately formed styrene epoxide is immediately inactivated to the corresponding diol by the enzyme epoxide hydratase. Styrene epoxide repre-sents an excellent substrate for epoxide-hydratase[6]. This example shows the limitations of structure-activity considerations.

212

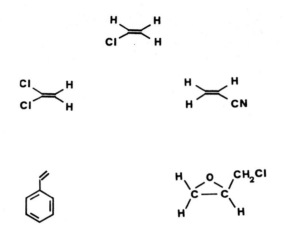

Fig. 7. Chemical structures of vinyl chloride, vinylidene chloride, acrylonitrile, styrene, and epichlorohydrin.

BINDING TO NUCLEIC ACIDS

It was shown mainly by the pioneering work of the Millers[1] that covalent binding of carcinogens is a crucial step during the course of tumour induction. In our laboratory much effort is spent on the elucidation of the biological significance of these reactions (for review see[7]). To study the interaction with DNA the chemical is administered in radioactive labelled form. The need for radioactive compounds represents the main disadvantage of our approach. Usually, radioactive pharmaceuticals, pesticides and food additives are used during the development of the compounds since they are synthesized for other purposes such as metabolic studies. However, non-proprietary drugs, industrial intermediates, environmental contaminants or natural toxins are hard to obtain in labelled form. After the administration of the compounds to the intact animal by routes where man is most likely to be exposed, one waits for several hrs for the absorption and metabolism to take place. The organs of interest are then excised, DNA is isolated and its radioactivity is determined after carefully purifying the DNA. One must be especially careful to avoid any contamination by labelled proteins. The degree of covalent binding of the xenobiotics to DNA is expressed by the so-called CBI (covalent binding index): This is defined as the damage to the DNA divided by the dose:

$$CBI = \frac{\mu mole\ chemical\ bound\ /\ mole\ DNA\text{-}phosphate}{mmole\ chemical\ /\ kg\ body\ weight}$$

The use of this approach is illustrated by the following examples: First, it is possible to determine dose-effect relationships of dose levels which are much lower than one needs for long-term animal studies. For example, with benzo(a)pyrene, dose levels in the range of mg/kg body weight must be given to elicit a tumour response, whereas with our technique it is possible to measure covalent binding even at levels of 10 - 40 µg/kg body weight[8]. In the low dose range we found a distinct step in the dose-effect relationship which would not have been predictable with other test systems (Figure 8).

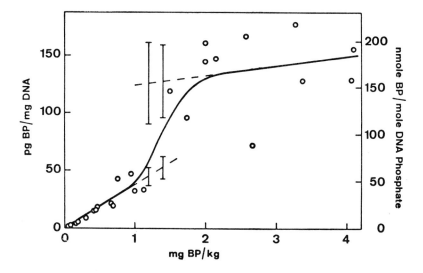

Fig. 8. Non-linear dose-response curve for the covalent binding of benzo(a)pyrene to rat liver DNA.

With this approach it is possible to come, by several orders of magnitude, closer to the likely exposure of man. Another application of the binding assay is the comparison of the binding potency of different suspected or known carcinogens. Quite a good correlation was found between the carcinogenic potency and the binding capacity of the compound[9] (Table 1).

TABLE 1

CORRELATION OF HEPATOCARCINOGENICITY OF CHEMICALS TO THEIR COVALENT
BINDING TO RAT LIVER DNA[9]

Compound	Route	Time (h)	CBI
Strong hepatocarcinogens			
Aflatoxin B_1	i.p.	6	16 500
Dimethylnitrosamine	i.p.	4	6 500
Moderate hepatocarcinogens			
2-Acetylaminofluorene	i.p.	16	560
N-Nitrosopyrrolidine	p.o.	12	170
Weak hepatocarcinogens			
Vinyl chloride	inhal.	24	240
4-Dimethylaminoazobenzene	i.p.	24	10
Urethane	i.p.	24	37

The binding capacity of strong hepatocarcinogens lies in the order of 100s
to 1000s. Whereas the binding of moderate hepatocarcinogens is by one or two
orders of magnitude lower, weak hepatocarcinogens only show a very weak binding
to DNA and the only compound where we so far have not been able to find any
binding to DNA was saccharin[2]. Based on recently published binding studies of
TCDD to liver DNA[10] we calculated a CBI of less than 0.1. This means that TCDD
would have to be classified as cocarcinogen or tumour promoter.
There are, however, several classes and substances where the correlation is
not as good as it has been shown here. This means that the binding assay has
to be refined. In addition to DNA binding other factors must be considered, such
as the persistence of the label on the DNA or the repair activity of the different
organs in relationship to the cell division rate. For instance, it has been
found that the CBI of aromatic amines are low compared to their carcinogenicity
while   the persistence of the label at the DNA is much higher than for other
compounds.

The covalent binding index can also be used for comparing the susceptibility
of different species to carcinogens. We recently determined the binding of
aflatoxin B_1 in rat, pig and mouse[11] (Table 2).

TABLE 2

COVALENT BINDING INDICES (CBI) OF ORALLY ADMINISTERED AFLATOXINS IN LIVER DNA
OF DIFFERENT SPECIES

Compound	Species	CBI
Aflatoxin B_1	rat	10 400
	pig	19 100
	mouse	240
Aflatoxin M_1	rat	2 100

The results are in agreement with the finding that mice are much less
susceptible to the carcinogenicity of aflatoxins. It is difficult predict
the position of man, but it is probable that man resembles rat and pig, because
mouse liver and metabolism of xenobiotics in mouse liver represent a very
special case and cannot be compared with other mammalians.

Another use of the test is to determine the potential carcinogenicity of
compounds chemically closely related to one of which long-term tests are
available. It is not possible to perform long-term tests with aflatoxin M_1, a
metabolite of aflatoxin B_1, occuring in milk , because it is found only at very
low levels. Therefore it would be difficult to isolate amounts of M_1 large
enough to perform long-term experiments. Aflatoxin M_1 also shows a high CBI
and therefore one can presume that its potential carcinogenicity also would
be quite high[11]. This compound most probably would be also fall in the class
of the very strong hepatocarcinogens.

Another application of results on the binding on metabolites to DNA for
predicting carcinogenicity was possible recently when the question of the
safety of the macromolecular metabolites of aflatoxin B_1 was raised. When
aflatoxin is given orally to animals about 10 % of the dose is bound to macromolecules of the liver[12]. The biological half-life of these metabolites is 1
to 2 weeks. These macromolecular bound aflatoxin residues are likely to occur
in the livers of meat animals, such as pigs or cattle while they are fed
ground-nut cakes contaminated with aflatoxins. We performed a so-called
relay experiment (Figure 9).

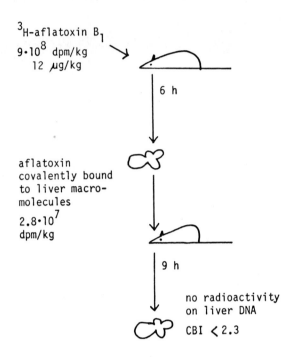

^{3}H-aflatoxin B$_1$
$9 \cdot 10^8$ dpm/kg
12 µg/kg

6 h

aflatoxin
covalently bound
to liver macro-
molecules

$2.8 \cdot 10^7$
dpm/kg

9 h

no radioactivity
on liver DNA

CBI < 2.3

Fig. 9. Binding to liver DNA of aflatoxin residues.

We administered orally aflatoxin B$_1$ to a first rat. We then isolated the macromolecules from the liver with the aflatoxin residues bound on the macro-molecules,and fed these macromolecules to a second rat[13]. No radioactivity was found in the liver DNA of the second rat. This shows that the macromolecular residues even after being digested in the second rat do not react with DNA and are therefore most probably devoid of any carcinogenic activity. Lastly, an example dealing with the determination of the binding of carcinogenic compounds which are only formed in the body. This is the case with those nitrosamines which are formed in the stomach by the reaction of nitrites and amines after administration of potassium nitrite together with a single oral dose of radioactive dimethylamine. A CBI of about 50 was found[14]. The CBI of dimethylnitrosamine was about 1900. From this data it can be concluded that about 3 % of the amine was nitrosated in the stomach. It would have been

very difficult to determine the yield of nitrosamine by other means because
at the same time as nitrosation occurs in the stomach, the products are
absorbed, distributed and rapidly degraded.

BIOLOGICAL TEST SYSTEMS

Many short-term tests have been developed in the past, most of them are
based on the induction of mutations in different *in vitro* systems. Recently
they were critically evaluated[15]; the currently used short-term tests have
been comprehensively reviewed[16]. Several criteria have to be met for such a
test to be useful, for example:

Predictive value

For this, it is necessary that the test is validated by quite a large
number of compounds belonging to different chemical classes. Many of the tests
which have been introduced and have been proposed in the past have not yet
been validated by a sufficient number of chemicals. This fact alone reduces
their usefulness.

Theoretical base

The end-point of the test should be linked as closely as possible to the
mechanism of tumour induction by chemicals. At first glance one
could argue that this is not an important point provided that it has been
shown that the test has a good predictive value. However, the probability
that this will happen and that the test will survive on the long run is quite
low if no such theoretical basis exists. In such a case, good correlation in
a given set of experiments is most likely due to factors such as chance, biased
compound selection, or unspecific cytotoxicity. Presumably, the test based on
inhibition of thymidine incorporation into DNA in the testis of living rodents
falls into this class[17, 18].

Reproducibility

The need for a useful test to be reproducible both within one laboratory
as well as in interlaboratory comparative studies is not disputable. However,
much effort is still needed to achieve this goal even for the most widely
used and simplest test systems. This last point still represents wishful
thinking.

Carcinogenic Potency

Development of means for prediction of the carcinogenic potency by short-

218

term tests is one of the most challenging and useful areas for future research
19, 20, 21, 22, 23. So far however, all the tests currently used do not predict the carcinogenic potency. This is not surprising when the enormous
biological differences between the non-mammalian single cell test systems and
the intact mammalian organism with its innumerable metabolic and kinetic possibilities for activation and inactivation of the chemicals are considered.

MUTATION TESTS

Table 3 lists those mutation tests which have been validated at liest to
some degree[15].

TABLE 3

VALIDATED MUTATION TESTS

- *S. thyphimurium*(gene mutations)
- *E. coli* (gene mutations)
- yeast (gene mutations)
- cultured mammalian cells (gene mutations)
- recessive lethals in *Drosophila*
- unscheduled DNA synthesis

Best-known among these is the famous Ames test. A validation has revealed
90 % correct answers for carcinogens and non-carcinogens[24]. However, it should
be borne in mind that only a limited number of chemicals have been studied and
that these compounds were not equally sampled from all chemical classes. The
correlation is best for strong carcinogens which do not require a species- or
organ-specific activation. A higher frequency of discordance is found for
compounds of low carcinogenic potency where little is known on the mechanism
of action. These compounds are important in real life and for them, not for
the strong model carcinogens like benzo(a)pyrene or benzidine, should short-
term tests be devised.

It has been shown that a combination of two different short-term tests
improves correlation and predictability[25]. This is partly a
purely statistical phenomenon but it has also some biological reasons.

The chromosomal structure of prokaryotes as they are used in the *Salmonella/*
microsome assay differs markedly from the chromosomal structure in eukaryotes
as in yeast and mammalian cells. Therefore, by combining the bacterial test
with another one based on eukaryotes, a quite important improvement in the

predictability is achieved. However, there is little evidence that by
further addition of test systems the predictability can still be improved.

Cell transformation and sister chromatid exchange

Although not much is known about different mechanisms leading to positive
results in these two test systems, concurrent answers are given for an extended
list of carcinogens and non-carcinogens[15]. It seems that with these systems
not only the typical DNA-attacking carcinogens but also those acting by other
mechanisms are detected. Saccharin was shown to be genetically inactive[2] although, at exceedingly high dose levels, evidence for tumour induction in animals
is available. Saccharin was positive in special assays for cell transformation[26]
and sister chromatid exchange[27]. Much research work is needed on the mechanism of these promising tests before their results can be used appropriately.

Tests on intact mammals

It has been shown that mammalian test systems for mutagenicity are quite
useful for predicting mutagenicity but they do not play an important role in
predicting carcinogenicity[15] (Table 4).

TABLE 4

TYPE OF GENETIC EFFECT

Type of test	Chromosome damage				Point mutations (incl. small deficiencies)
	Breaks → Losses ♂	♀	Rearrange-ment ♂	Non-Dis-junction	
Dominant lethal	+[a]				
Heritable translocation	+[b]		+		
Numer. sex-chrom. anomaly		+		+	
Micronucleus test	+	+			
Specific locus					+
Mouse spot test	(+)				(+)

[a] To compare sensitivity of different germ-cell stages

[b] Often more sensitive than the dominant lethal test, for meiotic and post-
meiotic stages

The dominant lethal test is too insensitive since only heavy chromosomal damages are measured but not point mutations. The same is true for the micronucleus test, the heritable translocation test and the test for numerical aberrations of sex chromosomes. Only the specific locus test and the mouse spot test detect point mutations in mammalians. So these tests theoretically would be suitable for predicting carcinogenic potential of the compounds. However, they are time consuming, they need much expertise and facilities and do therefore not fulfil the requirement for a short-term test which can be used routinely.

What is the situation for the short-term test?   It is certainly wrong to ask: Are you for or against the Ames test ? There is no doubt that results of the different short-term tests give valid information on the biological properties of the chemical. However, they are not at present and presumably not in the future able to replace long-term animal studies. They should not be used as the only base on which a decision regarding possible carcinogenicity can be taken. They have a definite place in the general evaluation of a compound when they are used together with other information on the properties of a compound such as structure, metabolism, degree of exposure. All these data should be combined to give the background on which decisions can be made. There might well be cases where one will drop the further development of a compound solely on positive results of short-term tests without proceeding to long-term tests. Such a decision is not taken because one regards the compound as a carcinogen but simply to avoid further expenses needed   for proving or disproving a suspicion of carcinogenicity. On the other hand, there will also be cases where, despite of a positive result of a short-term test, one cannot remove the compound from the environment. This is especially the case for many natural compounds. Provided that the exposure of man is so low that only a negligible risk is likely from this compound one will not even perform long-term tests. So it depends on the compounds, their use and the extent of exposure as to what value will be attached to the results of a short-term test.

REFERENCES

1. Miller, J.A. (1970) Cancer Res., 30, 559-576.

2. Lutz, W.K. and Schlatter, Ch. (1977) Chem.-Biol. Interactions, 19, 253-257.

3. Holland, V.R. et al. (1974) Tetrahedron, 30, 3299-3302.

4. National Cancer Institute (1979) Bioassay of Styrene, Technical Report Series No. 185,U.S. Department of Health, Education,and Welfare, Public Health Service, National Institutes of Health.

5. IARC, Monographs on the Evaluation of Carcinogenic Risk of Chemicals to Man (1976) 11, 201-208; (1979) 19, 275-283.

6. Oesch, F. (1974) Biochem. J., 139, 77-88.

7. Lutz, W.K. (1979) Mutation Res. 65, 289-356.

8. Lutz, W.K. et al. (1978) Cancer Res., 38, 575-578.

9. Lutz, W.K. and Schlatter, Ch. (1979) Arch. Toxicol. Suppl., 2, 411-415.

10. Poland, A. and Glover, E. (1979) Cancer Res., 39, 3341-3344.

11. Lutz, W.K. et al., submitted to Chem.-Biol. Interact.

12. Lüthy, J. et al., submitted to Fd. Cosmet. Toxicol.

13. Jaggi, W. et al., submitted to Fd. Cosmet. Toxicol.

14. Meier-Bratschi, A. et al., Meeting abstract submitted to Experientia.

15. IARC, Monographs on the Evaluation of Carcinogenic Risk of Chemicals to Man (1980, in preparation).

16. Hollstein, M. et al. (1979) Mutation Res. 65, 133-226.

17. Friedman, M.A. and Staub, I. (1976) Mutation Res., 37, 67-76.

18. Seiler, J.P. (1977) Mutation Res., 46, 305-310.

19. Meselson, M. and Russell, K. (1977) Origins of Human Cancer, Book C: Human Risk Assessment, Cold Spring Harbor Laboratory, pp. 1473-1481.

20. Clive, D. et al. (1979) Mutation Res., 59, 61-108.

21. Ashby, J. and Styles, J.A. (1978) Nature, 271, 452-455 274, 20-22.

22. Ames, B.N. and Hooper, K. (1978) Nature, 274, 19-20.

23. McGregor, D.B. (1978) Nature, 274, 21.

24. Rinkus, S.J. and Legator, M.S. (1979) Cancer Res., 39, 3298-3318.

25. Purchase, I.F.H., Proceedings of the Symposium on Quantitative Aspects of Risk Assessment in Chemical Carcinogenesis (in preparation).

26. Mondal, S. et al. (1978) Science, 201, 1141-1142.

27. Wolff, S. and Rodin, B. (1978), Science, 200, 543-545.

© 1980 Elsevier/North-Holland Biomedical Press
The Principles and Methods in Modern Toxicology
C.L. Galli, S.D. Murphy and R. Paoletti, editors.

TOXICOLOGIC PATHOLOGY: ISSUES AND UNCERTAINTIES

PAUL M. NEWBERNE AND ROBERT G. McConnell
Department of Nutrition and Food Science, Massachusetts Institute
of Technology, Cambridge, MA

INTRODUCTION

For one reason or another, be it to satisfy the innate curiosity of the scientist, the sincere interest of industry in a potential new product, or the regulations of government, many of us spend much of our time conducting investigations using laboratory animals.

A major goal of toxicity studies in animals is to characterize functional and morphological effects of a given chemical or drug. In attempting to delineate the effects of such an agent on biological systems, a whole host of determinations are used in the overall evaluation. These include the modes of action, the sites and severity of toxicity, age and sex differences, dose-response relationships, latency, progression and reversibility of effects and morphologic evidence of injury if such occurs. It is this latter aspect that often constitutes a stumbling block in deciding whether or not a given compound is worthy of further study and evaluation. It is also this area where the toxicologic pathologist spends the majority of the available time, evaluating tissues and other samples collected from experimental animals.

When should the pathologist, with his special expertise, be inserted into the process of experimental design of toxicologic investigation?; at an early point in the development of the protocol. This ensures pathology expertise from the outset, and enables the pathologist to incorporate those features necessary for proper development and assessment of the clinical and histologic material. In this regard, it must be emphasized that it is virtually always the histologic data that are used as a basis for final decisions regarding the safety or non-safety of a chemical agent.

The diagnosis of lesions in experimental animals is not an easy task, and requires considerable training, skill and experience. Whether or not a given drug or chemical will ever be used in human populations is determined in part by whether or not it causes specific kinds of organ toxicity and damage; more often however, a decision is made on the basis of whether or not it results in an increase in tumors or in the development of unusual types of tumors in experimental animals. Thus, the diagnosis of pathologic changes and particularly of tumors, becomes of paramount importance in the development of new chemicals and drugs for the benefit of society.

On the face of it, this goal of developing new chemicals would appear to be easily achievable, given the objective nature of the intelligent well-trained professional charged with the responsibility of evaluating data from safety studies in animals. However, in reality, to render an opinion on any given study that is entirely acceptable to a majority of the community of toxicologic pathologists is a very difficult task. Diagnoses of, and convictions about, pathologic lesions and their implications differ as widely as our background training and experience. It is this wide diversity of opinions among pathologists, regarding lesions induced in experimental animals, and of the implications of these lesions, that constitute many of the current controversial issues. The vagaries of the biologic test system employed, and how results are to be interpreted in light of risk - benefit equations, compound the uncertainties.

A. The Utility of Safety Assessment Studies in Animals

Results derived from animal toxicity studies often predict, or at least suggest, potential adverse effects in man and cannot be regarded merely as academic information bearing no relationship to human effects. We must also recognize, however, that direct extrapolation of animal toxicity data to man does have significant limitations.[1-4] Chemical or drug-related toxicity in animals may sometimes reflect an effect of the physiological or pharmacokinetic capabilities peculiar to that particular species, and thus the observations may not be applicable to man. Furthermore, toxicity manifested by subjective or symptomatic effects, -responses which are confined to man, -obviously cannot be predicted from studies in animals. While animal studies can never substitute for human exposure and the effects of a given compound on human populations, they are of considerable value in forecasting and characterizing possible adverse effects of a non-subjective nature in humans, and enable the setting of guidelines for those kinds of observations which will be relevant when human studies are subsequently performed.

B. Scientific, Regulatory and Sociopolitical Demands

One cannot question the intent of the Congress of 1906 that enacted the Pure Food and Drug Act as the first federal food and
drug safety law in the United States. The House Committee of that
Congress, commenting on the provisions of the Act, observed "the
question of whether certain substances are poisonous or deleterious to health, the bill does not undertake to determine, but
leaves that to the determination of the Secretary, under the guidance of proper disinterested scientific authorities, after most
careful study, examination, experiment and thorough research."
There was considerable faith implicit in the ability of "disinterested scientific authorities" to determine which substances
posed an unacceptable risk for society. This in fact was a naive
faith, and more than 70 years of regulation have brought this fact
into focus. The so-called disinterested scientists are no longer
delegated as the sole assessors of risk. In fact, the very concept of objectivity that is implied by "disinterested" has been
modified in recent years and, furthermore, there is little evidence that the scientific community has gained back any of the
confidence placed in it over 70 years ago.

Numerous regulatory agencies have been established in the United
States and around the world and, except for somewhat rare instances, the suggestions and comments of the scientific community are
accorded variable, generally minor, influence. Perhaps this is because of our frequent public displays of disagreement and lack of
objectivity in the assessment of the day-to-day problems that arise
in regard to the risk associated with various chemicals and drugs.
But then scientists do not agree on many things, and it is unrealistic to suppose that they do or that they should. An agreement
is usually for what is already established and a part of scientific
history. The ongoing aspect of science consists in part of an
active and quite often heated debate about data, ideas and safety
assessment, in what one might call a creative disagreement.[5] It
has been said that the scientific method is derived largely from
a reconstruction based on selected hindsights, while what goes on
in real life is much more a matter of trial and error, conjecture,
chance, and competition. Science does however answer to certain
constraints, including logical consistency, constructing testable

hypotheses, and exposing one's views and works to a peer review process.

The Congress of the U.S. must be given credit for its continuing efforts to accord the scientific community a place in the regulatory process. For example, in 1970, sixty-four years after the enactment of the Pure Food and Drug Act, the Congress passed an Act creating an agency for Occupational Safety and Health (OSHA), and directed that OSHA's standards be based on "research, demonstration, experiment" as well as "the latest available scientific data in the field." In contrast to this directive from Congress, a number of OSHA's regulations have been developed with very little scientific input and with more attention to legal and regulatory expediency.

Andre Cournand has recently published a cogent article on the Code of the scientist and its relationship to ethics.[6] In this paper he has quoted Paul Valery who, many decades earlier, had said "Never has humanity known so much power and so much confusion, so much worry and so much play, so much knowledge and so much uncertainty. In equal measure now anguish, and futility, command the hours of our days." Cournand has pointed out, and we are in agreement, that while this quote was made several decades ago, the words are probably even more appropriate today than when they were uttered. Science indeed is now in a state of seige with those who, having praised the scientist's contributions to human welfare in the past, are now questioning many aspects of his current scientific procedures. This is particularly true in the area of safety evaluation, where toxicologic pathology is intimately involved. The public is simply no longer willing to handle uncertainty in a rational manner. All citizens now want certainty and security in their jobs, their homes and their lives. However the very essence of our phenomenal technological advances in the past three decades have been a willingness to promptly utilize new technology enthusiastically, and to accept any accompanying increases in uncertainty. Roland Schmitt, vice-president for corporate research and development at General Electric, has placed this problem in some perspective.[7] He has noted that science advances by open and candid discussion of all possible alternatives, and has pointed out that if science, and in particular our own area of endeavor, becomes a center of political controversy, candid discussion will cease and

it will be difficult for the scientist to preserve scientific objectivity. Schmitt has alluded to the difficulties that the public
now faces in attempting to deal with the uncertainties that scientific knowledge continues to bring to society. He believes that
scientists need to change the way their work is presented to the
public, and should place more emphasis on the scientific process,
as well as on the results. Failures must be candidly acknowledged,
while emphasizing that it is only through mistakes that we learn;
there is no point in scientists displaying a seige mentality toward
the public, because the public is not against science. It is only
a very small extemely vocal minority of the public which provide
this impression. Nevertheless, disagreements amongst scientists
performing studies in the area of safety evaluation have left the
public confused and oft-times alarmed. It is the issues that we
are faced with, and the uncertainties that abound, which leave
experts in toxicology and especially in toxicologic pathology in
a highly vulnerable position today. In this presentation we will
point out a few of the pertinent issues and some of the problems
which contribute to these uncertainties.

C. Physical, Medical and Biological Sciences; the Role of
    Active Observation in Each.

The reliability of a chemical analytical measurement utilizing
principles of physical science is a function of the precision,
accuracy, dynamic range and freedom from interferences displayed
by the method.[8] The use of chemically-defined standard solutions
enables precise calibration of the measuring device and close control of analytic bias (accuracy); duplicate specimens and control
materials enable estimation of within-run and run-to-run analytic
variation. This results in a highly reliable quantitation of the
analyte measured. Observational error is minimized.

By way of contrast, scientific observations in clinical medicine
must, by their very nature, be considerably more subject to observer variance and inherently less reliable than those in the physical sciences. All observation, however, whether qualitative or
quantitative, is subject to error. And everyone makes mistakes,
not only in reasoning, but also in the observations on which judg-
ments are based. But the scope of the likely error differs remarkably between clinical medicine and physical sciences.

The clinician who posseses a retentive memory, a wide knowledge and experience of disease processes, and has developed a sound technique of clinical examination should produce reliable diagnoses, provided he also posseses an astute ability to reason from his observations. The complacency of highly experienced observers has been badly shaken in recent years, however, for it has been shown that inconsistency among them, however highly trained and experienced they may be, is quite common. Even the same man is liable to be inconsistent in his observations of the same thing on different occasions.[9]

These inconsistencies were not entirely of a quantitative nature, but were often qualitative. Abnormal shadows in a chest film were seen on one occasion, but not on another, simply due to faulty observation. This variability among experienced clinical observers attracted attention due to the increasing use of group experiments in which rigid diagnostic criteria were needed; as a result medical research workers are now quite aware of the possibility of errors of observation. The remedy, of course, has been to have the test done by two or more independent observers. Observer bias, that error introduced unconsciously when the observer knows what result he wants, is safeguarded against by not allowing the observer to know what results are favorable. And so the development of the double blind approach evolved.

The scientific and clinical basis of epidemiological research involves the measurement of the magnitude of causal effects in disease production. With the exception of clinical trials, epidemiology is basically an observational rather than a manipulative science, and thus is enormously susceptible to a wide range of variable parameters. Regarding data on the presence or absence of disease in individuals, the epidemiology data is often based on clinical-type observations, as discussed above, and incorporates their inherent variability.[10]

Animal toxicologic studies possess several components utilizing comparable observational techniques. In the antemortem phase, physical examination and digital palpation are relied on for detection of cutaneous and subcutaneous tissue masses (often improperly referred to as "tumors"), as well as certain disturbances of the neurologic, digestive, and special sense organ systems.

This data base is usefully supplemented by quantitative

measurements of selected chemical factors in body fluids or tissues.

The entire postmortem workup consists of a series of events employing trained observers; each event (gross necropsy; specimen trimming and processing for microscopic evaluation; histopathologic assessment), with few exceptions, generates a data base comprised entirely of observations by trained observers. These observations provide crucial data for safety assessment. Using experience in clinical medicine as an example, however, it is axiomatic that considerable observer variance will be encountered. As quoted previously from Stone, "---inconsistency among (experienced observers), however highly trained and experienced they may be, is quite common." Thus it is misleading and absurd to expect complete consistency in data generated by procedures based on trained observation. The confusion is further compounded by wide differences in the interpretation of such data. What potential impact does the data have on the morbidity and/or mortality of that species, and on other mammalian species? The state of the art in laboratory animal toxicology studies would be immeasurably improved if those involved would grasp the real nature of this problem, and then devise new means of successfully minimizing its impact. Only then might the expectations of other scientific disciplines and the general public be reconciled to the inherent limitations and the actual capabilities of the animal toxicology assessment team.

D. How much is safe?

The comparative strengths and weaknesses of individual components of the scientific process currently employed to determine which chemicals are noxious, and how to protect the public from them.

Safety assessment studies in laboratory animals provide data on adverse effects. Subsequently, to predict the risk of such effects occurring in humans, extrapolations from these animal data to the human species are performed. Limitations inherent in the lab animal database were identified and discussed above.

Pharmacokinetic and metabolism data in animal and man, as available, are assessed to determine the relative similarity with which the test agent is handled by these species. Although otherwise strong, the pharmacokinetics database usually is limited to a few individual subjects, may show considerable sample variance, and thus suffers from the real possibility of being a biased sample not truly representative of the test species population.

Again excepting rigorous prospective clinical studies, the detection and diagnosis of many human diseases incorporates observer variability of undefined, possibly large, magnitude. This weakens the clinical database, which in turn is employed by the epidemiologist in the characterization of the magnitude of chemical causality of a given disease entity. Thus, a potentially large component of observer variance repeatedly weakens the various databases employed in predicting and verifying human risk to a given chemical agent.

E.   The Relative Reliability of the Toxicologic Pathology Component of the Laboratory Animal Safety Database.

Presuming that properly trained personnel are employed throughout the entire postmortem assessment procedure of the animal toxicologic study, the probability of observer error should be similar to that occurring in opthalmoscopy, physical diagnosis, or similar clinical-type procedures performed during the antemortem phase. The absolute number of errors would be higher, if the number of observations is higher. Errors occurring during the postmortem workup may have greater impact on the total database, however, since no corroborating measurement offsets their effect. Thus, while histopathology data may supplement, complement, verify or refute antemortem data indicating an abnormality, no such backup is available for the pathologist. A lesion missed at necropsy is gone forever; a lesion overlooked or mis-diagnosed microscopically will remain uncorrected.

How might these weaknesses be averted? In the absence of established explicit training requirements for the pathologists' subordinate staff, correction is unlikely. Development of suitable certifiable training programs for each and every position, including necropsy prosector and specimen trimmer, would be a start. Maintaining highly motivated personnel is important. The routine use of structured, disciplined vocabularies for both gross and microscopic pathology would facilitate both intra- and inter- laboratory quality control programs. Meaningful continuing education requirements for all personnel would tend to maintain competence and stimulate career interest. These steps are long over-

due in toxicologic pathology. Lastly, the routine use of electronic data processing systems would notably reduce transcription errors, and greatly facilitate summary tabulation and manipulation
of anatomical pathology data.

The incessant scrutiny of the toxicologic pathologist's findings,
when conducted in a political arena as so often occurs when safety
issues are debated, requires that a major departure from conventional pathology assessment procedures be employed in research
studies supporting these activities. This will doubtless increase
the cost of such studies, but it is a necessary investment.

II. LIMITATIONS, PROBLEMS AND CHALLENGES OF TOXICOLOGIC PATHOLOGY.
  A. Diagnostic Difficulties:

Pathology is a subjective science and as such provides many opportunities for differences in opinion regarding specific lesions.
This is in particular the case with experimental pathology where
human lives are not immediately at stake. It is indeed unfortunate
that personal ambitions, lack of experience or discrimination and
other factors have, through inappropriate release of data not adequately reviewed, enhanced the divergence of opinions. This has
created in the minds of the public a cynical attitude toward legitimate efforts to identify potential toxic or carcinogenic chemicals in our environment. This is most obvious but not limited to
the unpublished reports of the Bioassay program of the National
Cancer Institute where an apparent lack of critical review has been
most obvious.

There will continue to be a divergence of opinion, a cynical view
of scientific studies in safety evaluation and a frustrated, confused public until or unless the scientific community, (government, academia, industry and others) agrees to cooperate in a
meaningful way toward a resolution of specific problems.
                    This must be accompanied by an adequate assess-
ment of results of studies (prior to releasing them) which are not
clearcut but which may have significant societal impact.

Adherence to simple professional ethics would resolve many of
the problems of disagreement in toxicologic pathology. In the
meantime those concerned about and charged with protecting the

public interest and safety, must continue to evaluate chemicals in
the most appropriate systems available, despite the fact that analytical expertise has far outstripped abilities to interpret results and correlate analytical and biologic data. In this presentation we will point out certain limitations, problems, and
challenges of toxicologic pathology. We will consider difficulties
in the diagnosis and interpretation of selected lesions, as model
examples, in a few organs about which there is frequent disagreement. Selected examples will include lesions observed, spontaneously or as a result of treatment in the liver, adrenal, thyroid,
and lymphoreticular system.

B. Liver

No single organ in comparative pathology has provided more controversy in toxicologic pathology than the liver of rodents. Perhaps this is in part because it has a limited number of morphologic expressions in response to injury and because it has a unique
propensity for replacing cells that are injured and lost from whatever cause. In addition the liver is the central focus for the
detoxification of compounds that are produced within the body and
those that are introduced from outside. Some of the confusing and
perplexing liver changes noted in animals exposed to drugs and
chemicals appear to be related in one way or another to attempts
by the liver parenchymal cell to dispose of foreign chemicals
through detoxification mechanisms residing in microsomal enzyme
systems. This is not to infer however that bile duct hyperplasia,
fibrosis, cholangiofibrosis, scarring, and other forms of morphologic expression of injury are not legitimate evidence of a response to toxic materials; many toxic agents are not enzyme inducers and the liver responds in other ways.

In the context of this presentation and in toxicologic pathology,
rodents are most important because they are most widely used, and
it is the liver lesions observed in these species that seemingly
create most problems and controversy in attempts to evaluate them.
Comments and illustrations presented here will therefore be restricted to the rat and the mouse as they are used in safety evaluations of drugs, foods and chemicals. Table 1 lists the incidence of spontaneous tumors in some strains of rats and although
all of these will not be addressed, the data may be useful from a
historical viewpoint.

TABLE 1

SPONTANEOUS TUMORS IN UNTREATED RATS USED IN CHRONIC SAFETY EVALUATIONS[1]

	Strain/Incidence/Number Affected/%							
	Fischer		O.M.[a]		S.D.[b]		C.R.[c]	
	M	F	M	F	M	F	M	F
	2370	2070	320	242	760	540	390	367
Lung	11.2	4.7	--	--	--	--	1.8	2.0
Liver	1.4	2.9	--	2.0	--	0.3	1.0	1.9
Kidney	0.2	0.2	3.0	3.2	3.2	--	1.4	--
Islets of Pancreas	0.9	0.8	2.2	1.6	0.7	0.6	2.5	1.1
Pituitary	12.5	31.6	7.2	24.1	10.4	35.0	36.2	60.4
Adrenal	10.4	3.8	9.8	3.6	1.2	3.1	8.2	5.0
Thyroid	6.6	7.3	5.4	12.1	2.1	1.7	3.5	2.1
Lymphoma/ Leukemia	12.1	10.2	1.8	2.0	3.5	4.5	2.5	1.8

[1] Compiled from studies in our laboratory and from National Cancer Institute Bioassay Reports.
[a] Osborne-Mendel.
[b] Sprague-Dawley.
[c] Charles-River.

Rat Liver.

The rat appears to be somewhat less responsive to the effects of chemicals and other noxious agents, in terms of liver changes, compared to the mouse. The rat liver will respond to a number of toxins and carcinogens in a rather predictable way. The usual response to a toxin that results in minimal if any liver cell necrosis is bile duct hyperplasia. Figure 1 is characteristic of a response of rat liver to a number of natural and synthetic toxins; this is not a specific lesion and will often regress or remain static if the inciting agent is removed. Bile duct hyperplasia is considered a non-specific response to exposure to toxins and in our opinion represents a physiologic mechanism designed to enhance the elimination of the toxin or its metabolites.

Nodular hyperplasia is a response of the parenchymal cells to injury and cell death. This can be considered compensatory hyperplasia resulting from a loss of parenchymal cells and replacement

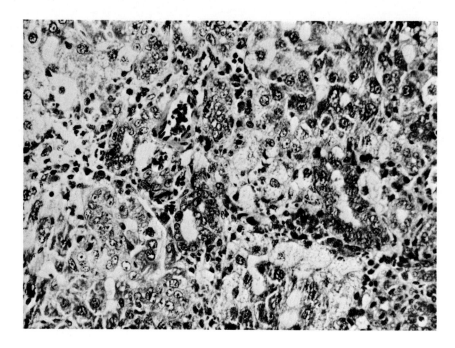

Fig. 1. Bile duct hyperplasia typical of response of the liver
to toxic materials.

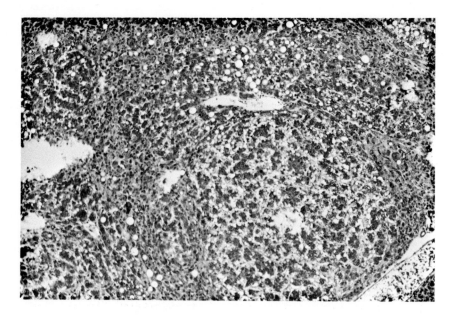

Fig. 2. Nodular hyperplasia, a benign lesion characteristic of a
response to injury and cell death; a compensatory device.

of these cells by physiologic mechanisms. (Figure 2). While based upon a pathologic change, namely cell injury, this lesion is benign and, at least in the rat, if the noxious agent is removed hyperplastic nodules will often regress. The nodules are not transplantable and do not meet standard criteria for neoplasia. Such nodules have been induced by phenobarbitone, a substance not considered to be a carcinogen,[11] and by a whole host of chemicals usually given in high doses which result in liver necrosis.

Whether hyperplastic nodules can be induced by noncarcinogenic chemicals other than phenobarbitone is not known. Dietary deficiencies can induce nodular, hyperplastic liver (cirrhosis) in rats but do not appear to produce hyperplastic nodules. The distinction is that hyperplastic nodules are hyperplastic in comparison to the remaining liver parenchyma whereas the hyperplasia in precirrhotic and cirrhotic liver of deficient rats is diffuse and increased cell division and numbers are present in both nodular and non-nodular parenchymal cells.

The nodular hyperplasia that is induced by dietary means[12] has been shown to regress if the diet is supplemented and further, even under the most severe dietary stress, the nodules never progress to liver cell carcinoma.[13]

In our experience, nodular hyperplasia is neither a necessary nor sufficient change to result in the induction of liver cell carcinoma. This is not to infer however that it may not be a step toward development of liver cell carcinoma, and the question about whether or not nodular hyperplasia is a pre-neoplastic lesion is unresolved.

A discussion of the sequence of events that may lead to liver cell carcinoma has been reviewed and illustrated using aflatoxin B_1 as the model system.[14] We believe that liver cell carcinoma can arise directly from the parenchyma without prior nodular hyperplasia (Figure 3). On the other hand, we also feel that some liver cell cancers do arise within hyperplastic nodules, probably as an event associated with but not necessarily dependent upon nodular hyperplasia. Transformed cells are likely present in nodular and non-nodular regenerating areas alike and some from either focus can go on to carcinoma. Liver cell carcinoma may be found in three generally distinct morphologic forms, namely, well-differentiated hepatocellular carcinoma, trabecular carcinoma and anaplastic carcin-

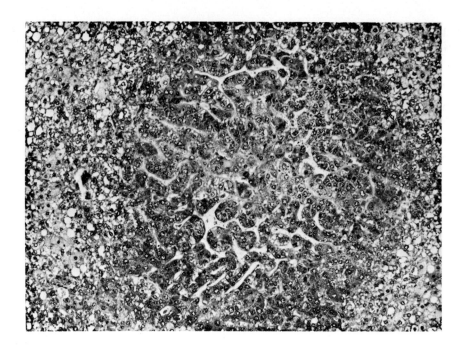

Fig. 3. A liver cell carcinoma arising from parenchyma without progressing through nodular hyperplasia.

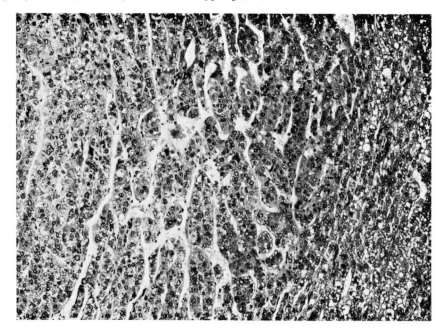

Fig. 4. Trabecular carcinoma most often encountered in rodent liver. These tumors are intermediate in malignancy but often metastasize.

oma. In our experience, it is the trabecular carcinoma (Figure 4)
that is most common in the rat as a result of exposure to liver
cell carcinogens. There are disagreements among pathologists as
to the nature of some liver lesions in the rat (such as distin-
guishing between hyperplastic nodules and adenoma), but in general,
disagreements in diagnosis of hepatocellular carcinoma, are minimal. Experienced pathologists have little difficulty in arriving
at a diagnosis. There is a tendency, however, for some pathologists to overdiagnose liver lesions, perhaps to avoid controversy
and because they feel that potentially pre-neoplastic lesions always become tumors. The practice of referring to hyperplastic
nodules and adenomas as "neoplastic nodules"[15] is regrettable;
there is nothing to be gained by inventing new terms to describe
lesions, the descriptions of which are well ingrained in pathologic nomenclature historically. There may be some utility however, for regulatory agencies to lump all nodules together and
classify them as "neoplastic" since this facilitates assigning a
chemical to the category of a carcinogen, even though this may not
always be justified.

Mouse Liver

   Mouse liver nodules are controversial; they occur in most strains
of mice, either as spontaneous or induced lesions. Hyperplastic
nodules occur in the liver of mice just   as in rats, and the
same criteria for assessment and diagnosis should apply to the
mouse as to the rat. Hyperplastic nodules are comprised of proliferating cells, derived from the parenchyma, and are related
for the most part to necrosis and compensatory hyperplasia. In
the case of the mouse, however, compared to the rat there seems to
be a greater propensity to overrespond with consequent formation
of a nodule. There is an abundance of convincing evidence which
clearly indicates that hyperplastic nodules in the mouse do not
necessarily progress to liver cell carcinoma any more than they
do in the rat. Table 2 lists a classification of liver lesions
in $B_6C_3F_1$ hybrid mice used for NCI Bioassay studies with heptachlor. The disagreement amongst contract laboratory pathologists,

NCI pathologists and others led to a request for the
National Academy of Sciences to assemble a group of independent
qualified pathologists to give their opinion of the lesions.
According to the classification of this group, hyperplasia of the
liver increased with increasing dose of heptachlor but there was
not a concomitant increase in hepatocellular carcinoma. This would
seem to indicate that the necrosis incurred by high dietary concentrations of heptachlor resulted in compensatory hyperplasia and
nodule formation but that this hyperplasia did not go on to carcinoma.

TABLE 2

CLASSIFICATION OF LIVER LESIONS IN $B_6C_3F_1$, MICE, NATIONAL ACADEMY
OF SCIENCES PIREC, ASSOCIATED WITH HEPTACHLOR

Heptachlor Concentration	Hyperplasia		Hepatocarcinoma[1]	
	M	F	M	F
None (Control)	3/19	1/10	2/19	0/10
Low Dose	11/45	3/44	3/45	0/44
High Dose	22/45	21/42	2/45	2/42

[1] In reviewing studies in this strain of hybrid mouse in our laboratories and from the NCI Bioassay Program, incidence of spontaneous liver tumors ranges from 8 to 49%.

Recent studies in our laboratory have shown that necrosis
(table 3) resulting from an excessive level of another pesticide
resulted in a dose related hyperplasia but did not increase liver
carcinomas. This is in agreement with the data in table 2.

There are other factors which can influence the incidence of
nodules. Gellatly[16] has shown that spontaneous mouse liver nodules can be increased significantly by an increase in the amount
of dietary fat (table 4), but that carcinoma increased only when
a carcinogen was superimposed.

The question of the influence of necrosis is still an open and
important one. It is interesting to note that a concern for the
role of injury and repair or chronic irritation in the etiology of
cancer, has been around for more than fifty years.[17,18] This concept has recently attracted renewed interest and a variety of types

TABLE 3.

EFFECT OF PESTICIDE LEVEL, NECROSIS, HYPERPLASIA, AND HEPATOCELLULAR CARCINOMA IN MICE[1]

| Dose Level | Necrosis | Incidence, Hepatocellular | |
		Hyperplasia	Carcinoma
None	0/20	0/20	1/20
Low	0/20	0/20	0/20
Medium	8/20	6/20	0/20
High	20/20	17/20	1/20

[1]Following 54 weeks exposure.

of injury have been related to an enhancement of liver carcinogenesis.[12,19,20] This has been referred to as the principle of "secondary carcinogenesis" and may be one of the consequences of non-specific tissue damage. This often occurs when the maximum tolerated dose of a chemical is administered; such mechanisms may account for the results seen in some carcinogenesis studies, particularly those in which the maximum tolerated dose (MTD) is used. In fact, this concept was used by the Food and Drug Administration in its deliberations as to whether or not to allow the addition of selenium to animal foods. Selenium is an essential trace element for animals, but at high doses it has been associated with liver damage and hepatocellular carcinoma.[22,23]

The principle of secondary carcinogenesis may well be applied in a much broader way when sufficient knowledge about it is available. Its implications have not been adequately explored but the production of cancer by secondary mechanisms is an instance where the end result is not necessarily an indication of the potential of a compound for producing cancer. In considering the case for selenium for example, the Commissioner of the Food and Drug Administration alluded to the consumption of alcohol and pointed out that this "is associated with a higher incidence of liver cirrhosis which in turn is associated with a higher incidence of liver cancer. Other common agents, at high levels, may produce the same result," and the Commissioner concluded that such substances "are not by reason of their capacity to induce liver damage when abused by being consumed at high levels, properly classified as carcino-

genic because of their potential association with a higher rate of
liver cancer." We believe that this same phenomenon may well be
operating in some of the mouse carcinogenesis studies particularly
with those compounds which induce microsomal enzymes and which, at
high dietary levels result in marked necrosis of the liver paren-
cymal cells. We have in fact, conducted studies in rats which
support the Commissioner's views about selenium (table 5).

TABLE 4.

DIET, BUTTER YELLOW AND HEPATIC NODULES IN MICE

Type of Diet	Type of Nodule	
	Types 1&2 (Benign)	Type 3 (Malignant)
Natural Product Type Diet	9	3
Semi-purified Diet, Groundnut oil 5%	30	2
Semi-purified Diet, Groundnut oil 10%	62	5
Semi-purified Diet, +0.06% Butter Yellow	100	79

From Gellatly in Butler & Newberne, 1975. % Survival with nodules.

TABLE 5.

SECONDARY EFFECT OF SELENIUM IN RATS ON LIVER CARCINOGENESIS BY
AFLATOXIN B_1

Group	Treatment (PPM) AFB$_1$	Selenium	Liver Injury	Nodular Hyperplasia	Hepatocellular Carcinoma
1	–	0.05	0	0	0/20
2	+	0.10	0	0	0/20
3	+	0.50	0	0	0/20
4	+	1.00	0	0	0/20
5	+	2.00	0	1/20	0/20
6	+	3.50	+	3/20	0/20
7	+	5.00	+	20/20	14/20

Aflatoxin B$_1$ was administered after eight weeks on diet, 5 daily
doses of 10 micrograms each. Rats were kept on respective diets
for 12 months.

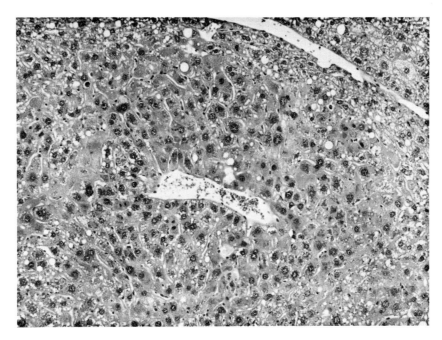

Fig. 5. Centrilobular hypertrophy, pleomorphism of nuclei and hepatocellular necrosis in mouse liver exposed to a potent enzyme inducer.

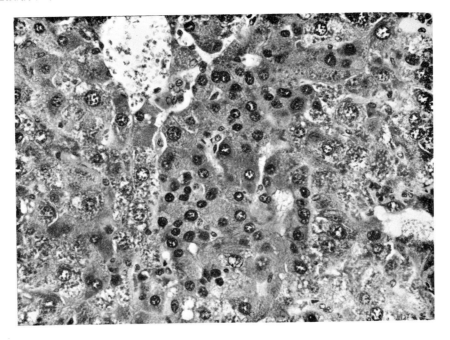

Fig. 6. Centrilobular zone of liver of mouse. Hypertrophy and necrosis is followed by focal hyperplasia of parenchyma, the early beginning of nodule formation.

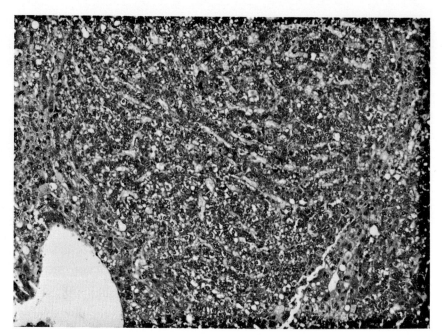

Fig. 7. Hyperplastic nodule of mouse which developed adjacent to
the central vein where hypertrophy, necrosis and parenchymal cell
proliferation can be identified.

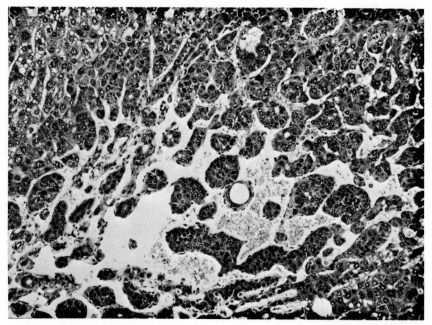

Fig. 8. Trabecular liver cell carcinoma induced by aflatoxin B_1 in
a hybrid mouse. These tumors often metastasize and exhibit other
criteria of malignancy. Most tumors associated with centrilobular
hypertrophy and necrosis in the enzyme induced mouse liver do not
appear malignant nor do they satisfy other criteria of neoplasia.

There is very little disagreement amongst experimental pathologists and those dealing with carcinogenesis about the liver lesions
that occur in animals exposed to true carcinogens. The disagreement is about those lesions that appear histologically benign, are
different morphologically from classical liver cell cancer and generally do not fulfill criteria which most of us believe necessary
to establish that a tumor is malignant. The chlorinated hydrocarbons are examples of chemicals which induce lesions difficult
to interpret; the enzyme inducer pehnobarbitone is another.[11,27]
Phenabarbitone not only produces extensive centrilobular hypertrophy, a result of enzyme induction, but also at high doses, results in significant necrosis, after a sufficient time period. It
has also produced liver cell carcinoma in the mouse, but not in
the rat.[11] It appears that phenobarbitone produces a low grade
liver injury with focal necrosis and bile duct proliferation; eventually, small focal areas of hyperplasia develop, usually in the
centrilobular zone where enzyme induction, hypertrophy and necrosis has occurred. These lesions are identical morphologically to
those seen in animals fed one of several of the chlorinated pesticides; this is also the case with other chemicals which induce
microsomal enzymes. We have found a similar pattern of enzyme induction, centrilobular hypertrophy, necrosis, and nodular hyperplasia in the centrilobular zone, associated with a chemical, a potent enzyme inducer, used in some chronic studies recently in our
laboratory. These lesions are clearly different from those produced by known hepatic carcinogens, such as the nitrosamines or
the aflatoxins. A sequence of morphologic changes appears to precede formation of hyperplastic nodules. First, there is a marked
centrilobular hypertrophy (Figure 5) nuclear pleomorphism, and
necrosis. After a period of time, this is followed by focal hyperplasia of the parenchyma (Figure 6). With continued exposure to
the chemical these foci become nodules (Figure 7) and may be sufficiently large to distort the architecture of the liver. Whether
or not these are the progenitors of liver cell carcinoma is not
clear at this time. There is however a clear difference in the
morphology between lesions such as these and those such as trabecular carcinoma that are produced by aflatoxin or some of the
nitrosamines (Figure 8). Therefore, one should use caution in the
interpretation of lesions that occur in livers of mice where

enzyme induction, cellular necrosis and compensatory proliferation
are common and concommitant findings.

C. Thyroid

Table 1 lists the incidence of tumors observed in four strains
of untreated rats. Variation in the incidence of thyroid lesions
in the several strains is notable. The types of lesions that are
usually observed in the thyroid of rats are divided roughly into
two groups, based on derivation namely, follicular (figure 9) and
interstitial or "C" cell tumors.

There is a secondary mech-
anism of carcinogenesis in the thyroid gland. Table 1 illustrates
that thyroid tumors in untreated rats of the various strains
ranges from around 2% to as much as 12%. Obviously, this would be
of concern when examining the effects on rats of a chemical that
might be related to thyroid function.

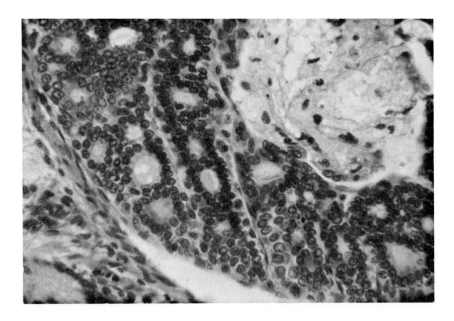

Fig. 9. Thyroid adenocarcinoma found in an untreated rat. While
this neoplasm had not metastasized, many of them do.

It is a simple matter to produce thyroid hyperplasia in rats by dietary goitrogens, sulfonamides, and other anti-thyroid agents.[28] It is well-known that if anti-thyroid action is continued long enough there will be thyroid follicular epithelial hyperplasia; this in turn can lead to neoplasia, the mechanism by which simple iodine deficiency elicits thyroid cancer in rats.[26,27] While this mechanism of iodine deficiency results in thyroid cancer in rats, it apparently does not lead to thyroid cancer in people.[26]

In view of these observations, some strains of rats are unsuitable for studies of thyroid hyperplasia and carcinogenesis, the results of which are expected to be extrapolated to man. Based on what is known at this point, we cannot use thyroid hyperplasia to predict development of thyroid carcinoma. This is borne out in studies that show that cessation of exposure to anti-thyroid agents usually will result in regression of hyperplasia.[29] These hyperplastic conditions are dose dependent and the etiological agents fall into the same category as many toxicological agents.

D. Adrenal Gland

The adrenal gland is subject to hyperplasia of either the cortex or the medullary zone, this may be spontaneous or under the influence of known stimulating agents. It is a difficult matter to assess the effects of a given chemical on the adrenal gland of most strains of rats because of the high incidence of these lesions in untreated rats. For example, in our experience the Fischer rat has an incidence of about 10% in the male and about 5% in the female (table 1). Osborne-Mendel rats have an incidence rate of about 10% in male and about 3% in female. The Charles River CD strain has an incidence rate of about 8% in male and 5% in female. For this reason it is a difficult task to separate out the effects of a chemical on the incidence of such lesions from the lesions that would be there spontaneously in untreated animals. Hyperplasia of the cortex of the adrenal is a common phenomenon and is usually accorded little significance. Pheochromocytomas (figure 10) or lesser degrees of medullary hyperplasia, are often noted in publications but from photographic illustrations these lesions range anywhere from minimal hyperplasia to a characteristic tumor replacing most if not all of a medullary zone. It therefore is difficult, if not impossible to assess from the literature what

246

actually has been observed; for this reason we attach little significance to the designation of adrenal tumors. We have as well
concluded that they are non-functional tumors in the rat and of
little importance. In some cases however, such as those where
an agent is a depleter of catecholamines (reserpine) one might
expect to observe medullary hyperplasia.

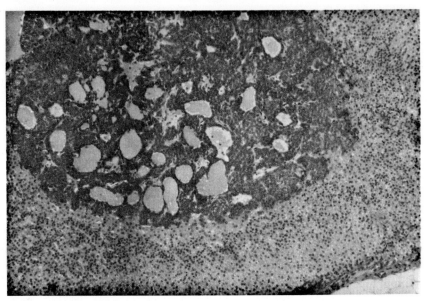

Fig. 10. Pheochromocytoma of the adrenal of the rat. These
tumors are not rare in the rat but the biological significance is
obscure.

E.   Lymphoreticular and Hematopoietic System Tumors

These are tumors of the spleen,   lymph nodes and bone marrow.
In mice the thymus gland is a frequent site. Lymphoreticular tumors can develop at any site where lymphatic cells are found
(spleen, liver, bone marrow, Peyers patches, and thymus). Table 1
lists the incidence of leukemia and/or lymphoma in various strains
of rats and it is obvious that most of them have a significant
spontaneous incidence. For example, the male Fischer rat has about
12% and the female about 10%; other strains range anywhere from
about 2% to 5% incidence. Thymic lymphoma, myeloid leukemia and
reticulum cell sarcoma are most common forms observed in various
strains of mice.[30] This means that there is a background incidence
of significance and that   rodents will develop lymphoma and
lymphoreticular tumors without imposing any type of treatment.

These are important types of neoplasms but as yet they have been very poorly studied in the rodent, except in those cases where they have been used for carcinogenesis investigations. For this reason we have litte information on initiation, progression and overall implication of lymphoreticular tumors in regard to the safety of chemicals. Dunn[31] has provided the best description of tumors of the reticular tissue in mice; Squire et al have described the disease in rats.[32]

Recently we have shown that the administration of sodium nitrite markedly increased the incidence of lymphoreticular tumors in Sprague-Dawley rats.[33] There was about 4% incidence in controls and up to 15% incidence in treated rats. The results need confirmation in other rat strains and other species because the potential impact is significant. Classification of the tumors, which differ in some respects from the spontaneous lymphoreticular tumor in rats, and morphologic identification of precursor lesions are areas of experimental pathology in which we are interested and plan to perform studies.

III. SUGGESTIONS: MANAGEMENT OF HISTOLOGIC EVALUATION OF SOCIO-
    ECONOMICALLY SENSITIVE TESTS.

In view of the critical nature of the subject and a necessity to assume a positive approach, we propose, as an alternative to current practice a procedure for conducting a joint histopathologic assessment of necropsy findings in every animal toxicologic study with expected broad socio-economic impact:

1) The Director, National Toxicology Program will identify each animal toxicology study which has broad socio-economic impact, based on recommendations by the study sponsor and/or the study Pathologist, or by the government regulatory agency(s) to whom the study report is to be submitted. This joint histopathology assessment procedure, and this procedure only, will apply to each such study.

2) All histopathologic sections (slides) from such a study will be independently evaluated and reported by the designated study Pathologist and by a second Pathologist selected by the study Sponsor, with the concurrence of the study Pathologist. This second Pathologist will not be an employee of the study Sponsor. A

single agreed-on diagnostic syllabus will be employed by both Pathologists. Each pathologist will prepare a final draft report of
histopathologic findings for such study, and submit each report
promptly to the Pathology Referee (item 3, below).

3) The study Pathology Referee will be selected by joint concurrence of the two study Pathologists, from a list of several can-
didate pathologists prepared independently and exchanged by the
two Pathologists. The role of the Pathology Referee involves
identification of each diagnostic disagreement between the two
final draft pathology reports, and reconciling those disagreements
by joint discussion sessions between the two pathologists; this
assures that acceptable professional ethics are used throughout.
No information regarding the nature of the histopathologic findings of the study is to be released by anyone in any form prior to
the completion of the final joint pathology report (see item 4,
below).

4) The goal of this entire procedure is to produce a final pathology report reflecting the combined scientific expertise of two
pathologists initially working independently and subsequently
working jointly to eliminate apparent but unsubstantial differences of diagnostic opinion, and to reduce to a minimum and to
clearly identify those scientific disagreements that were ir-
reconcilable, if such exist. The Pathology Referee does not provide independent scientific judgement regarding diagnostic dis-
putes, but rather arbitrates such matters, thus assuring the Pathologists involved and ultimately the study Sponsor, interested
and involved government institutions, and the general public that
proper professional ethics were adhered to throughout the diagnostic data reconciliation process.

5) A single final histopathology report will be prepared, signed
and dated by the two Pathologists and the Pathology Referee, and
submitted to the study Sponsor. At this point the Pathology Referee will notify the Office of the Director, NTP that the joint
pathology report for this study has been compiled, as required,
and will return the two draft final pathology reports to their
respective authors.

6) After completion of step 5, above, the pathology report may be
divulged by the study Sponsor, consistent with regulatory requirements affecting such study.

7) The cost of this joint histopathologic assessment will be borne
entirely by the study Sponsor.

   Contrary to initial impression, it is expected that implementation of this procedure would reduce, rather than increase, the
total cost of scientific evaluation and reporting of histopathology
data from an animal study having broad socio-economic impact. It
would accomplish this through eliminating the confusion and discordance related to apparent, but unsubstantive, diagnostic differences and by minimizing errors or omissions due to oversight
or momentary lapse by a single pathologist. Completion of the
final study report would not be notably delayed for those studies
identified promptly, since joint histopathologic review will proceed essentially in parallel.

   The primary purpose, however, is to provide the Pathologist and
the public with assurance that professional ethics and due care
were exercised throughout the entire histopathology process which
culminated in submission of the joint pathology report. Likewise,
both pathologists could be jointly available for subsequent con-
sultation with regulatory agencies or other interested parties,
as appropriate. We believe that implementation of this process,
or a suitable modification thereof, deserves the prompt attention
of relevant professional organizations as a high priority item.
Such procedures would significantly reduce the problems and con-
troversies which now surround reports from government sponsored
studies and eliminate or at least control those concerned with
personal interests as opposed to the public good.

IV. PROCEDURAL RECOMMENDATIONS IN CONDUCTING THE POSTMORTEM WORKUP
   There are a number of procedural problems in handling the experimental animal once it has reached the end of the study and is
ready for necropsy, processing, and completion of the necessary
histologic evaluation and final reports. A number of general constraints are in effect, some obvious and some not so obvious. In
the following pages we will lead the reader through the major considerations and concerns involved in moving the animal and its
invaluable tissues through the chain of events from necropsy to the
final report. Figure 11, by use of specific impact points of procedures, illustrates in a graphic manner the major compartments,
as we see them, which are essential to successful completion of

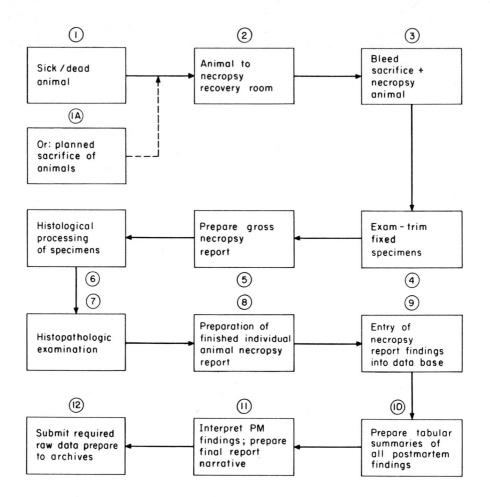

Fig. 11. Procedural problems in conducting the post-mortem workup at end of study include a number of activities and special personnel needs. At each step, significant procedures must be conducted accurately in moving the animal and its valuable tissues through the chain of events from necropsy to final report. A gap at any point can result in loss of invaluable data necessary for an accurate, acceptable report. The text describes the individual steps in detail.

the final process. The following considerations are worthy of comment, relating to the requirements and the expertise essential to completing the process.

General Constraints

A. The ready availability of personnel with demonstrated competence for performing each link in the chain of events contributes immeasurably toward achieving a high quality operation and result.

B. Involvement of the same multi-skilled individuals for performing successive procedural steps increases the risk of introducing errors, through reducing the number of independent checks on accuracy.

C. The use of personnel not possessing demonstrated competence for any of the procedural steps markedly increases the risk of error and notably reduces the liklihood of achieving even a medium quality operation.

D. The availability and use of job training manuals for each procedural step, with personnel certification following demonstration of stipulated skills to professional staff, enables proper assignment of personnel. Professional staff are thus responsible for the adequacy of training manuals and the skills certification procedures. Certification by appropriate professional organizations may eventually replace, totally or in part, the need for on-site certification of skills.

Using figure 11 as a guide, we can go through procedural processes step-by-step. In each step we'll identify key functions included, and key personnel required.

Step 1. Sick or dead animal observed. This step includes; identification of the animal; comprehensive review of prior clinical observations records; a professional decision regarding sacrifice; preparation of a clinical findings summary, a necropsy record form; and deletion of the animal from the antemortem database. It requires: availability of an experienced animal research technician and a professional staff member. The incomplete summary of prior physical examinations may result in failure to examine in detail and comment on a particular anatomical site at necropsy. For manual systems, a master diagram of cage rack layout should be stored with the prepared necropsy forms; the technician initials and dates   the diagram in the appropriate cage box upon removal of the necropsy form.

Step 1A. Planned sacrifice of many animals. This step <u>includes</u>: identification of each animal; preparation of a clinical findings summary and a necropsy record form for each animal; deletion of each animal from the antemortem database. It <u>requires</u>: the same personnel as in step 1, above. The availability of several personnel facilitates immediate cross-checking of the accuracy of each activity.

Step 2. Delivery of the animal to the necropsy receiving room. This step <u>includes</u>: verification of animal identification and necropsy form accuracy; a decision regarding animal preservation prior to necropsy; review of project protocol; preparation of necropsy instruments and supplies package, including labeling of specimen containers. It <u>requires</u>: the availability of a necropsy assistant trained in reviewing project necropsy protocols, preparing necessary specimen containers and instruments, and in identifying animals. The project protocol, through inclusion of Standard Operating Procedures (SOP) must stipulate dead animal storage conditions in case the necropsy cannot be performed immediately.

Step 3. Bleed, sacrifice, and necropsy the animal. This step <u>includes</u>; the need to identify the animal; perform body fluid collection techniques; perform gross prosection and lesion description procedures. It <u>requires</u>; the availability of a necropsy prosector with established ability to detect and describe gross lesions, and to select appropriate specimens; a pathologist to provide supervision/consultation, as necessary. This is the most crucial single step in the postmortem process; if improperly performed, the loss cannot be rectified. This step delimits what the pathologist will examine microscopically.

Step 4. Examination and trimming of fixed tissues. This step <u>includes</u>: a need to read and understand descriptions of fresh gross lesions; to accurately identify fixed specimens of normal organs and/or lesions; to properly trim, orient, and package specimens according to nature and pre-determined procedure; to detect, describe, and select specimens from previously undetected gross lesions. It <u>requires</u>: the availability of personnel competent in identifying gross specimens; trimming them as necessary for optimal predescribed orientation; detecting and describing previously unrecorded lesions; packaging specimens in stipulated sequence; and reliably ascertaining the presence/absence of all specimens required by the necropsy protocol. The mechanical skills for this job are available in experienced histology technicians; to acquire both mechanical and judgemental skills neccessary, an experienced necropsy prosector must be specially trained. This step provides an excellent opportunity for a Quality Assurance (QA) check on each necropsy prosector's performance; records from such routine performance evaluation are a suitable data source for auditing the quality of the postmortem procedure to this point. This specimen trimming step, if improperly performed, will place severe limitations on subsequent histopathologic examination and interpretation.

Step 5. Prepare a report of gross necropsy findings. This step includes: a need to read, transcribe, and proof-read longhand accurately, when manual data reduction and transcription are employed; an ability to process a machine-readable form when an electronic data processing system (e.g. mark-sense) is employed for data reduction. It requires: the availability of an experienced typist for data transcription, and a pathologist for data proofreading and sign-off, if a manual system is employed; an experienced technician to process machine-readable input forms, and a pathologist to review and approve by sign-off, if an electronic data processing (EDP) system is employed. Risk of data-handling error is markedly reduced by use of machine-readable records. Approved gross necropsy records are filed with the histology laboratory supervisor.

Step 6. Histological processing of specimens. This step includes: a need to dehydrate, embed, section, mount, and stain tissue specimens, and to maintain appropriate records. It requires: an availability of histology technicians with demonstrated competence. This step is highly vulnerable to specimen mix-up errors, and to loss of small lesions due to improper orientation during embedding or to destruction of the face of the block during sectioning. Additionally, the quality of the preparation examined by the pathologist is, in large part, determined during this step. A meticulous inventory of the number and nature of tissue slides per animal should be completed prior to releasing the slides for histo-

pathologic assessment. Missing specimens should be clearly indicated on the gross necropsy report for that animal.

Step 7. Histopathologic examination. This step includes: a need
to accurately diagnose lesions microscopically and record findings.
It requires the availability of a competent pathologist. A diagnosis or other statement must be recorded for each lesion observed
grossly; missing specimens must be indicated.

Step 8. Preparation of the finished individual animal necropsy
record. This step includes: a need to transcribe longhand or dic-
tated histopathologic findings to a typed report; a need to accurately proof-read such report against the draft copy; comparison
of gross vs. microscopic findings for errors of omission or commission; substantiate the validity of the report by initialing
and dating. It requires: the availability of a competence typist
and proof-reader pathologist, if manual data handling is employed;
machine-readable input requires only a data-input technician, and
the pathologist to read the report. Irrespective of method, the
pathologist must reconcile gross and microscopic findings, correct
any oversights or errors, and substantiate the validity of the
necropsy report by initialing and dating. This latter step, if
properly performed, will eliminate much confusion and will markedly up-grade the quality of the postmortem operation. If not
properly performed, it may cause confusion and even suspicion of
the entire postmortem process. This data reconciliation procedure
is a crucial step in assuring the integrity and quality of the
postmortem report on each animal.

Step 9. Entry of necropsy report findings into the database.
This step includes: the need to convert the histopathologic findings per animal into machine-readable form for entry into a computer database, if an EDP system is employed; or submission of the
finished individual necropsy reports to the project librarian,
if a manual system is employed. It requires: the availability of
a data-input technician if a computerized system employing natural
(English) language terminology is used; a project librarian, if a
manual system is employed.

Step 10. Preparation of tabular summaries of all postmortem findings. This step includes: the need to tabulate the incidence of
histopathologic lesions and a number of specific organs examined,

per sex and per dose level, etc. It requires: the availability of
a data-input technician, if a computerized system and a pre-determined tabular format and content are used; or experienced
clerical personnel familiar with pathology terminology, if manual
data handling is employed. This is a crucial step, and manual
accuracy can best be assured by independent development of the
entire tabular summary by independent personnel or groups, under
the supervision of the pathologist.

Step 11. Interpretation of postmortem findings and preparation of
the final report narrative. This step includes: a need to detect
and interpret underlying pathologic processes, based on discrete
lesions of various organs; a need to assess and determine causality
between test agent and lesions observed; performance of statistical evaluations, if indicated; preparation of a typed report. It
requires: a pathologist, a typist, and may require a statistician.
Professional judgement is the primary resource here.

Step 12. Submission of the required raw data and final report to
the Archives. This step includes: a need to select and assemble
records, as required by the project protocol and/or government
regulation, for submission to the Archivist for permanent storage.
It requires: the availability of a project Librarian, with assistance as needed from the Necropsy, Histology and Pathology Super-
visors.

CONCLUSION

The toxicologic pathologist today, in contrast to the recent
past, is even more at a pivotal point in the overall evaluation
of the safety of foods, drugs and other chemicals. It is the histologic evidence most often used as a basis for decision making.
More stringent requirements occasioned by regulatory mandates are
absorbing resources which should be directed toward understanding
the response to a chemical. Indeed, as Golberg has pointed out,[4]
at a time when we seem to be entering a new era in toxicology where
we probe the inner workings of the animal in attempts to understand
underlying mechanisms for morphologic expression, we stand to suc-
cumb to progressive asphyxiation by proliferating regulatory requirements. A few are good and will contribute to the quality of
scientific testing. Many are burdensome and will reduce scientific

productivity. We need to use our experience and expertise to design better, more efficient studies and to come to agreement among
ourselves on terminology, diagnosis and methods of quality control.

   If the pathologist is to provide optimum input into a safety
evaluation, such input must be inserted from the very beginning
and continue throughout the study to the assessment of tissue lesions. At that point as we see it, there is a critical need to
gain agreement among toxicologic pathologists on nomenclature for
lesions in experimental animals; such agreement should be at both
the national and international levels. Further, there must be some
additional emphasis placed on the value of adequately assessing
the data, its biological significance (as opposed to statistical)
and its implications prior to public release of a report. A necessity for scientific rigor is greatest when scientific evidence
is to be used as a basis for public policy. The pathologist who
views histologic material generated by studies with broad socio-
economic impact has the responsibility to see that the histopathology results are confirmed, reported as required and published in
the scientific literature. Handler has pointed out that a decade ago
 it may have been desirable to flag public attention to potential
hazards and proceed as if each were a clear danger, but "it is
time to return to the ethics and norms of science so that the political process can proceed with greater confidence." Scientists
best serve public policy by living within the ethics of science,
not those of politics. The toxicologic pathologist has an important role in keeping science an integral part of safety evaluation.

REFERENCES

1. Balazas, T. (1976) Advances in Modern Toxicology 1, 141.
    Mehlman, M., Shapiro, R. and Blumenthal, H. eds., John Wiley
    & Sons, New York.

2. Peck, H.M. (1968) Importance of Fundamental Principles in
    Drug Evaluation. Tedeschi, D. and Tedeschi, R. eds. Raven
    Press, New York, 449.

3. Zbinden, G. (1976) Progress in Toxicology, Vol. 2. Springer-
    Verlag, New York.

4. Golberg, L.   Proceedings of the Workshop on Cellular
    and Molecular Toxicology. Fawcett, D. and Newberne, J. eds.
    Pharmacological Reviews (in press).

5. Harnad, S. (1979) Bulletin The New York Academy of Sciences
    19, 18. New York, New York.

6. Cournand, A. (1977) Science 198, 699.

7. Schmitt, R. (1979) Chemical and Engineering News, editor's
    page 5.

8. Statland, B.E. (1979) American Journal of Pathology 95, 243.

9. Stone, K. (1966) Evidence in Science, p. 68. John Wright &
    Sons, Ltd.

10. Rogan, W. and Brown, S. (1979) Federation Proceedings 38,
    1875.

11. Butler, W.H. (1978) British Journal of Cancer 37, 418.

12. Newberne, P. et al. (1966) Laboratory Investigation 15, 962.

13. Newberne, P. et al. (1969) Cancer Research 29, 230.

14. Newberne, P.M. (1976) Cancer Research 36, 2573.

15. Squire, R.A. and Levitt, M. (1975) Cancer Research 35, 3214.

16. Gellatly, J. in: Mouse Hepatic Neoplasia (1975). W.H. Butler
    and P.M. Newberne, eds. Elsevier, p. 77.

17. Deelman, H. (1927) Proceedings Royal Society of Medicine 20,
    19.

18. Berenblum, I. (1944) Archives of Pathology and Laboratory
    Medicine 38, 233.

19. Craddock, V. (1971) Journal National Cancer Institute 47,
    899.

20. Craddock, V.M. (1975) Chem.-Biol. Interaction 10, 313.

21. Federal Register (1974) Selenium in Animal Feed 38, 10458;
    39, 1355.

22. Kolbye, A.C. Jr. (1976) Ontology 33, 90.

23. Peraino, C. et al. (1971) Cancer Research 31, 1506.

24. Peraino, C. et al. (1973) Journal National Cancer Institute
    51, 1349.

25. Rossi, L. et al. (1977) International Journal of Cancer 19,
    179.

26. Doniach, I. (1970) Tumors of the Thyroid Gland, p. 73.
    E.N.S. Livingstone, Edinburgh.

27. Lupuleschu, A. and Petrovich, (1968) Altered Structure of
    the Thyroid Gland, p. 36. Williams & Wilkins, Baltimore.

28. Astwood, E. et al. (1943) Endocrinology 32, 210.

29. Jemec, B. (1977) Cancer 40, 2188.

30. Cosgrove & Upton (1965) Pathology of Laboratory Animals,
    W. Ribelin and J. McCoy, eds. Charles C. Thomas Co.,
    Springfield, Ill., p.21.

31. Dunn, T.B. (1954) Journal of the National Cancer Institute
    14, 1281.

32. Squire, R.A. et al.(1978) Pathology of Laboratory Animals,
    K. Benirschke, Garner, F. and Jones, T.C. eds., Springer-
    Verlag, New York; chapter 12.

33. Newberne, P.M. (1979) Science 204, 1079.

34. Handler, P. President, National Academy of Sciences (1979)
    Dedication Address Northwestern University Cancer Center.

© 1980 Elsevier/North-Holland Biomedical Press
The Principles and Methods in Modern Toxicology
C.L. Galli, S.D. Murphy and R. Paoletti, editors.

THE CHOICE OF ANIMAL SPECIES IN EXPERIMENTAL TOXICOLOGY

A. Mondino, Istituto di Ricerche Biomediche "Antoine Marxer" S.p.A. - RBM, Casella Postale 226, 10015 Ivrea, Italy.

As a person concerned with toxicologic matters and as a consumer, I am particularly pleased to observe that the choice of animal species in experimental toxicology has, of late, come to the fore as a topic of major concern both to people directly involved in toxicologic examinations and to the decision makers through whom the results of "in vivo" studies must pass.

Even regulatory bodies in many countries are now attempting to deal with the problem by establishing regulations and guidelines on this subject.

To explain why such great interest has only now arisen, several historical considerations are in order.

Until relatively recently, most toxicologic studies were acute and subacute, designed merely to determine if chemicals were literally "poisons" to man and animals by assessing the immediate toxic effects after a high dose. It was generally held that most toxic reactions, when not lethal, were reversible and that if sublethal exposures were given, no lasting harm would (in most cases) be done to the subject. Hence, little attention was paid to adverse cumulative effects that might occur after chronic exposure to low doses of the chemical which, in the acute trials, did not elicit untoward effects.

Personally, I recall that not many years ago, still in the fifties, a new drug could be registered without any particularly exhaustive preclinical chronic examination.

We have to realize that as little as 40 years ago, not everybody was in agreement on the fact that a chemical could originate a cancerous process in an organism.

At regulatory level, the need for toxicologic documentation exploded after the thalidomide disaster, in the early sixties, and after Rachel

Carson's emotional book "Silent Spring" had become a bestseller.

Unfortunately Carson, waging her own personal battle with a tumor, did not live to see the tremendous effects her passionate book was to have on public opinion and on the authorities, to the point that the United States President's Scientific Advisory Committee in its report dated May 15, 1963, stated that the time had come for the appropriate Federal Departments and agencies to initiate programs of public education describing the use and the toxic nature of pesticides. Moreover, they explicitly said (I am quoting) that public literature and the experience of Panel members indicate that, until the publication of "Silent Spring" by Rachel Carson, people were generally unaware of the toxicity of pesticides.

So the so-called "safety explosion" took place, involving as we know apparently conflicting interests, often on an emotional rather than on a scientific basis at economic, industrial, political, and regulatory levels, spreading from the United States all over the world. But despite the multiplicity of the bandwagons, both past and still to join, we should in my opinion view such an awakening positively. Among other emerging sciences, experimental toxicology, as we know it today, chiefly intended as safety evaluation, is an offspring of the late fifties and, interesting to note, its birthplace was not in Academia, but in the Regulatory Agencies, mainly of the United States of America.

Actually, until around 1940, few if any routine animal bioassays had been specifically designed to test for effects of long term chronic exposure including carcinogenicity. Major credit must be granted to the U.S. Department of Agriculture and the U.S. Food and Drug Administration for introducing such procedures. The landmark study by Wilson et al., in 1941, revealed the pesticide 2-acetylaminofluorene to be a potent carcinogen and its introduction for general use was consequently witheld.

FDA investigators subsequently studied many compounds in the long term, according to the two-year rat study model developed by Lehman and coworkers in 1955 that became standard with the toxicologist of those times and is still followed today without major changes, reported in the "Appraisal of the Safety of Chemicals in Foods, Drugs and Cosmetics", that little booklet considered the toxicologists' Bible.

But - and now to return to my title - if the objectives of experimental toxicology have been broadened from acute investigations to long term chronic observations, the real purpose has always been to acquire knowledge conducive to forewarning us of possible hazards to man. The safety test should then be focused toward this aim and hence tailored to the intended use of the new drug or chemical. Consequently, the toxicologic investigation should permit the widest latitude with respect to choice of species, number of animals, route and method of administration and kinds of pre- and post-mortem observations to be made.

Particularly, the choice of the test animal should always be made considering that many toxic reactions can be species-dependent, as we can see from some examples:

Compound	Toxicity	Reactive species	Non-reactive species
Beta-naphthylamine	carcinogen	dog,man	rat
Aflatoxin B1	carcinogen	rat,trout	monkey,mouse
Phenylthiourea	pulmonary edema	rat	rhesus monkey
Norbormide	respirat.failure	rat	cat,dog,mouse
DDT	weak carcinogen	mouse	hamster
3-methylcholantrene	carcinogen	mouse,rat	rhesus monkey
Thalidomide	teratogen	rabbit,man	hamster, rat, mouse

In daily practice, we have observed that the choice of species is too often overlooked, and what is worse, it is practically predetermined without any precise rationale, rather for reasons of availability or economy or because that particular species is explicitly required by too dogmatic a guideline.

Thus the animal of choice has come to be the rat, rendering the investigator very like the fellow in the story, who, having lost his car keys on a dark night, searched for them under the streetlight, not because he thought he had lost them there but because that was the only place he had hopes of seeing a little.

In so stating, my intention is not to denigrate this valuable experimental model, for I am convinced that few people, as a teacher of ours used to say, have not benefitted in some way – even for survival – by studies made on the rat.

In the United States alone, it is calculated that in 1977 some 18 million rats were used in medical, psychological, and toxicological studies.

Their credentials as experimental animals are impressive. Curt Richter of Johns Hopkins recently made an apt profile I would like to quote:"The dietary habits of man and rat are almost identical, except that we eat by day and the rat by night. Its short life span aids in studies of growth and aging, and in following inheritance through many generations in a short time. Also, it is stable, reliable – and just the right size to work on. Given the power to create an ideal lab animal, I could not possibly improve on the Norway rat."

Nevertheless, I do not believe that "in primis" the Norway rat was chosen for all these features from among the world's some 4,000 mammalian species, as an experimental animal. I worked back in time to find the answer in scientific literature and, explicit help not appearing forthcoming, I evolved my own hypothesis which may seem to have rather more to do with the history of custom that with toxicology itself.

People have always hesitated to harm mammals in research. The Italian Law number 924 of June 12, 1931, which with some changes is still in force, opens by stating that vivisection and all experiments on vertebrate, warm-blooded animals, mammals and birds is forbidden except when the objective is the promotion of progress in biological and experimental medicine.

Hence (the law does not state this, but we can deduce it), reptiles, which are cold-blooded, a feature shared by other vertebrates such as the amphibians, can be chopped up with a clean conscience. Popular custom has viewed these animals as close to diabolic or accessories to witchery, the devil, in biblical cosmogenesis taking the form of a snake. So, extrapolating to past times, lizards, newts and frogs as experimental models would hardly have been considered defensible.

Certainly, it was no chance that Luigi Galvani, at the end of the eighteenth century, made his revolutionary discovery, experimenting on frogs, whose cold heart, indifferently plucked out, also served as a model for extensive pharmacologic studies on the isolated heart.

In 1874 in England a law was issued, "intended as an amendment of the law relating to cruelty to animals by extending it to the cases of animals which for medical, physiological or other scientific purposes are subjected when alive to experiments calculated to inflict pain." These are words of the law, simply called the "Cruelty to Animals Act", which in clause 22 states that it is not applicable to invertebrate animals.

But if we peruse this Act, we notice that the animals to be protected are actually those considered man's friends, to which he customarily talks. Dogs and cats are explicitly mentioned, along with horses, asses, and mules that can be used only when "no other animal is available for such experiment". Among the "other animals", obviously the rat, the lapdog of the devil, could be included.

As a matter of fact, even before 1874, when the use of animals in experimental medicine had not yet been regulated, we can suppose that if a scientist in England wished to experiment on mammals without raising remonstration from certain factions, his surest prospect was the Norwegian rat as an experimental subject.

It appears almost certain that the Norway rat came into captivity as the albino. Albinos probably trace their ancestry to the grisly passtime known as rat baiting. This was a popular sport in England and France as early as 1800 until its prohibition some seventy years later. In this sport, between 100 and 200 recently trapped wild rats were placed in a pit and a trained terrier was let loose among them. The spectators bet on the time required by different terriers to kill the last rat. Large numbers of rats had to be caught and held in readiness for these spectacles. Richter (1954) writes of records indicating that albinos were selected from such groups and retained for breeding and exhibition. From these prosaic beginnings, it was likely that individuals found their way into laboratories. The albino was not so disagreable as its grey brother and, as the albino trait is dominant, it was very easy to start a colony after having found either a

white-coated male or female. If the animals had been frequently handled
from birth, they were likely to be semi-tame and relatively tractable for
experimental purposes.

According to Richter, the first paper dealing with the use of rats in the
laboratory was by Philipeaux (1856): on the effects of adrenalectomy, and
the animals were referred to as albino.

Forgive me if I have been a little iconoclastic or at least have treated
my topic thusfar rather unscientifically. No doubt we all agree, however,
that seldom have rats, or for that matter dogs, been chosen as models for
man upon scientific bases:that is upon comparative anatomical, physiological or biochemical criteria, but rather upon factors such as availability,
convenience and cost.

We know that very few chemicals when introduced in man or in animals
are excreted unchanged; the majority of them undergo transformations in
the organism which usually increase the rate of excretion. In general,
metabolism converts drugs or foreign compounds from relatively lipid
soluble materials into relatively water soluble products. The reactions
involved can be conveniently divided into two phases, as Williams was the
first to indicate:

PHASE I includes:

-   oxidations and reductions catalysed by liver microsomal
    enzymes
-   oxidations not catalysed by liver microsomal enzymes
-   hydrolyses – some catalysed by liver microsomal enzymes
    and others catalysed by various liver and plasma enzymes
-   miscellaneous, such as ring opening or ring formation

PHASE II includes the following conjugations:

glucuronide formation
glycine conjugation
glutamine conjugation
mercapturic acid synthesis
ethereal sulphate synthesis
O- N- and S-methylations
acetylation
thyocyanate formation

These reactions are in general common to the different mammalian
species, including man. There are only a few examples of metabolic
reactions apparently unique to one species. Despite the general similarity,

there are species and interindividual differences that may arise mainly from different rates of metabolism along a common pathway.

Let us consider some interesting examples of interspecies differences or similarities.

The formerly mentioned pesticide 2-acetylaminofluorene is a potent carcinogen, the activity of which Miller (1969) and coworkers brilliantly demonstrated was due to the development of a proximate carcinogen following a N-hydroxylation reaction. The parent compound is carcinogenic in a variety of species which all form the carcinogenic metabolite. It is not however carcinogenic in the guinea-pig or the steppe-lemming, which fail to form the active N-hydroxy derivative.

Species	Carcinogenicity	N-hydroxylation % of the dose
rat	+	8
rabbit	+	21
hamster	+	17
dog	+	5
guinea-pig	−	0
steppe-lemming	−	trace
man	?	9

Irving (1975), studying the toxicity of this N-hydroxy derivative, found that its LD_{50} by intraperitoneal injection in various strains of rats was dramatically different according to the strain.

ACUTE TOXICITY (LD_{50}) OF N-HYDROXY-AAF IN VARIOUS STRAINS OF RATS

Strains	Source	LD_{50} mg/Kg	M/F ratio
Sprague-Dawley			
Female	Holtzman	315(241-413)	6.3
Male	Holtzman	50(42-58)	
Sprague-Dawley			
Female	Carworth CFE	506(372-689)	7.4
Male	Carworth CFE	68(54-86)	
Wistar			
Female	Carworth CFN	116(76-175)	2.2
Male	Carworth CFN	52(32-83)	
Fischer 344			
Female	Charles River	52(34-80)	0.9
Male	Charles River	61(38-97)	

Another example, given by Smith (1974), of species variations in response to a toxic chemical is the following, related to the acute toxicity of alpha-naphthylthiourea:

ACUTE TOXICITY (LD$_{50}$) OF ALPHA-NAPHTHYLTHIOUREA IN VARIOUS SPECIES

Species	LD$_{50}$ mg/Kg Intraperitoneal	Approx. Relative Toxicity (Rat=1)
Rat	8	1
Dog	16	2
Mouse	56	7
Guinea Pig	350	44
Rabbit	400	50
Cat	500 *	63
Chicken	2500	313
Monkey	4250 *	532

* oral

These examples show how important and desirable it would be, when developing an animal model for evaluating the toxicological hazard of a chemical to man, to find a species or strain that metabolizes the chemical in a way similar to him. Ideally, a complete animal model should be similar to man with regard to the rate of chemical absorption, effect of intestinal bacteria, distribution throughout the body, rate and route of metabolism, rates of excretion and reabsorption and with regard to the molecular receptor sites.

Unfortunately no species, even the subhuman primates, is exactly like man in its response to all chemicals, but certain effects that occur in the common laboratory animals generally occur in man and many of the effects that are produced by chemicals on man can in retrospect be produced in some species of common laboratory animals.

Notable exceptions are those toxicities that occur in man and are dependent on immunogenic mechanisms. Most such sensitization reactions are notoriously difficult or even impossible to induce in laboratory animals.

If the immunogenically based toxicities are excluded, the differences between man and laboratory animals in toxic responses that are observed are in most cases more quantitative in nature than they are qualitative.

Hence, thorough and intense conduct of toxicity tests on more than one animal species provides information that frequently can be qualitatively transposed to humans.

With the aim of estimating the utility of safety studies intended to disclose potential hazards of new drugs to man, Litchfield (1962) selected six drugs chemically unrelated – namely an antibiotic, a synthetic antibacterial agent, a tranquilizer, a central nervous system depressant, a chemical blocking alcohol oxidation, and a glucocorticoid – which had been studied in detail in rats, dogs, and man. In both rats and dogs, each drug had been studied for acute toxicity and subacute short term feeding of 30 to 90 days.

In addition each drug had been given to dogs for at least 6 months and to rats for 1 year.

Clinical summaries were available on 500 or more human cases for each drug. All six drugs had been studied on man within a 6-year period under closely comparable conditions.

The available data for each drug on the three species including man were examined and the incidence of 89 different effects caused by the six drugs were evaluated, discarding those symptoms that could not, for specific physiological reasons, be common to all three species, such as headache, tinnitus, metallic taste and others demonstrable only for man, and vomiting, of which the rat is incapable.

From the data pertaining to the rat and dog, he predicted the occurrence or absence of each effect in man by following two rules: first, if a sign was found in both rats and dogs, it was predicted to occur in man, and second, if a sign was found in either the dog or rat, but not in both, it was predicted that the sign would not occur in man. Since he already knew the effects of the drugs in man, he set up a table of each drug and tabulated the number of items that he had predicted correctly or incorrectly.

Prediction in man	correct	incorrect	total	% correct
occurrence	26	12	38	68
absence	38	10	48	79
total	64	22	86	74

Of 86 predictions for the six drugs, 26 of 38 positive predictions and 38 of 48 negative predictions were correct. Litchfield pointed out further that predictions made on the basis of flipping a coin would be expected to yield 50 per cent correct results, but the probability of obtaining 74 per cent correct predictions by the coin flipping method is very small.

In this example, therefore, animal studies permitted, to some degree, prediction of drug effects in man based only on the theory that a drug action that is seen in both the rat and the dog probably involves a common physiologic mechanism that is likely to be present in the human, whereas an effect seen in only one of two species indicates that the effect is peculiar to that species and is less likely to be present in the third species. Such evidence shows the importance of using at least two species in the animal tests and the value of animal tests for predicting the effects of chemicals in man.

But if the number of species were elevated to three, including a subhuman primate, the transposition of the results from animal to man would become more appropriate.

Smith and Caldwell (1976) have recently surveyed the metabolism by primate species of a variety of drugs and concluded that primates are more likely to provide a better metabolic model for man than non-primate species. They attempted to summarize from scientific literature as follows the adequacy of the rhesus monkey, the rat and other non-primate mammalian species, as metabolic models for man.

PRIMATES AS METABOLIC MODELS FOR MAN

Compound	Species		
	Rat	Other* non-primate	Rhesus monkey[+]
Amphetamine	invalid	fair(D)	good
Phenmetrazine	invalid	poor(G)	good(M)
Chlorphentermine	invalid	good(G)	good
Norephedrine	invalid	invalid(R)	good(M)
Phenylacetic acid	invalid	invalid(D)	good
Indolylacetic acid	invalid	invalid(D)	good
1-Naphthylacetic acid	poor	fair(R)	good
Hydatropic acid	good	good(R)	good
Diphenylacetic acid	good	good(R)	good
4-Hydroxy-3,5-diiodoben- zoic acid	invalid	invalid(R)	good
Sulphadimethoxine	poor	poor(D)	good
Sulphadimethoxypyridine	poor	invalid(R)	good
Sulphamethomidine	invalid	invalid(R)	good
Sulphasomidine	fair	good(D)	good
Isoniazid	–	poor(D)	good
Indomethacin	poor	poor(D)	fair
Halofenate	poor	poor(D)	good
Oxisuran	good	fair(D)	fair
2-Acetamidofluorene	good	poor(D)	fair
Nalidixic acid	–	fair(D)	fair
Methotrexate	poor	good(D)	good
Phencyclidine	poor	fair(D)	poor
Morphine	fair	fair(D)	fair

* D = Dog; G = Guinea-pig; R = Rabbit.   [+]M = Marmoset

Where the similarity is close, a 'good' rating is given and where the pathways are quite different an 'invalid' rating is applied. A 'fair' rating implies that the metabolic pathways are similar but that there are significant interspecies differences in the amounts of metabolites produced by the different pathways. It can be seen that for the 23 compounds quoted the best metabolic model for man is provided by the monkey species on 17 occasions. By contrast the rat provided a good model on only 4 occasions and was invalid for 8 of the compounds.

It has to be emphasized that the comparisons have been made on the basis of metabolic pathways and do not take into account kinetic or excretion differences. Actually, for the choice of an animal model for man in safety evaluation, differences in rates of drug metabolism are less important than differences in pathways of metabolism. This is because differences in rates of metabolism can be largely compensated for by different dosage schedules in accordance with the pharmacokinetic patterns whereas it is not possible to compensate for actual species differences in the pathways of metabolism.

Considering the present state of the art, I would say that we have reason to be optimistic, since general acceptance of the value of such metabolic studies is becoming more and more widespread as methodologies improve and regulatory requirements begin to make the provision of metabolic information mandatory. It is my feeling that very soon it will be unacceptable to take an animal "a priori" and say that the safety evaluation must be made on it unless it can be established that the metabolic fate and the total handling of the compound in this animal is at least somewhat similar to man.

With pleasure, I see that the FDA Good Laboratory Practice Regulations enacted in the U.S. on December 22, 1978, and implemented in June 1979 request that the reason for selection of the test animal be indicated.

The "Notes for guidance on pharmacokinetic studies in the safety evaluation of new drugs", prepared by the working party of the CPMP (Committee for Proprietary Medicinal Products of the EEC) give better specification with regard to the previous norms and protocols and point to the philosophy of this research, which is:

a) to obtain information on the relationship between target organ toxicity and body fluid and organ concentration of a drug

b) to assess drug cumulation

c) to choose, where possible, the animal species to be used on the basis of their similarity to man.

Furthermore, in this same document, a very important statement was made to the effect that a preliminary study of the kinetics of a drug in a few human subjects could provide useful information in choosing the animal species for chronic toxicity study. Moreover, the notes specify that the study of the time course of pharmacodynamic effects may provide useful additional information but can not substitute a formal pharmacokinetic study; this fact reflects the increasing sensitivity of modern methods of quantitative determination of substances in body fluids (gas-chromatography, gas-mass, HPLC, radioimmunoassay, radioreceptor assay). This same reason is behind the request of characterizing, whenever possible, the pattern of metabolites and of identifying the major metabolite(s) and of studying their kinetics, which represents actually more a field of research than of routine analysis of a given drug.

But this document does not cover all the aspects of pharmacokinetics which need to be investigated in the case of a new drug. Other aspects of pharmacokinetics are mentioned in other European "notes", that is, in those requiring the assessment of drug absorption and of its levels during chronic toxicity studies and the evaluation of the level in fetuses in reproduction studies.

Another document I would like to recall is the proposed "Health Effects Test Standards for Toxic Substances Control Act Test Rules" published in the Federal Register of July 26, 1979 by EPA. These have just been discussed in a public hearing on October 15 and 16, 1979 in Chicago and are about to become U.S. law. They also contain a detailed regulation concerning general metabolism test standards. It is explicitly stated that (I quote)" these proposed standards may be used to estimate the extent to which the test substance and/or its metabolites are absorbed, distributed and bioaccumulated. The information will be used in the assessment of species selection, route of administration and dose selection rationale for long-term studies". Moreover, it recommends, the "report should include a discussion section in which the authors indicate clearly how they relate the metabolic and pharmacokinetic data to toxicologic observations in animals, and also to risks, if any, to human health. When the authors conclude that these relationships cannot be made on the basis of existing data, they should meet with Agency personnel to decide upon the design of additional studies."

And here is the indication of what is meant by additional metabolic studies:

"Some areas for possible further study include: Binding by macromolecules in the blood, liver, gonads, and other tissues; placental transfer; entrance into breast milk; biotransformation by specific organs or tissues; absorption by dermal or inhalation routes of exposure; and measurement of levels of the test substance and its metabolites in the gonads. Plasma binding studies can be conducted, usually, "in vivo" with plasma. Placental transfer of a test substance can be determined readily by dosing pregnant rodents with radioactively labeled test substance and assaying their fetuses for radioactivity. Entrance of a test substance into breast milk can be determined similarly in rodents. Biotransformation studies can be performed, usually, with whole liver homogenates or liver fractions such as microsomes or cytosol."

Such a position at regulatory level proves the greater consciousness of the value and applicability of these studies, which has led to the recognition that metabolic and pharmacokinetic data are not merely ancillary information but constitute fundamental knowledge of the compound, to be used in planning both the strategy and tactics to approach safety evaluation.

As we observe in another very important publication, entitled "Proposed system for food safety assessment", prepared by the Scientific Committee of the Food Safety Council, "metabolic and pharmacokinetic information is central to the design of protocols, leading to proper species selection, definition of dose regimens and the appropriate conduct of both "in vivo" and "in vitro" tests. Intelligent application of metabolic and pharmacokinetic information is one of the principal tools that permits the selection of appropriate tests and conditions specifically tailored to the characteristics of the individual compound under study. Thus in the plan of investigation, metabolic comparability between man and the animal species proposed for use in a long-term test are to be established before any such test is initiated.

How, in practice, can such a recommendation be adopted? If the product under study is a drug, we know that many regulatory bodies permit passage to preliminary clinical studies in man after the acute and subacute tests in animals have been performed and (I must cite the Italian regulation) after a battery of mutagenesis tests has been run. In this case, even on patients and/or on healthy volunteers, it is possible to do a preliminary investigation regarding the plasma kinetics of the unchanged drug, which will be paralleled by similar studies on more than one animal species. A study like this is of great interest and generally provides good information by itself in orienting the species selection for the long term studies.

But it is easy to realize that a kinetic study on humans at that early stage is not always possible when dealing with a food additive, and absolutely unfeasible when dealing with an industrial chemical, an intermediate or, last but not least, a pesticide. In these cases, it is nevertheless possible at present to obtain some information about the way man will handle the new product. I refer to the relatively new methodologies regarding the covalent binding of the chemically reactive metabolites into which many foreign compounds are converted, which either uncouple integrated biochemical processes in cells or combine covalently with various cellular components including proteins, glycogen, lipids, DNA and RNA. The capacity of the compound under investigation to form chemically reactive metabolites is key information that can provide insight into its toxic potentialities, with particular reference to "irreversible" effects, knowledge of which is essential for products such as food additives, pesticides and industrial chemicals which constitute great concern for carcinogenesis bioassays.

Rather than enter into further detail, I refer those interested to the works of Gillette, Ehrenberg, Van Duuren, Meleke, and others. It is, however, important to point out that these studies can be conducted both "in vitro" and "in vivo" and usually great sensitivity can be achieved, in that the parent compound is appropriately labeled with a radioactive tracer. It is possible, when working "in vitro" to use human tissues, as we observe more and more frequently in literature. From a recent article in "Science", we understand that in Sweden, along with the kidneys donated for transplants, livers are also donated for this kind of study. Obviously, similar research conducted on a human tissue "in vitro" can be paralleled by the same research conducted on animal tissues "in vitro" and then "in vivo" with the goal of choosing the appropriate animal species for the long term bioassay or of understanding the species and strain differences in toxicity, contributing especially to the extrapolation of test results from animals to man.

Clearly, such an approach is far from being or becoming routine. It is, however, a contribution that will help the practice of safety evaluation develop into scientific endeavour performed by dedicated people who will refuse to blindly apply what generic guidelines set forth. We need such a revolution; otherwise chemical testing is in danger of becoming a meaningless formal ritual, irrational rather than scientific, far from assessing the real hazards to man and environment.

REFERENCES

1. Galvani L. (1791), De Viribus Electricitatis in Motu Musculari. De Bononiensi Scientiarum et Artium Instituto atque Academia Commentarii. Tomus Septimus.

2. Philipeaux (1856) in Robinson R. (1965), Genetics of the Norway Rat, Pergamon Press, Oxford.

3. Wilson, R.H., F. DeEds and A.J. Crox (1941), The toxicity and carcinogenic activity of 2-acetaminofluorene, Cancer Res. 1:595.

4. Richter C., in Canby,T. (1977), The Rat, Lapdog of the Devil, National Geographic, 152, 1, 60.

5. Lehman A. J., W.I. Patterson, B. Davidow, E.C. Hagan, G. Woodard, E.P. Lang, J.P. Fawley, O.G. Fitzhugh, A.R. Bourke, J.H. Draize, A.A. Nelson and B.J. Vos (1955), Procedures for the Appraisal of the Toxicity of Chemicals in Foods, Drugs and Cosmetics. Food Drug Cosmetic Law Journal 10: 679.

6. Editorial Committee of the Association of Food and Drug Officials of the United States (1959), Appraisal of the Safety of Chemicals in Foods, Drugs and Cosmetics. Topeka, Kansas.

7. Litchfield J.T. (1962), Evaluation of the Safety of New Drugs by Means of Tests on Animals,. Clin. Pharmacol. Therap., 3, 665.

8. Miller E.C., J.A. Miller and M. Enomoto (1964), The Comparative Carcinogenicities of 2-acetylaminofluorene and its N-hydroxy metabolite in Mice, Hamsters and Guinea-pigs, Cancer Res. 24, 2018.

9. Loomis T.A. (1968), Essentials of Toxicology, Lea and Febiger, Philadelphia

10. Smith (1974), in NCTR Advanced Course for Investigators: Bio-research Monitoring Nonclinical Studies, 1978.

11. Irving (1975), in ibid.

12. Smith R.L. and J. Caldwell (1977), Drug Metabolism in Non-human Primates, in Drug Metabolism from Microbe to Man, Editors.D.V.Parke and R.L. Smith, Taylor and Francis, London.

13. Dring L.G. (1977), Species Variations in Pre-Conjugation Reactions of Non-primate Mammals, in ibid.

14. Gillette J.R. (1977), The Phenomenon of Species Variations: Problems Opportunities, in ibid.

15. Smith R.L. (1978), Extrapolation of Animal Results to Man, in Drug Metabolism in Man, Editors J.W.Gorrod and A.H. Beckett, Taylor and Francis, London.

16. Rollins D.E., C. von Bar. H. Glaumann, P. Moldeus, and A. Rane (1979), Acetaminophen: Potentially Toxic Metabolite Formed by Human Fetal and Adult Liver Microsomes and Isolated Fetal Liver Cells, Science 205, 1414.

17. Segre G. (1979), Pharmacokinetics, International Symposium on Scientific Criteria and Methods for Drug Assessment, Rome, July 5, 1979.

18. Shubik P. (1979), Identification of Environmental Carcinogens: Animal Test Models in Carcinogens: Identification and Mechanisms of Action, Ed. A.C. Griffin, Raven Press, New York.

© 1980 Elsevier/North-Holland Biomedical Press
The Principles and Methods in Modern Toxicology
C.L. Galli, S.D. Murphy and R. Paoletti, editors.

ASSESSMENT OF THE POTENTIAL FOR TOXIC INTERACTIONS AMONG ENVIRONMENTAL POLLUTANTS.

SHELDON D. MURPHY

Division of Toxicology, Department of Pharmacology, University of Texas Medical School, P. O. Box 20708, Houston, Texas, 77025, U.S.A.

INTRODUCTION

For purposes of this discussion, a *toxicological interaction* is defined as a condition in which exposure to two or more chemicals results in a qualitatively or quantitatively altered biological response relative to that predicted from the action of a single chemical. Such multiple-chemical exposures may be simultaneous or sequential in time and the altered response may be greater or smaller in magnitude.

With thousands of natural and synthetic chemicals in use today, it is logical to assume that humans and other desirable organisms will be exposed to two or more potentially injurious chemicals, simultaneously or close in time. The exposure dosages in man for each such chemical may range from repeated exposures near the doses causing adverse effects singly (as might be expected with some occupational exposures, gross contamination of the environment or self administered chemicals) down to minimal and occasional exposures to low doses contained as legal residues or contaminants in food, air and water. Desirable organisms, other than humans, may be directly exposed to mixtures of chemicals in relatively high concentrations resulting from deliberate application to wide areas of the environment (e.g., with pesticides) or from incidental environmental contamination associated with waste disposal practices; or they may be indirectly exposed through bioconcentration of chemicals in food chains. An understanding of the potential for toxicological interactions is, therefore, important for assessing chemical hazards to the environment as a whole as well as hazards to human health.

Unfortunately, chemical technology has advanced more rapidly than our abilities or resources to adequately assess the toxic hazards of the products of that technology as even single-chemical exposures. It would be virtually impossible to undertake comprehensive toxicological testing of the myriad combinations of chemicals to which humans may conceivably be exposed under conditions which may result in toxicological interactions. Therefore, in

order to make any attempt at assessment of the potential for toxic interactions among environmental pollutants it is essential to develop a systematic approach to the problem, even if that approach is theoretical with respect to the current knowledge base. One approach might be to merely identify
combinations of chemicals to which the greatest number of individuals are the
most likely to be exposed simultaneously or close in time to concentrations
at which at least one of the chemicals is at (i.e., drugs) or near (i.e.,
hazardous occupations) a biologically effective dose. Such combinations
could then be subjected to conventional toxicological assessments according
to a priority scheme derived from estimates of either the greatest numbers
at risk or, if knowledge permits, greatest likelihood of toxic interaction.
This second criteria "greatest likelihood of toxic interaction," is, in
itself, the ultimate objective for prediction. In order to make this prediction it will be necessary to consider the various mechanisms by which toxic
interactions may occur and then to collect or assemble the appropriate data
for each of the chemicals involved.

In its broadest sense, the subject of toxic interactions among environmental contaminants would include physical-chemical interactions in the
environment that alter the biological activity of the contaminants, as well
as reactions that occur within the tissues of test organisms. This discussion
will be primarily concerned with toxicological interactions occurring *in vivo*.
However, the broad view should not be lost since products of photochemical
and physical-chemical reactions in the environment may differ markedly in
toxicity from the chemicals that are emitted at the source of pollution or
that are initially added to the environment for economic reasons. Examples
of such environmental *toxification* reactions would include: the photochemical
formation of the potent lung irritant ozone derived from relatively non-
irritant precursors in automotive exhaust emissions[1], the formation of
carcinogenic nitrosamines from inorganic nitrite and naturally occurring
(as in foods) or synthetic amines[2], the oxidation of phosphorothionate
insecticides to their more toxic oxygen analogues by the action of sunlight
and oxygen on foliage or other surfaces[3], and the adsorption and/or
oxidation of irritant gases and vapors on particulates to result in enhanced
bronchoconstriction[4]. Of course many, perhaps most, reactions of chemicals
that occur in the environment, external to the organism, render the chemicals
less toxic or less accessible for human exposures.

MEASUREMENT AND DESCRIPTION OF INTERACTIONS

Toxicological interactions, as defined above, would include only those responses to mixtures which differ qualitatively or quantitatively from expected actions of individual chemicals acting alone. It has, however, been common practice to classify the quantitative joint action of chemicals by three general terms: *Addition* - when the toxic effect produced by two or more chemicals in combination is equivalent to that expected by simple summation of their individual effects, *Antagonism* - when the effect of a combination is less than the sum of the individual effects, and *Synergism* - when the effect of the combination is greater than would be predicted by summation of the individual effects. The term *potentiation* is sometimes used synonymously with synergism. The distinction, in meaning, if any, between these two terms requires considerable knowledge of the mechanism by which greater-than-additive effects are produced. Veldstra[5], argued that the term "potentiation" should not be used since it implies that one compound endows another with power, a phenomenon which Veldstra felt was not possible. However, in the two and one-half decades since Veldstra made that proposal it has become amply clear that one compound can alter body processes in manners which allow the body to transform a chemical to one with more "power", i.e., biological activation. In this sense, then perhaps "potentiation" is an appropriate term.

Considerations of statistical methods for experimentally identifying and measuring the intensity of interactions have generally dealt with acute toxicity end points and for situations in which two or more chemicals are given simultaneously or within a short (few minutes) time interval. Two essential conditions must be fulfilled, that is, there must be a quantitatively definable effect for each compound involved and dose response information for this effect must be available. A method described by Finney[6] for predicting the acute toxicity of mixtures of chemicals has frequently been used[7,8]. This model is as follows:

$$\frac{1}{\text{Predicted LD}_{50} \text{ of Mixture}} = \frac{\text{P of A}}{\text{LD}_{50} \text{ of A}} + \frac{\text{P of B}}{\text{LD}_{50} \text{ of B}} \; - - -\text{etc.}$$

"P" is the proportion (as a decimal part of 1) of each constituent (A, B, etc.) in the mixture. The model assumes additivity of action of the constituents and with all values on the right hand of the equation known, a predicted LD_{50} for a mixture can be calculated and compared with the actual, experimentally-determined LD_{50} of a mixture, containing the specified proportions of each constituent. From this information a conclusion can be made as to the quality and intensity of interaction, if any, by calculating the ratio of the *predicted* LD_{50} of the mixture to the *observed* LD_{50} determined experimentally. Thus, if this ratio exceeds one, the combination can be classified as synergistic and if it is less than one as antagonistic. The size of the ratio is often used to quantify the interaction. The Finney method has usually been considered applicable only in situations where the components of the mixture have similar mechanisms of action and where their dosage-mortality curves are parallel. However, Smyth et al[8] found this model reasonably satisfactory for testing acute interactions among randomly selected chemicals, and Dunnett[9] has described a modification of the method that does not require parallel dose-response curves. The example described above identifies the LD_{50} as the quantitatively defined response. The same method could be applied for other quantal end points of response and a modification has been recommended for calculating threshold limit values for mixtures of industrial air contaminants when it is expected that the actions would be additive[10].

When only one constituent of a mixture is capable of producing the particular effect under consideration, the problem of detecting joint action and providing a quantitative estimate of the degree of altered action is simplified. The dose of an active compound "A" required to produce a certain level of response in the presence and absence of an inactive compound "I" are compared. The altered potency of the active compound can be expressed as a ratio of the dose of "A" alone to the dose of "A" in the presence of "I" that will cause the same degree of response. Ratios greater than one represent synergism and ratios of less than one antagonism.

Frequently, the joint action of chemicals is investigated by merely measuring an altered intensity or duration of a response at a standardized dosage level. This approach, although less quantitative, is useful if certain criteria are fulfilled: i.e., only one of the compounds produces the response at the dosage levels or times employed and the dose-response characteristics for the active chemical, by itself, are known.

Graphic methods (isobolograms) for depicting the different types of interactions among biologically active chemicals are illustrated in Figure 1 adapted from others[11]. They are useful from a theoretical standpoint, but the experimental construction of isobolograms requires such an extensive testing program that they are not generally used for practical evaluations of interactions of chemicals.

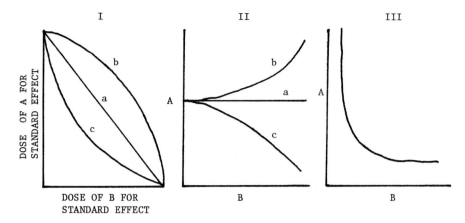

Fig. 1. Isobolograms: I. both A and B are active in producing the same effect, II. only A produces effect, and III. Neither A or B alone produce an effect.

In this illustration, each point on the curves would be constructed from the intersecting dosage points for two chemicals at which a specified, quantitatively identified effect occurs. In graph I, line a represents the line for additive action, line b for antagonistic action and line c for synergistic action when both chemical A and chemical B produce the measured effect. In graph II, only chemical A produces the effect at the dose represented by the point of intersection with the abscissa. Isobol a represents no effect of B on A, isobol b describes B acting as an antagonist to A and line C describes B acting as a synergist to A. In graph III the isobol line represents a situation in which neither compound, by itself is capable of producing a specified effect. Although this may seem an unlikely possibility, such a condition is conceivable for cases of weak carcinogens and cocarcinogens.

EXPERIMENTAL DESIGN OF TESTS FOR INTERACTIONS

Temporal considerations. Most theoretical and applied screening tests for consideration of toxicologic interactions have dealt with interactions occurring when chemicals are administered simultaneously. This type of experimental design may greatly limit the ability to detect potential interaction or it may lead to the wrong conclusion. As a theoretical

282

example, two chemicals may affect the same cellular mechanism to produce
a manifestation of injury, but have significantly different times of onset
and of maximum effects. If a critical threshold of reversible cellular
injury is required for the injury to be come manifest at the organism level,
tests of acute toxicity of combinations given simultaneously may indicate
antagonism while additive action may be manifest if the dosing were spaced
to coincide with maximum action. This is illustrated by the schematic in
Figure 2.

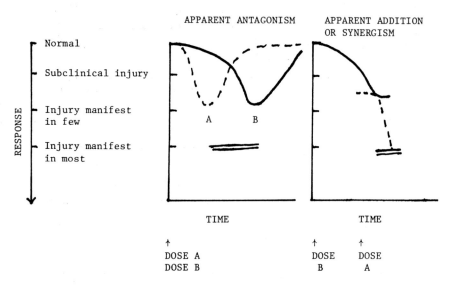

Fig. 2. Illustration of importance of temporal factors in detecting
interactions.

Several other time related and sequence related determinants of interactions
can be envisioned. For example, if chemical A is synergistic with chemical
B because B inhibits the enzyme that rapidly detoxifies A, then administration of B after administration of A may be less synergistic than if B were
given before or simultaneously with A.

Another classic example of where temporal order of exposure is critical
is the interaction between initiators and promoters of chemical carcinogens[12]
where skin exposure to an initiator chemical, as a polynuclear aromatic
hydrocarbon, must precede the exposure to the promoter, croton oil, for the

interaction to become manifest. Similarly, sequence of exposure is critical when one chemical acts to synergize the injury produced by another chemical by altering normal cellular repair processes. Such is the case where repeated exposure to 100% oxygen after a single dose of butylated hydroxy-toluene (BHT) prevented normal repair of BHT-induced lung injury which resulted in lung fibrosis. This effect was only seen when the oxygen ex-posures followed the BHT[13].

Dosage considerations. In addition to proper timing of administration of compounds for purposes of detecting interactions, it is essential to select dosages somewhere near the mid-point of a dose response curve. For screening purposes this may allow rather rapid determination of the quality of potential interaction, i.e., whether antagonism or synergism is likely. The sometimes-used expedient of administering one-half the LD_{50} of each of a pair of compounds, to determine if the combination is lethal to more or less than 50 per cent of the test animals, has serious limitations even for screening purposes. This can be appreciated by considering the shape of dose-mortality curves. One-half the LD_{50} of a chemical which has a very steep dose-response curve may be much below the response threshold dose while it may exceed the threshold for a chemical with a flat dose-mortality curve. Detection of small degrees of synergism and antagonism will be more likely in such simplified test schemes if one chooses equal response doses, e.g., combinations of LD_{25} for each chemical. In any event, quantitative consideration of interactions will require rather extensive dose-response data for the combination as well as for each individual compound.

Response end-point consideration. A third important consideration in the design of interaction studies is the quantifiable end-point of response that is chosen. Most toxic chemicals have multiple effects and the nature of the interaction may vary depending upon the response or injury end-point chosen. Thus, a chlorinated insecticide and a halogenated hydrocarbon solvent might be expected to both produce liver injury independently and to be additive or synergistic in this regard when combined. On the other hand, the insec-ticide could be expected to be a central nervous system stimulant and the solvent a CNS depressant; hence, an antagonistic quality of interaction would be expected in the central nervous system.

PREDICTING INTERACTIONS

   Although in the short term it may be necessary to assess toxicological
interactions by an empirical experimental approach, a goal for toxicologists
to pursue is the development of an adequate data base for each chemical which
will permit reasonable predictions of the potential for interactions.

   Basic principles concerning the kinetics of reaction of chemicals with
primary sites of *action* (tissue recepter sites) and with secondary tissue
sites of *reaction* are important to a consideration of the joint toxic action
of chemicals. Most of these were succinctly reviewed by Veldstra[5] twenty-five
years ago, but have received additional detailed consideration in more recent
reviews[14,15]. With respect to the joint action of chemicals, three factors
were identified by Veldstra as being most important: (1) relative affinities
(taken as the net of the association and dissociation rate constants) of the
individual chemicals for *sites of action* (e.g., target enzymes, neuro-effector
sites or other vital target sites), (2) relative affinities for *sites of loss*
(e.g., detoxifying enzymes, non-vital tissue binding sites, pathways of
excretion and storage sites), and (3) the *intrinsic activity* of the compounds
at their sites of actions. It is also important to keep in mind the concept
that there are a limited number of sites of action or sites of loss within
any organism. Therefore, there will be a limiting dosage range within which
synergism or antagonism can be demonstrated. Although when Veldstra published
his review there were few known examples of biological activation of chemicals,
this phenomenon is now well established and therefore *sites of activation*,
as well as sites of loss and sites of action, are identified as reaction loci
for toxic interactions.

   The injury produced by a chemical in a living organism is proportional
to the quantity of the biologically active form of that chemical available
to react with critical, responsive cellular macromolecules. Thus toxicological interactions can be perceived, in general, as taking two forms: (1) the
quantity of an active form of one or more chemicals available to the pool
of critical cellular macromolecules is altered by the presence (or past
presence) of one or more other chemicals, or (2) the reactivity of the
critical macromolecules with the active form(s) of exogenous chemicals is
altered by the presence (or past presence) of one or more other chemicals
which may or may not themselves be capable of eliciting a response. The
first case can be said to involve primarily *sites of loss* (i.e., sites of

detoxification, excretion, storage or neutralization) or *sites of activation* of a chemical and case two represents interaction at *sites of action*. In the latter case either affinity for or intrinsic activity at the site of action may be altered.

At least three general mechanism of reactions among chemicals are involved in toxicological interactions.

Chemical-chemical. Either following absorption or in the fluids bathing the site of entry (i.e., in the G.I. tract or lung) one chemical may react directly with another such that potentially injurious forms never reach macromolecular reaction sites in cells. Numerous examples might be cited ranging from neutralization reactions among acids and bases to chelation reactions with heavy metals. Other reactions between organic molecules that actually lead to degradation of one or more of the reactive molecules, such as direct reaction of organophosphate insecticide with aldoximes, can also be included. Such chemical-chemical reactions are generally thought to be antidotal or protective in nature. Thus, reduced injury might be expected if workers were exposed to two or more such cross-reacting chemicals. However, enchanced injury or altered form of injury might also occur. A case in point would be the formation of nitrosamines from secondary amines and nitrites in the stomach. The fact that many nitrosamines are carcinogenic would seem to classify this chemical-chemical interaction as one yielding enhanced risk of injury.

Chemical competition at macromolecules. This general mechanism deals primarily with the question of relative affinities of exogenous chemicals for a limited number of reaction sites on cellular macromolecules. These cellular macromolecules for which exogenous chemicals compete may be sites of: absorption, activation, detoxification, injurious action or excretion. Competition for binding or reaction at these various sites may result in either enhanced or reduced toxicity. Knowing the nature of the individual chemicals and the kinetics of their reactions at these sites will permit logical prediction of the toxicological consequences of competition for reactions with these cellular macromolecules. This type of mechanism for toxicological interactions generally requires that the interacting chemicals or their reactive derivatives be present in the organism at the same time. However, the actual form present may be only a small residue of the original molecule that is bound to one or more reactive sites.

Altered cellular reactivity or responsiveness. A third general mechanism
for toxicological interactions is one in which cells and tissue are altered
by one chemical in such a way that the tissue's response to a second chemical
is altered, even if the first chemical is no longer present. This type
of toxicological interaction is more likely to result when exposures are
separated in time. The interaction of chemicals that initiate and promote
carcinogenesis would be included in this classification. Induction of
biotransformation enzymes for one chemical by exposure to another could be
another example, and alterations by one chemical of the repair of a cellular
lesion induced by another represents still a third sub-class of this general
mechanism.

The toxicological consequences of one chemical reacting with or otherwise
altering various critical biological reaction sites for another compound are
summarized in Table 1.

TABLE 1

THEORETICAL TOXICOLOGICAL CONSEQUENCES OF INTERACTIONS OF TWO COMPOUNDS
(A AND B) AT BIOLOGICAL REACTION SITES

Biological Loci of Reaction	Effect of B	Consequence to Toxicity of A
Site of Action	B's affinity > A	Reduction likely unless B's intrinsic activity > A's.
	B's affinity < A	Additive
Site of Loss	B's affinity > A	Enhancement likely
	B's affinity < A	Lesser enhancement (or none)
	Induction/Activation	Reduction
	Destruction/Inhibition	Enhancement
Site of Activation	B's affinity > A	Reduction
	B's affinity < A	Lesser reduction (or no effect)
	Induction/Activation	Enhancement
	Destruction/Inhibition	Reduction
Sites of Repair of A-induced injury	Induction/Activation	Reduction
	Destruction/Inhibition	Enhancement

Additional factors that must be considered in attempting to predict or to understand mechanisms of toxicological interactions are shown in Table 2.

TABLE 2

SOME ADDITIONAL DETERMINANTS OF INTERACTIONS

---

1. Criticality of altered sites and mechanisms of activation and/or loss to toxic action.
    a. Presence of alternative reactions.
2. Proximity of sites of action to altered sites of activation and loss.
3. Temporal "Opportunity factors".
    a. Oportunity to be activated.
    b. Opportunity to accumulate at site of action.
    c. Opportunity for reversal of injury.
    d. Opportunity for loss to occur.

One compound may alter the number or the activity of either sites of activation or sites of loss of a second compound. But the extent that this will be manifest in an altered susceptibility of the total organism to toxic action of the second compound will depend upon whether the altered sites and pathways are *rate limiting with respect to the toxic action*. If alternative and unaffected pathways or sites of activation or loss are present the predicted interaction may not develop; or it may be modulated in its intensity.

The proximity of sites of action to the critical sites of activation or loss may be an important determinant of toxic interactions. Thus, the induction of an activation enzyme in liver cells may have unexpectedly little effect on acute toxicity that is mediated through a target enzyme (i.e., the site of action) located in the brain, if the active metabolite produced by the liver is so reactive that it irreversibly binds to noncritical molecules in liver cells (where it is produced) or if it is detoxified as rapidly as it is produced. Thus, with multiple pathways of metabolism which both activate and detoxify organic chemicals, and with multipe sites of action which may vary widely in their criticality to life, it is often necessary to consider the so called opportunity factors in predicting or understanding the mechanisms of toxic interactions. Opportunity for a certain critical reaction of one compound to occur in the face of other competing macromolecular reactions can be dramatically altered by other chemicals. That is, if one compound, as a mixed function oxidase inducer, increases the concentration of microsomal sites of detoxification as well as microsomal sites of activation, will the induction of the detoxifying system effectively reduce the *opportunity* for the parent compound to be activated to a tissue-reactive form? Another time related *opportunity* relates to the rate of reversal of the injury, or the binding of an active metabolite to a primary site of action in relation to the net rate at which the active metabolite can accumulate at the site of action.

ILLUSTRATION OF SOME PRINCIPLES OF INTERACTION WITH SPECIFIC CHEMICALS

   Phosphorothionate insecticide metabolism and action. Several of the principles discussed above can be illustrated by a discussion of toxic interactions involving organic phosphorothionate insecticides.

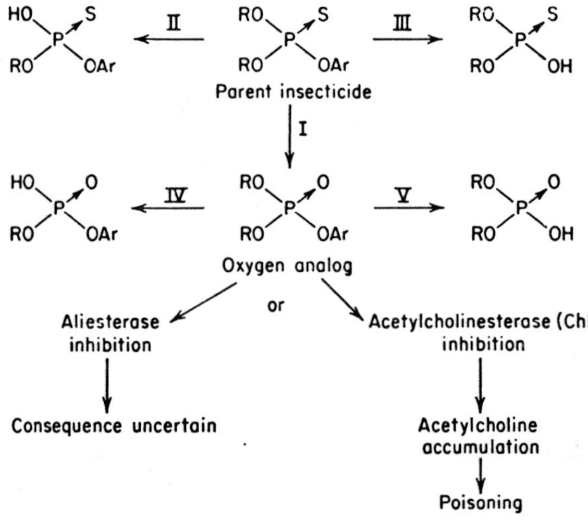

Fig. 3. General scheme of metabolism and mechanism of toxic action of dialkyl, aryl phosphorothioates.

As indicated in Figure 3[16] acetylcholinesterase of nerve tissue is the primary *site of action*; but this site is only reactive with a biotransformation product of the parent compound formed via reaction I. The *site of activation*

is in liver endoplasmic reticulum (microsomes) and to a much smaller extent
in other tissues including nerve tissue[17]. Reactions II through V are all
detoxification reactions and hence may be considered *sites of loss*. Reaction
III has cofactor and oxygen requirements and distribution (both intracellular
and in tissues) characteristics closely resembling, if not identical to those
of reaction I. Hence the site of activation and at least one site of detoxification have very similar properties. Reaction V is catalyzed by
hydrolases widely distributed in mammalian tissues including plasma. React-
tions II and IV are catalyzed glutathione alkyltransferase for some compounds
(usually when R is methyl), and by oxidases for a very few compounds. A
second *silent* target is carboxyl esterase (Aliesterase). The toxicological
significance of this reaction is not known except when animals are exposed
to additional ester-containing toxic compounds for which carboxylesterase
is a *site of loss*. Then phosphate esters that inhibit carboxylesterases
enter into toxicological interactions with these ester containing compounds.

A few years ago we were struck by the observation that piperonyl butoxide,
an important insecticidal synergist and known inhibitor of mixed function
oxidases, had not been very thoroughly investigated with respect to its
effect on the mammalian toxicity of phosphorothionate insecticides, known
to be both activated and detoxified by mixed function oxidases. We under-
took studies in mice which showed that piperonyl butoxide and SKF-525A,
both mixed function oxidase inhibitors, potentiated the intra-peritoneal
toxicity of diethyl substituted phosphorothionates but they protected against
the toxicity of the *dimethyl* substituted homologues (Table 3).

TABLE 3

EFFECT OF PIPERONYL BUTOXIDE AND SKF-525A ON DIMETYL AND DIETHYL PHOSPHORO-
THIONATE TOXICITY IN MICE

Insecticide Challenge	24 Hour LD_{50} (mg/kg)[a]		
	Pretreatment		
	Corn Oil (1 ml/kg)	Piperonyl Butoxide (400 mg/kg)	SKF-525A (50 mg/kg)
Methyl Parathion	7.6	330	220
Ethyl Parathion	10.0	5.5	6.1
Methyl Guthion	6.2	19.5	11.8
Ethyl Guthion	22.0	3.4	9.1

[a]Mice were given pretreatment compounds, i.p. 1 hour before injection,
(i.p.) with graded doses of the challenge insecticides. Data adapted
from Levine and Murphy[18].

We then investigated the major biochemical pathways of metabolism in appropriately fortified liver homogenates using both parathion and methyl para-
tion as substrates.

The pathways studied are illustrated schematically on Figure 4.

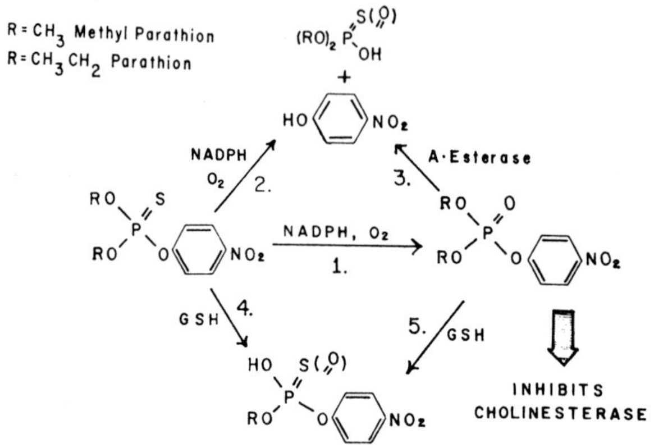

Fig. 4. Metabolism and action of methyl parathion and parathion. Reaction
products derived from the oxygen analog are indicated by (⟋0).

Note that reaction #1 is an activating reaction and the availability of its
product, the oxygen analog, to react with the target enzyme, acetylcholinesterase, at critical sites in nerve tissue is generally accepted as the
limiting factor in the acute mammalian toxicity of this class of insecticides.
All other reactions shown in Figure 4 are detoxification reactions.

Table 4 summarizes the results of a large number of experiments, which
have been published in detail elsewhere[19]. These studies were conducted
as part of our search for an explanation for the marked protective effect of
piperonyl butoxide on methyl parathion toxicity as opposed to the mild
potentiation of ethyl parathion. In each case methyl parathion and ethyl
parathion were compared in each system. With respect to both oxidative
activation and oxidative cleavage (or detoxification), there were no
striking differences in enzyme kinetic data nor in piperonyl butoxide's

inhibitory potency with respect to the two pesticide substrates. Although the Vmax for hydrolysis of the oxygen analogue of methyl parathion was only about 1/3 that for parathion oxygen analog, the Km values were nearly identical and furthermore this detoxification pathway was not inhibited by piperonyl butoxide.

On the other hand, we found, as have others, that methyl parathion detoxification by glutathione alkyl transferase was infinitely greater

TABLE 4

COMPARATIVE IN VITRO REACTIONS FOR METHYL PARATHION AND PARATHION

Oxidative Activation (liver)	Methyl Parathion/Parathion[a]
Km	1.16
Vmax	0.62
Ki for Piperonyl Butoxide	1.07
Oxidative Cleavage (liver)	
Km	0.84
Vmax	0.50
Ki for Piperonyl Butoxide	0.91
Hydrolysis of Oxon (liver)	
Km	0.91
Vmax	0.37
(not inhibited by Piperonyl Butoxide)	----
Glutathione Transfer (liver)	∞
Reactivation Rates (Kr) of Inhibited Che	
Brain	7.50
Diaphragm	7.67
Plasma	(none reactivated)

[a]Values are ratios of values obtained when methyl parathion/parathion were tested in the system indicated. Original data from which ratios were calculated are in Levine and Murphy[18,19].

than for ethyl parathion. Thus, this alternate pathway of detoxification which was not inhibited by piperonyl butoxide provided an opportunity for the methyl compound to be detoxified. This alternative was not available to parathion which is not deethylated by glutathione transferase.

Furthermore, the reactivation rate of inhibited acetylcholinesterase was markedly more rapid with methyl parathion than with ethyl parathion. Thus with oxidative activation inhibited by piperonyl butoxide, the reduced rate of methyl paraoxon production did not give an *opportunity* for accumulation of injury (i.e., cholinesterase inhibition) at a rate sufficient to exceed the rate of reversal of injury at the site of action. With parathion, even though oxon production was slowed, there was no alternative detoxication pathway to the oxidative cleavage which was also inhibited. Finally, because reversal of cholinesterase inhibition was very slow with paraoxon, the inhibition could accumulate sufficient to cause fatalities at lower doses of parathion even though the poisoning was somewhat delayed in onset.

This example represents but one example of numerous cases of toxicological interactions involving organophosphate insecticides[16] observed under laboratory conditions. It is illustrative, however, from the standpoint of emphasis of the complexities of interactions among chemicals which have multiple pathways of metabolism some of which are toxifying and some that are detoxifying. Furthermore, it illustrates that the dynamic relationships between *sites of activation, sites of loss* and *sites of action* must be thoroughly understood before accurate predictions can be made regarding the action of one chemical on the toxicity of even chemically and toxicologically closely related compounds.

Another mechanism of potentiation of a few organophosphate insecticides, which contain carboxy ester linkages, involves the inhibition of carboxylesterases by certain other organophosphates often at doses less than those required to react significantly at the usual site of toxic action, i.e., acetylcholinesterase. This mechanism to explain the potentiation of malathion, O, O-dimethyl S-(1,2-dicarboethoxy) ethyl phosphorodithioate, was well established experimentally twenty years ago[20,21]. Initially the observation and elucidation of the mechanism of potentiation of malathion toxicity by other organophosphates led to regulatory requirements, on the part of the U.S.F.D.A., for specific tests for potentiation for any new anticholinesterase insecticides. However, about ten years later, this requirement was dropped. It is interesting to note, however, that this mechanism of toxic interaction has recently been called forward to explain the poisoning of several thousand spraymen in Pakistan during 1976[22]. It was demonstrated that the spraymen using a batch of technical malathion which contained the greatest quantities of certain impurities suffered greater red blood cell cholinesterase inhibition than those using less contaminated malathion. Four years previously, Pellegrini and Sante[23] had demonstrated that several of the contaminants (eventually found in some samples of malathion used in the Pakistan mosquito control program) were capable of synergizing the toxicity of purified malathion. These observations were more recently confirmed by Umetsu et al[24], and by Miles et al[25]. Talcott et al[26], recently demonstrated that these impurities were rather selective inhibitors of malathion carboxylesterase.

The opportunity for malathion's toxicity to be synergized by other chemicals was well documented by laboratory studies at least two decades before it apparently "came home to roost" as an incident of mass occupational poisonings. At least two very practical principles are illustrated. One, as stated in the outset, the actual occurrence of toxicological interactions in the human population is most likely in those who have greatest risk of exposure to nearly-effective doses (e.g., occupational exposures). The second practical principal relates to safety considerations in the design of bioactive compounds, namely if man chooses to depend upon the detoxication system of non-target species to protect them against biocides for target species, then it is essential to know the characteristics of the detoxification system in great detail so that any condition that disrupts this system can be predicted. Another lesson to be derived from this example is that tox-icological interactions need not involve specifically separate products, but can occur between so called *minor contaminants* and the *active ingredient* as well. Finally, it illustrates that knowledge cannot assure safety, diligent *application* is required.

REFERENCES

1. Pitts, J.N. (1969) J. Air Poll. Cont. Assn., 19, 658-667.
2. Mirvish, S.S. (1977) J. Toxicol. Environ. Hlth., 2, 1267-1277, 1977.
3. Crosby, D.G. (1969) Ann. N.Y. Acad. Sci. 160 (Art. 1), 82-96.
4. Amdur, M.O. and Underhill, D. (1968) Arch. Environ. Health 16, 460-468.
5. Veldstra, H. (1956) Pharmacol. Rev. 8, 339-387.
6. Finney, D.J. (1952) Probit Analysis: A Statistical Treatment of the Sigmoid Response Curve. 2nd Ed. Cambridge University Press, London, pp. 1-318.
7. DuBois, K.P. (1961) Advances in Pest Control Research IV, 117-151.
8. Smyth, H.F., Weil, C.S., West, J.S. and Carpenter, C.P. (1969) Toxicol. Appl. Pharmacol. 14, 340-347.

294

9. Dunnet, C.W. (1968) Selected Pharmacological Testing Methods, A. Burger, Ed., Marcel-Dekker Inc., N.Y., pp. 1-515.

10. American Conference of Governmental Industrial Hygienists (1977) TLVs, Threshold Limit Values for Chemical Substances and Physical Agents in the Workroom Environment, ACGIH, P.O. Box 1937, Cincinnati, OH, pp. 45-49.

11. Gaddum, J.H. (1957) Proceeding of a Symposium on Drug Antagonism Pharmacol. Rev. 9, 211-268.

12. Ryser, H.J.P. (1971) New Eng. J. Med. 265, 721-734.

13. Witschi, H. and Côte, M.G. (1977) Chem.-Biol. Interactions 19, 279-289.

14. Gillette, J.R. and Mitchell, J.R. (1975) Handbuch der experimentellen Pharmakologie - New Series, Eds. O. Eichler, A. Farah, H. Herken, A. D. Welch, Springer-Verlag, Berlin, pp. 359-381.

15. Schand, D.G., Mitchell, J.R., and Oates, J.A. (1975) Handbuch der experimentellen Pharmakologie - New Series, Eds. O. Eichler, A. Farah, H. Herken, A.D. Welch, Springer-Verlag, Berlin, pp. 272-314.

16. Murphy, S.D. (1969) Residue Rev., 25, 201-221.

17. Neal, R.A. (1967) Biochem. J., 103,183-191.

18. Levine, B.S. and Murphy, S.D. (1977) Toxicol. Appl. Pharmacol. 40, 379-391.

19. Levine, B.S. and Murphy, S.D. (1977) Toxicol. Appl. Pharmacol. 40, 393-406.

20. Murphy, S.D. and DuBois, K.P. (1957) Proc. Soc. Exp. Biol. Med. 64, 813-818.

21. Frawley, J.P., Fuyat, H.N., Hagan, E.C., Blake, J.R. and Fitzhugh, O.G. (1957) J. Pharmacol. Expt. Therap. 121, 96-106.

22. Baker, E.J., Zack, M., Mites, J.W., Alderman, L., Warren, M., Dobbin, R.D., Miller, S., Teeters, W.R. (1978) The Lancet, Jan. 7, 31-34.

23. Pellegrini, G., and Santi, R. (1972) J. Agric. Food Chem. 20, 944-950.

24. Umetsu, N., Grose, F.H., Allahyari, R. Abu-El-Haj, S., Fukuto, T.R. (1977) J. Agric. Food Chem. 25, 946-953.

25. Miles, J.W., Mount, D.L., Staiger, M.A. and Teeters, W.R. (1979) J. Agric. Food Chem. 27, 421-425.

26. Talcott, R.E., Mallipudi, N.M., Umetsu, N. and Fukuto, T.R. (1979) Toxicol. Appl. Pharmacol. 49, 107-112.

© 1980 Elsevier/North-Holland Biomedical Press
The Principles and Methods in Modern Toxicology
C.L. Galli, S.D. Murphy and R. Paoletti, editors.

TOXICOLOGY OF IMMUNITY

ANGELO NICOLIN, ANTONIO COSCO, ORNELLA MARELLI and FILIPPO SARRA
Institute of Pharmacology, School of Medicine, University of Milan, Via
Vanvitelli 32, 20133 Milan (Italy)

SUMMARY

   A variety of diseases have been associated or have been closely related to
alterations of the immune system. Abnormal immune reactivity either below or
above the physiological level could be involved in pathogenetic mechanisms.
Moreover, the altered reactivity can be determined, in many circumstances, by
disordered interactions among cell subsets collaborating for the antigen
response. In this chapter special emphasis is placed on the review of chemical
or physical agents capable of selectively depressing or enhancing the activity
of one cell subpopulation among those responsible for the regulation of the
immune response. Methods for mass screening are critically discussed following
the studies recommended by the Seveso Medical Committee to evaluate the immunological alterations among people contaminated by the Dioxin at Seveso. Recent
theoretical and experimental findings that might further the actual understanding of immunological mechanisms and their possible alterations are also
discussed in brief. The lack of assays that closely fit the needs of immuno-
toxicology, technical difficulties, the still incomplete knowledge of the
basic mechanisms of immunity, and finally, the actual limits of this topic as
well as the realistic expectations are pointed out.

INTRODUCTION

   The pressing needs of society and the tremendous progress of technology have
forced the tumultuous development of all biomedical studies. Among the youngest
and fastest developing disciplines, toxicology and immunology are worthy of
special mention. This impetuous growth might in part account for the scant
attention toxicologists and immunologists have regarded each other. More than
other studies, toxicology is in need of borrowing concepts and methodologies
from other disciplines. Moreover, the fast accumulation of new information
makes it necessary to make continuous changes in basic concepts and in experimental procedures. The concomitant growth and changes in the expectancies of
people who are responsible for public health might contribute to disturb a
mediate settlement of the matter. For instance, a few years ago, toxicology

was called upon with dramatic urgency to deal with teratogenesis, whereas it is now enjoined to find out simple and reliable methods to identify environmental carcinogens.

Although in the fastest stage of development, toxicology and immunity have sometimes had the opportunity to come in contact. However, an intimate collaboration in objectives and purposes has not yet been established. Not even epidemiology has brought a systematic collaboration to toxicology in discovering the environmental influence on diseases of immunological pathogenesis. Many studies on professional hypersensitivity have not been, until recently, associated with satisfactory investigations on the mechanisms of action, nor has the genetic background or the immunological status of the population at risk been evaluated. In spite of the fact that drugs used in therapy are required to undergo complex toxicologic studies before licensing for marketing, present laws do not forecast any kind of immunological assays.

Although damages produced by anticancer agents and corticoid hormones on the immune system have been extensively investigated[1] and studies on different compounds, for instance antiinflammatory drugs[2], have also been performed, the peculiar interest of toxicologists was not properly considered. Some studies dealing with oral contraceptives might be cited among the rare studies devoted to toxicology of the immune system[3].

The immunosuppressive effects of carcinogenic compounds might have been underestimated. Although the direct correlation between immunodeficiency and cancer has been experimentally proved only for viral oncogenesis[4], the increased incidence of cancer in immunodepressed patients is well known. Special emphasis should be focused on the new findings now emerging from studies on immunity. An aspecific depression is no longer the only damage that might be exerted on the immune system. Aspecific and, likely more relevant, specific and fine mechanisms regulating immune reactions throw new light on the damage the immune system may undergo as well as on diseases caused by an alteration of immune reactivity.

It is now time for the birth of a new scientific branch: toxicology of the immune system.

PRINCIPLES

Immunological responses are distinguishable from other recognition processes by their possession of three cardinal features, namely specificity, memory and amplification. Specificity and memory will not be discussed in this chapter.

Amplification, although not an exclusive feature of immunologic responses, is a unique event in the sense of a qualitative change in the reactive material.

Apart from particular situations, immune response does not occur operatively in the absence of amplification. Features like the magnitude or the temporal extension of amplification are in turn regulated by cells, or their soluble products, which belong to the immunological compartment. Imbalance in the complex interactions among effector cells and regulatory cells is actually responsible for a variety of alterations in the immune functions[5]. The fundamental mechanisms of immune regulation and the immunological disorders as a consequence of altered interactions among immune cell subsets will be briefly discussed.

CELLS OF THE IMMUNE SYSTEM

ANTIGEN SPECIFIC

B		ANTIBODY
LYMPHOCYTE		
		CML
	T_e	CMI DTH
		GVH
T		Lymphokines
	$T_h - T_s$	B and T
	T_a ?	B and T

ANTIGEN NOT SPECIFIC

MONOCYTE		⌈ Antigen presentation
MACROPHAGE		| Immune Regulation
		⊣ Phagocytosis
		| Pharmacological active
		⌊ factors
	NEUTROPHIL	⌈ Phagocytosis
		⊣ Pharmacological active
		⌊ factors
GRANULOCYTE	BASOPHIL	⌈ Histamine
		⊣ S R S - A (Leukotriene C)
		⌊ Enzymes
	EOSINOPHIL	⌈ Prostaglandins
		⊣ Perossidasis
		⌊ SRS inactivator

Precursor effector cells undergo definitive maturation to competent cells upon contact with the antigen and amplifying cells, or their products, which are in turn activated by the relevant antigen. Opitmal immunogen presentation is a necessary step provided by the macrophage compartment[6]. Because of the absence of specific receptors for antigens, antigenic presentation and accessory activities of macrophages lack specificity, although collaboration is restricted to cells sharing the macrophage genotype[7]. Toxicologic studies have been almost disregarded because of the assumption that macrophages can resist, better than lymphocytes, physical and chemical damage. This is in contrast with the fact that macrophages are susceptible to exogenous damage. For instance, the specific toxic effects of carrageenan[8] or silica[9] have been shown to deplete macrophages, which allows establishment of their role in immune reactions in living animals. Cytotoxic compounds have exhibited antimacrophage activity not associated with lymphocyte toxicity. Therefore, environmental specific toxicity to the macrophage pool can no longer be excluded. There is no doubt that regulatory T lymphocytes are of the greatest interest for toxicology. The major regulatory T cells are T-helper and T-suppressor lymphocytes, the effects of which are evidently opposed. A great deal of work is now devoted to characterization of their functional properties and their surface markers. A third subpopulation of T cells, the amplifying cells[10], has been identified, but their role in the immune response is not yet well defined and is likely to be less relevant. A receptor specific for the antigen and products coded for by genes in the major histocompatibility complex (MHC)[11] determines the specificity and the genetic restriction of the collaboration.

Specific phenotypic markers expressed on the T_h cell surface[12], identified by proper antibodies, make their recognition feasible. T_s lymphocytes carry surface markers[13] specific for the subset and express products coded for by genes in the MHC; the latter is likely responsible for the suppressor effect[14]. In the correct balance between the opposing activities lies the safety of immune response. At the occurrence of an antigenic stimulus, T_h clones specific for the relevant antigen should be activated before T_s cells are ready to play their part. The antigenic load is also important; for instance, an overdose of the immunogen enhances the T_s cell activity[15].

The idea that the intensity and the duration of the immune response might be under the control of a mechanism other than T_h-T_s cell interaction has found some experimental support. Following the hypothesis of the immunological network[16], an autologous immune reaction against the receptor for the antigen might contribute to modulate immune reaction. Since the antibody itself is the B lymphocyte receptor and the T lymphocyte receptor behaves like the antibody combining site, an immune reaction to the very peculiar amino acid sequence that binds a specific antigen, the idiotype, inhibits effector immune cells by a simple feedback-like mechanism.

REGULATION OF IMMUNE REACTION

T HELPER   ↑ humoral and cell
                          mediated immunity

T SUPPRESSOR   ↓ humoral and cell
                          mediated immunity

IMMUNOLOGICAL NETWORK   antibody and CMI to
                                  effector cell idiotype

The immunological network needs further studies and, in the present formulation, does not appear specifically influenced by physical or chemical treatment.

The great influence on immune response exhibited by the helper-suppressor cell system might capture the interest of toxicologists, because an imbalance in the physiological interactions is associated with a number of diseases and because a selective damage by radiation or by chemical compounds on a regulatory subset has been clearly documented. Specific pathologic disorders have not been joined to an altered helper activity; however, strains of mice genetically defective of the T_h compartment are now extensively studied[17]. In contrast, an abnormal activity of T_s cells has been demonstrated in the pathogenetic noxa of a number of experimental diseases[18]. Exaggerated suppressor activity, either genetically encoded or determined by alterations in the soma, as occurring, for instance, in old age, has been evidenced in a few strains of mice[19]. Diseases like experimental thyroiditis[20], or augmented oncogenic viruses in the blood[21] or in the tissues, followed by the development of lethal tumors, have been related to the prevalence of T_s cells. Other strains of mice, defective of the T_s functions and therefore immunologically hyperactive, are very susceptible to a number of pathologic alterations, leading to the appearance of autoimmune diseases.

The major interest for toxicology in these facts lies in the particular susceptibility of suppressor cells to chemical or physical inhibition, which indicates the capacity of exogenous factors for unbalanced T_h-T_s activities per se responsible for illness. Cytotoxic compounds, under proper dosages and opportune schedules of treatments, selectively inhibit suppressor cell activities. The potentiation of a specific immune response by limiting the involve-

EFFECTS OF IMBALANCED REGULATION

↑ HELPER		I	Anaphylaxis	
	HYPERSENSITIVITY	II	Antibody and Complement	
↓ SUPPRESSOR		III	Immune complex	
		IV	CMI	

↓ HELPER		Bacteria	↓ Ab
	INFECTION	Viruses	↓ Ab or CMI
	SUSCEPTIBILITY	Fungi	↓ CMI
↑ SUPPRESSOR		Protozoa	↓ Ab or CMI

CANCER ?   ↓ CMI

ment of the T_s lymphocytes has therefore become possible. Most effects exerted by the immune system, either through the humoral or the cell-mediated mechanisms, can be enhanced in this way. Delayed type hypersensitivity[22], immediate allergic reactions[23], graft versus host[24] and transplantation reactions[25] and, in short, all responses elicited by molecular or particulate antigens can be strengthened. For this purpose, among other compounds, cyclophosphamide is noteworthy. Following reports from the literature, others and our laboratory have been able to paradoxically increase host reactivity to a syngeneic tumor cell by treatment with the immunosuppressive drug cyclophosphamide. Suppressor cell activity was potentiated by exposure to low doses of x-rays[26] through a preferential damage to the T_h compartment.

SELECTIVE MODULATION OF HELPER OR SUPPRESSOR ACTIVITY

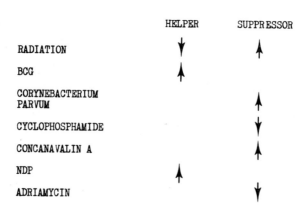

	HELPER	SUPPRESSOR
RADIATION	↓	↑
BCG	↑	
CORYNEBACTERIUM PARVUM		↑
CYCLOPHOSPHAMIDE		↓
CONCANAVALIN A		↑
NDP	↑	
ADRIAMYCIN		↓

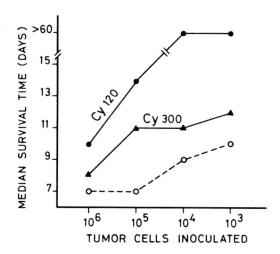

Fig. 5. CD_2F_1 mice, untreated (O) or treated on day -3 with cyclophosphamide (Cy), 120 mg/kg i.p. (●), or 300 mg/kg i.p. (▲), were challenged on day 0 with a graded number of L1210 leukemic cells, as indicated, and 10×10^6 L1210/DTIC leukemic cells. L1210/DTIC is a subline of L1210 leukemia, which has been found to induce host resistance to L1210 parental leukemia. The experiment shows that L1210/DTIC vaccination did not increase host survival. In contrast, the Cy pretreatment, by enhancing the immune response elicited by L1210/DTIC cells, increased the survival time of the mice.

Since a variety of agents can preferentially damage suppressor cells rather than other lymphoid subpopulations, concern should be directed to the effects on immunity of environmental compounds. Even in the lack of ad hoc studies and considering the complexity of the origins, the increased morbidity from infectious agents, in spite of the improved hygienic conditions (such as winter fever in children) might in part be due to temporary alterations in the regulatory cells of immunity. Yet the augmentation of allergic and autoimmune diseases might find in the environment similar pathogenetic mechanisms. It should be pointed out that, although discussing the hypothetical hazards, the potential dangerousness should justify the setting up of specific toxicologic and epidemiologic studies.

METHODOLOGY

Immunology has been exploiting numerous laboratory tests and experimental

assays in animals and humans to dissect and disclose the complexity of the
immune reactions. In studying the toxicology of immunity, methods actually
available are only those developed for these purposes. Toxicology therefore
needs to adopt, among a variety of immunological methods, those assay systems
that might help in the settlement of its requirements. In addition to dealing
with improper technology, difficulties lie in selecting the optimal experimental systems for each purpose. For instance, toxicology might be asked to
establish whether a compound might alter in some way immune functions or
whether, in a large group of compounds, toxic agents might be identified by
screening procedures. In the former case, the finest methods should make clear
the nature and the step(s) of the alteration; in the latter case, few and easy
assays are the most suitable.

Studies on toxicology of the immune system carried out in consequence of the
Dioxin (2,3,7,8-tetrachlorodibenzo-p-dioxin) (TCDD)) accident in Seveso will
be discussed in some detail. This dramatic event required that toxicology
consider, besides many and new problems, the occurrence of immunological alterations in people exposed to Dioxin. Since wide and persistent damage to the
immune system of different animal species was well known from the literature,
in the absence of immuno-toxicology scientists, immunologists have been charged
to identify immunological alterations and associated diseases. Laboratory and
in vivo tests adopted by the Medical Committee to study and monitor Seveso
patients will serve for a survey on the most popular immunological assays and
for a comment on the information that might be obtained.

For the purpose of this paper, groups of patients and control groups,
selected for immunological studies, or relevant aspects that do not strictly
concern technical features, will not be discussed. Immunologists decided to
investigate both humoral and cellular properties with special emphasis on the
latter, since experiments in animals have indicated that cell-mediated immune
reactions were more susceptible than antibody productions to Dioxin damage [27-29].
The immunological tests adopted for the Seveso large-scale population study
might fall into two groups: the first one contributing to delineate a quantitative image of cells and products on the immune system, and the second one
indicating the capacity to react to stimuli.

The contents of gamma globulin in the serum of patients were determined by
a well-known electrophoretic method, which is used routinely in all clinical
analytical laboratories. The total amount of circulating gamma globulins and
the relative amount of IgG, IgM and IgA antibodies can be determined by use of
this method. Only gross alterations in circulating antibodies can be assessed.

If their level is above normal, serious diseases are often associated; if
below, a deficit in the antibody-producing machinery has occurred. The dosage
of antibody contents in the serum is an essential, preliminary step, although
not sufficient to reveal specific or fine alterations of humoral immunity.
The serum level of IgE, the antibody class responsible for immediate allergic
reaction, has been evaluated by radioimmunoassay. An IgE level above normal
indicates the presence of an allergic status or a susceptibility to undergo
sensitization, although the allergen cannot be revealed by this assay. Complement, a group of circulating proteins, exhibits many accessory activities of
the immune system following its cascade activation by antigen-antibody reaction.
The amount of hemoglobin released in the supernatant by antibody-coated red
blood cells in the presence of the serum under investigation is indicative of
complement activity. The evaluation of only one of many activities, although
the most significant in that it needs the activation of all the complement
constituents, might increase the concern about gamma globulin dosage.

Leucocyte formula is a fundamental assay in all hematologic analyses. White
blood cells are specific cells or accessory cells of immunity. The number of
circulating lymphocytes might be preferentially reduced by toxic agents,
because of their particular susceptibility in respect to the other white cells.
Subtle alterations by exogenous agents obviously cannot be evidenced by determining, at the microscope, the leucocyte formula. Blood analyses so far
described, simple to perform, allow a quantitative although rough picture of
components of the immune system in the blood. These preliminary analytical
studies very seldom offer the chance to discover environmental damages to the
immune system. Immuno-toxicologic studies can evidence fine but not less
harmful alterations in the cells, in the products, and in the functions of
immunity, which complex techniques might only partially detect.

Lymphocyte enumeration, in the case of Seveso studies, has been integrated
by lymphocyte rosetting[30], a relatively simple experimental assay not yet in
general use. Human T lymphocytes bind sheep red blood cells (SRBC) on their
surface, whereas B lymphocytes, through receptors for the third component of
complement, bind SRBC previously coated with anti-SRBC antibodies and complement. At the microscope, lymphocytes surrounded by three or more SRBC, hence
the name "rosette", are respectively T or B lymphocytes. By the rosetting
assay an alteration in the proportion of T and B lymphocytes in the blood can
be easily established. Since a number of agents can act selectively on T or B
lymphocytes without obvious alteration in the total number of circulating
lymphocytes, the rosette assay greatly improves the study of human lymphocytes.

To complete the survey of immune characteristics, histocompatibility antigen (HLA) typing, a quite sophisticated and specialistic assay, has been proposed. The MHC, HLA in humans, like similar systems in animals, is a genome segment in chromosome 6, which codes for a large yet undefined number of surface molecules antigenically specific for each patient. The individual HLA, recognized by immune cells of an unrelated individual in the species, are fundamental for the rejection of transplanted tissues. Moreover, HLA codes for a number of activities not entirely identified yet very relevant in the regulation of the immune response. Surface molecules strictly associated with helper and suppressor activity, similar but not identical with those previously known, have been recently recognized[31]. Lastly, the absolute importance of the MHC in all immunological functions determines the association of a defined histocompatibility genotype with susceptibility to certain diseases[32]. The serological identification of the surface HLA (i.e., tissue typing) requires precise methodology, good experience, and the battery of antisera made available only to laboratories dedicated to these studies. HLA typing can therefore only be afforded by highly specialistic laboratories and, at present, can only be adopted in very special circumstances. The test might furnish data of maximum relevance.

An alteration in the expression of surface antigens, although not frequent, would reveal a mutation that has occurred in the area of genoma corresponding to the MHC. Some kind of autoimmune disease, i.e., an immune reaction against autologous cells, might be triggered by a mutation of the genoma or by an alteration of the HLA. The intensity of immune reactions might also be modified as a consequence of an alteration in the molecular structure of the surface antigens. Moreover, the susceptibility to the effects of exogenous agents in some instances is under genetic control. It means that the histocompatibility genotype might influence susceptibility to toxic agents like Dioxin. HLA typing might reveal a relationship between the expression of a HLA and the occurrence of a toxic effect. Tissue typing would establish whether a patient expressing specificity A might be susceptible, more easily than patients who express specificity B, to a toxic event. In this case, patients expressing specificity A could be submitted to preventive care. One might reasonably predict that in the future, thanks to a new technology in raising monoclonal antibodies, people will be typed at birth.

The assays described can give the quantitative variations of the physiological constituents of the immune system. The immunological reactivity and the integrity of physiological functions have been tackled in a second set of

analytic methods. An altered synthesis of specific antibodies was studied by
the aid of two serological tests. Both tests can detect the binding of natural
antibodies (natural means not induced by exogenous antigenic stimulation) to
red blood cells. The natural alloreactivity test measures the antibody binding
capacity (hemagglutinin titer) of the serum from a group A blood sample to red
blood cells of type B. Natural heteroreactivity detects specific antibodies
to SRBC. From the literature it is known that the titer of anti-red blood cell
antibodies, as evaluated by the above assays, might predict, at least in part,
patient capacity to synthesize and release specific antibodies.

The macrophage-monocyte system contributes, by the antigenic presentation,
to optimize immune reactions and exhibits a number of collateral, although
relevant, immunological activities. Unfortunately, macrophage studies in man
require a large amount of blood samples, which has discouraged the Medical
Committee of Seveso, since the concern has been mainly related to pediatric
patients. New miniature experimental procedures might overcome this problem.

Experiments have been set up with the final aim to establish whether or not
lymphoid cells can, under appropriate stimulus, proliferate. By the use of
mitogenic studies, the functional integrity of the afferent arch of the immune
response, the recognition and the proliferative phase, can be assessed. The
amount of [^{3}H]thymidine incorporated into the DNA of lymphocytes, although in
principle not strictly related to proliferation, has been widely accepted as
an index of the proliferative rate. Human T lymphocytes can be polyclonally
stimulated (which means not specifically) to synthesize DNA by lectins, such
as concanavalin A or phytohemagglutinin. In contrast, human B lymphocytes
obviously cannot be induced to proliferate in vitro. Polyclonal stimulation
with pokeweed mitogen has been adopted because of its capacity to stimulate
both B and T lymphocytes. Products like staphylococcal protein A bound to
Sephadex behave like B polyclonal stimulators, although their use has not yet
received wide enough experimentation.

The in vitro culture (MLR) of lymphocytes (responders) with metabolically
inert allogeneic cells (stimulators) indicates the capacity of responding
lymphocytes to recognize foreign cells, which in turn trigger the proliferative
reaction. By similar laboratory procedures the cytolytic activity against
stimulator cells exhibited by responding lymphocytes can now be evaluated.
The in vitro evaluation of MLR and cell-mediated cytotoxicity (CML) will give
a wide range of important T lymphocyte functions. In most instances, in vitro
lymphocyte reactivity may in part be correlated with in vivo tests for cell-
mediated immunity. Among a number of substances, old tuberculin, protein

purified derivative, streptokinase-streptodornase, and tricophytin, upon
scarification or contact with the skin, elicit an inflammatory reaction not
hazardous to patients, the amplitude of which might predict the degree of the
host cell-mediated reactivity. However, skin tests deal with a complex
reaction in which many cell types are involved. An altered response cannot be
used to show a precise site of disreactivity. Moreover, the execution and
the reading of the test, in the opinion of the experts, is not as easy as one
might suppose.

However, the technical difficulties and the quality of information obtained
with the methods adopted to study immunologic alterations in a large number of
patients should be pointed out. A few other assays more recently developed
might further complete the screening procedures. In addition, CML mentioned
in discussing MLR, lymphotoxins and products released upon lymphocyte activation might accurately predict the status of activities not obviously related
to those already studied at Seveso. Sera reacting with a lymphocyte subpopulation can be now used to evaluate the percentage of lymphoid cell types and,
by the use of a cell sorter, their fractionation allows studies on purified
populations.

Techniques are now available to assess suppressor cell activity. A few
methods actually adopted do not give entirely reproducible data. The information obtained on regulatory T-lymphocyte populations and the efforts in this
field will aid in the evaluation of suppressor and helper activities for
screening purposes.

In conclusion, immunological methods can aid to detect fine alterations of
immunological functions in humans. A careful immunological screening requires
a battery of complex tests, which are time consuming and costly. Furthermore,
to verify data the Seveso Medical Committee has decided on a double-blind
performance of the assays in two different laboratories.

ENVIRONMENTAL TOXICANTS TO THE IMMUNE SYSTEM

Discussing in very general terms its features, toxicology of the immune
system has been presented as a new branch of toxicology in a way to stand up
alone under the pressure of environmental events. Extensive studies are
therefore not reported in the literature, and data actually available have
been obtained from various fields. From these disseminated studies a few
examples of environmental products that cause immunological alterations will
be reported and discussed in brief.

The well-known carcinogen aflatoxin has been described to exhibit the capacity to depress protein synthesis[33], as well as to inhibit both humoral and cellular immunity[34]. Cell-mediated immunity seems the most susceptible to aflatoxin, although studies have been performed on a limited number of animal species, and experiments actually available are rather few[35]. Mico-toxin-treated target cells have shown increased resistance to the cytotoxic damage of the hepatocarcinogen aflatoxin[36]. The basis for the resistance is unknown, and it will not be discussed here. However, this and other experimental evidence indicate that cell resistance to immunological damage might be modified by environmental agents. For instance, virus-infected cells or cancerous cells might enhance their resistance to immunological attack or, in contrast, target cells might increase their susceptibility to effective immune response under environmental exposure. The altered target cell fragility might mimic the effects induced by modulators of immune mechanisms.

Perturbation of the physiologic course of the immune response by heavy metal ions has been reported. Unlike aflatoxin, lithium has been found to strengthen some immune cell functions. The matter requires more extensive studies, since contrasting observations have been reported. Lithium seems to stimulate lymphocyte and macrophage activities[37] and shows a positive effect in inducing resistance to infections[38], whereas it improves the sympto-matology in asthmatic patients[39]. In another study, thymus hypoplasia has been observed following lithium treatment[40]. Neither of these studies has been sufficiently confirmed. The capacity of lithium to stimulate granulo-poiesis in vitro and to enhance the recovery of neutropenic patients, although extensively studied, has not yet been definitely proved. The precise bound-aries of lithium activity on the immune system cannot be defined, although a stimulatory activity on some cells with immune functions is a possibility. In addition, lithium studies have been run with "pharmacologic dosages", and it is possible that lithium can modify the delicate balance of immune mechanisms. As discussed before, irrespective of the immunological circum-stances, lithium might exhibit therapeutic or toxic effects.

Lead or zinc have also been shown to modulate the strength of the immune response. Zinc deficiency was associated with severe immunodeficiency, abnormalities of thymus morphology, and T-dependent areas in lymphoid tissues of animals[41] and man[42]. In the course of these studies, animals fed with a zinc-enriched diet had a higher level of thymic hormone[43] than the control group.

The chemokinetic migration of resting human T-lymphocytes has been stimu-lated in vitro by arachidonic acid in a dose-related manner[44]. By increasing random locomotion, migration, homing and accumulation of lymphocytes, one might find a way to alter the immunological reactivity in the tissues.

The extraordinary septic complications in acute thermal injuries are well known. Thermal injury has been shown to affect various cellular-immune functions[45]. In dissecting the activity of a cell population from burned mice, the immunological impairment has been shown to be mainly localized in the expansion of T-suppressor cell activity. In this impressive study, removal of the T-cell fraction followed by reconstitution with normal, syngeneic T cells brought about normal functioning of the immunological machinery of burned animals[46].

Although not strictly related to toxicology, it might be worth mentioning that nutritional deficiencies impair the developemnt and function of the immune system. In addition to aspecific deterioration associated with protein deprivation, certain nutritional deficiencies also have deleterious effects. Vitamin B6 deficiency has been widely reported to reduce the capacity of lymphoid cells[47] to respond to certain antigenic stimuli or to reject foreign tissues. Dramatic depletion of thoracic duct lymphocytes, severe alteration in the thymus, depletion of lymphocytes, and the relative increase in epithelial cells and macrophages are normally found in congenital vitamin B6-deficient animals.

CONCLUSIONS

Minor modification in the physiologic course of the immune response might be, in most instances, a pathogenetic event. Immunological methods will reasonably indicate the cellular subpopulation or the mechanism mainly targeted by the perturbing agent. Although not properly developed for toxicological studies, immunological methods are becoming miniaturized, easier to handle, cheaper and, not less relevant, quite reproducible. This does not mean that the immunological screening of a large group of people or the effects of environmental chemicals on the immune system can be easily faced. In the meantime, knowledge of the immune machinery and the pathogenesis of immunologic disorders does not yet allow an exact indication of the relevance of a toxic event for the health of people.

How immunology has developed, most of its functions and mechanisms of action, and its role in maintaining the physiologic homeostasis as well as hindering foreign invasions have been discussed. The damage on immune activities by environmental agents has been, in some cases, proved and in many others reasonably suspected. Toxicologists are called upon to assume a new responsibility, since theoretical and technical instruments are actually available to individualize agents toxic to the immune system.

REFERENCES

1. Hersh, E.M. (1975) Immunosuppressive agents. In: Handbook of Experimental Pharmacology, vol. 38/1, Springer Verlag, Berlin.

2. Godwin, J.S., Bankurst, A.D., and Sellinger, D.S. (1978) Clin. Res., 26, 12-18.

3. Vecchi, A., Tagliabue, A., Mantovani, A., Anaclerio, A., Barale, C., and Spreafico, F. (1976) Biomedicine, 24, 231-237.

4. Stutman, O. (1975) Adv. Cancer Res., 22, 261-422.

5. Talal, N. (1976) Transplant. Rev., 31, 240.

6. Nelson, D.S. (1976) In: Immunobiology of the Macrophage, Academic Press, New York, pp. 1-253.

7. Rosenthal, A.S., and Shevach, E.M. (1973) J. Exp. Med., 138, 1194-1212.

8. Keller, R. (1977) J. Natl. Cancer Inst., 59, 1751-1753.

9. Davies, P., Allison, A.C., Dym, M., and Cardella, C.J. (1975) In: Infection and Immunology in the Rheumatic Diseases (D.C. Dumonde, ed.), Blackwell, Oxford.

10. Okada, M., Klimpel, G.R., Kuppers, R.C., and Henney, C.S. (1979) J. Immunol., 122, 2527-2533.

11. Katz, D.H. and Benacerraf, B. (1976)   The Role of Products of the Histocompatibility Gene Complex in Immune Responses, Academic Press, New York.

12. Cantor, H. and Gershon, R.K. (1979) Fed. Proc., 7, 2058-2064.

13. Jandinski, J., Cantor, H., Tadakuma, T., Peavy, D.L., and Pierce, C.W. (1976) J. Exp. Med., 143, 1382-1384.

14. Clark, D.A., Philips, R.A., and Miller, R.G. (1977) Cell. Immunol., 34, 25-37.

15. Tada, T., Taniguchi, M., and Takemori, T. (1975) Transplant. Rev., 26, 106-129.

16. Raff, M. (1977) Nature, 265, 205-207.

17. Shultz, L.D. and Green, M.C. (1976) J. Immunol., 116, 936-943.

18. Steinberg, A.D. (1974) Arthritis Rheum., 17, 11-18.

19. Barthold, D.R., Kysela, S., and Steinberg, D. (1974) J. Immunol., 112, 9-13.

20. Dauphinée, M.J. and Talal, N. (1979) J. Immunol., 122, 936-941.

21. Kende, M., Stephenson, J.R., and Kelloff, G.J. (1978) Nature, 273, 383-386.

22. Katz, S., Parker, D., and Turk, J. (1975) Cell. Immunol., 16, 396-403.

23. Staykova, M. (1978) Ann Immunol, 129, 415-417.

24. Miller, J.F.M. (1977) Clin. Haematol., 6, 277-298.

25. Steel, G. and Pierce, G.E. (1974) Int. J. Cancer, 13, 572-578.

310

26. Lawrence, D.A. (1978) Cell. Immunol., 36, 97-114.

27. Bun-Hoi, N.P., Pham-Hun, C., Azum-Gelade, M.C., and Saint Ruf, G. (1972) Naturwissenschaften, 4, 174-177.

28. Vos, J.G., Moore, J.W., and Zinkl, J.G. (1973) Environ. Health Perspect., 5, 149-159.

29. Voss, J.G., Kreeftenberg, J.G., and Kater, L. (1978) In: Dioxin, Toxicological and Chemical Aspects (F. Cattabeni, A. Cavallaro, G. Galli, eds.), Spectrum Publ. Medical & Scientific Books, New York, pp. 163-175.

30. Lay, W.H., Mendes, N.F., Bianco, C., and Nussenzweig, V. (1971), Nature, 230, 531-532.

31. Cullen, S.E., David, C.S., Schreffer, D.C., and Nathenson, S.G. (1974) Proc. Natl. Acad. Sci., 71, 648-652.

32. Rose, N. (ed.) (1978) Genetic Control of Autoimmune Diseases, Elsevier North-Holland, Amsterdam.

33. Pai, M.R. (1978) Toxicon, 16, 283-289.

34. Giambrone, J.J. (1978) Aust. J. Vet. Res., 39, 305-311.

35. Peir, A.C. (1977) Ann. Nutr. Aliment., 31, 781-791.

36. Judah, D.J., Legg, R.F., and Neal, G.E. (1977) Nature, 265, 343-345.

37. Shenkman, L. (1978) Clin. Immunol. Immunopathol., 10, 187-192.

38. Shapira, (1977) Arthritis Rheum., 20, 1556-1561.

39. Nasr, S.J. (1977) Am. J. Psychiatry, 134, 1042-1045.

40. Perez Crouet, S. (1977) Experientia, 32, 646-647.

41. Brummerstedt, E., Basse, A., Flagstad, T., and Andersen, F. (1977) Am. J. Pathol., 87, 725-728.

42. Julius, R., Schulkind, M., Sprinkle, T., and Revvert, O. (1973) J. Pediatr., 83, 1007-1012.

43. Iwata, T. and Incefy, G.S. (1979) Cell. Immunol., 47, 100-105.

44. MacCarty, J. and Getzl, E.J. (1979) Cell. Immunol., 43, 103-112.

45. Markley, K., Smallman, E.T., and La John, L.A. (1977) Proc. Soc. Exp. Biol. Med., 154, 72-76.

46. Miller, C.L. and Claudy, B.J. (1979) Cell. Immunol., 44, 201-208.

47. Willis-Carr, J.I. and Pierre, R.L. (1978) J. Immunol., 120, 1153-1159.

© 1980 Elsevier/North-Holland Biomedical Press
The Principles and Methods in Modern Toxicology
C.L. Galli, S.D. Murphy and R. Paoletti, editors.

GOOD LABORATORY PRACTICE

GIOVANNI FALCONI

Farmitalia Carlo Erba, Via Imbonati, 24, Milan (Italy)

BACKGROUND

Some years ago the Food and Drug Administration discovered that some studies submitted in support of the safety of regulated products were not conducted in accordance with acceptable practice. Consequently the American Agency decided to develop good laboratory practice regulations, analogous to the existing good manufacturing practice regulations. A preliminary text was prepared and published in the Federal Register of November 19, 1976 with the title "Nonclinical Laboratory Studies. Proposed Regulations for Good Laboratory Practice". Subsequently a pilot inspection program began in December 1976 and covered a representative sample of testing facilities. The outcome of these inspections was evaluated and published as "Results of the Nonclinical Toxicology Laboratory Good Laboratory Practice Pilot Compliance Program" in the Federal Register of October 28, 1977.

Concurrently the Food and Drug Administration analyzed the comments submitted by many interested persons, such as: manufacturers of regulated products, associations, medical centers, private testing or consulting laboratories, educational institutions, government agencies, animal breeders, computer industries, and foreign regulatory authorities. The main criticisms on the proposed regulations were the following ones: lack of precision, lack of flexibility, risk of stifling the research, doubt that one person alone (i.e. the study director) may possess all the expertise required in multidisciplinary studies, unclear professional background for the quality assurance unit, possible leakage of confidential data, excessive requirements, inquisitional trend, abuse of check lists, difficulties in auditing raw data from on-line entry systems, legal authority of Food and Drug Administration to disqualify the research facilities, and, last but not least, the excessive cost of all the operation.

The above comments have been considered by the Food and Drug Administration in preparing the final regulations, published in the Federal Register of December 22, 1978 as "Nonclinical laboratory Studies. Good Laboratory Practice Regulations". These regulations are preceded by a long preamble where the reasons for accepting or rejecting the various criticisms are discussed.

These regulations were effective from June 20, 1979 and they must be complied by all laboratories conducting nonclinical studies that support or are intended to support applications for research or marketing permits for products regulated by the Food and Drug Administration.

FINAL REGULATIONS

In order to recall and comment the main points of the final regulations, the various paragraphs (numbered in parentheses) will be summarized in parallel with the relevant parts of the preamble.

The scope (58.1) of these regulations is to assure the quality and the integrity of the safety data for the products regulated by the Food and Drug Administration. The safety data include mutagenicity tests, while the range-finding experiments are excluded. Although inspections of a foreign facility may not be made without the consent of the facility itself, the Food and Drug Administration will refuse to accept any study submitted by any facility that does not consent to inspection.

Most of the definitions (58.3) of the terms used in the text are self-explanatory, while others are better clarified in the preamble. The definition of "control article" includes the carrier materials given to control groups as well as the articles used as positive controls. The data generated on-line are considered "raw data" provided that the computer memory and program are accompanied by a procedure that precludes tampering with the stored information.

In the case of studies performed under contract (58.10), the sponsor shall notify the contractor that the study shall be conducted in compliance with the good laboratory practice regulations.

The inspection of a testing facility (58.15), to be performed by Food and Drug Administration officers, shall not apply to the quality assurance unit records of findings and problems, as was required in the proposed regulations. The confidentiality of the quality assurance unit reports is granted in order to keep its inspections candid and complete.

A controversial point concerns the criteria for assessing the qualification of the personnel (58.29). In fact the degree of education, training and experience adequate to perform the assigned functions is not always easy to assess. Similarly, it may be difficult to evaluate the compliance to the requirements concerning health precautions designed to avoid contamination of test articles and test systems. A number of comments said that the disclosure of medical records is an invasion of privacy.

The responsibility of the testing facility management (58.31), which was not defined in the proposed regulations, consists mainly in: 1) appointing the study director, 2) designating the quality assurance unit, 3) taking the corrective actions suggested by the quality assurance unit, 4) assuring the identity of the test article.

The study director (58.33) has the overall responsibility for the technical conduct of the study according to the protocol approved by the sponsor. The study director is also responsible for the interpretation of the experimental data.

The quality assurance unit (58.35) is a new function in research. This unit refers to management and must be independent of the study director. The quality assurance unit shall maintain: 1) the master schedule sheet, reporting the status of each study, and 2) a copy of all protocols pertaining to the studies for which the unit is responsible. The quality assurance unit has to: 1) in spect each phase of a nonclinical laboratory study to assure the compliance to the protocol, 2) review the final study report to assure that the reported results reflect the raw data, and 3) pre- pare and sign a statement to be included with the final study report which shall specify the dates inspections were made and findings reported to the management and to the study director. The Food and Drug Administration shall inspect the standard oper- ating procedures of the quality assurance unit but not their rec- cords of findings and problems. A certification of compliance to the good laboratory practice may be requested by the Food and Drug Administration from the management. The quality assurance unit qualification should be determined by the management and will vary according to the type of facility and study. The functions of the quality assurance unit may be performed by outside consultants. The quality assurance unit should not attempt to evaluate the scientific merit of the final report.

The facilities (58.41) shall be of a suitable size, construc- tion, and location to facilitate the proper conduct of the study. Many comments requested a more detailed definition of the facili- ties, but the Agency said that the broad variety of test systems precludes the establishment of specific criteria for each situa- tion.

The animal care facilities (58.43) shall have a sufficient number of rooms or areas to assure the separation of species, test systems, biohazardous articles, diseased animals, animal waste, etc. Many comments asked for the recognition of the accred itation system for animal care facilities, but the Food and Drug Administration does not like to delegate its responsibility to an organization over which they have no authority.

The animal supply facilities (58.45) shall have storage areas for feed, bedding, supplies, and equipment.

The facilities for handling test and control articles (58.47) shall be separate from areas housing the test system and shall be adequate to preserve the identity, strength, purity, and stability of the articles and mixtures.

The laboratory operation areas (58.49) shall include areas for aseptic surgery, intensive care, necropsy, histology, radiography, handling of biohazardous materials and space for cleaning, sterilizing, and storing equipment and supplies.

The specimens and data storage facilities (58.51) shall consist of archives the access to which is limited to authorized personnel only. Concern was expressed regarding the limited access but, according to the Food and Drug Administration, the potential for misplaced data and specimens is too great to allow unlimited access to the archives.

Areas shall be provided for administrative and personnel facilities (58.53).

The equipment design (58.61) shall be adequate for the protocol and suitably located for operation, inspection, cleaning, and maintenance. Exact design and capacity requirements for each piece of equipment are clearly beyond the scope of the regulations.

The methods for the maintenance and calibration of equipment (58.63) shall be set forth in sufficient detail in written standard operating procedures. The standard operating procedures shall designate the person responsible for each operation, and for each operation written records shall be maintained. Comments suggested that the manufacturer's instructions should be sufficient, but, according to the Commissioner, textbooks and manufacturer's literature are not necessarily complete. It is in fact highly unlikely that such materials can be used without modifications to fit a particular laboratory's needs. This material may be used, however, as a supplement to and reference for standard operating procedures. If maintenance is subcontracted, this fact does not relieve the facility of the responsibility for maintenance.

The standard operating procedures (58.81) shall be authorized by the management, while all deviations from them in a particular study shall be authorized by the study director. Written standard operating procedures shall be established in detail for a series of routine and repetitive laboratory operations concerning: animal rooms, animal care, test and control articles, test system, laboratory tests, moribund or dead animals, necropsy, histopathology, specimens, data handling, equipments, etc. Each laboratory area shall have the standard operating procedures on hand. A historical file of standard operating procedures shall be maintained. Several comments said that the requirements for the standard operating procedures are unnecessary and burdensome, but, according to the Food and Drug Administration, this requirement will prevent the introduction of systemic errors in the generation, collection and reporting of data. The quality assurance unit is no longer required to maintain copies of the standard operating procedures. Textbooks may be used as supplements to written standard operating procedures.

All reagents and solutions (58.83) shall be labeled to indicate identity, titer or concentration, storage requirements, and expiration date.

The animal care (58.90) methods shall be described in standard operating procedures. Newly received animals shall be placed in quarantine until their health status has been evaluated. Several comments stated that quarantine is unnecessary when animals are obtained from a reputable source. According to Food and Drug Administration the supply source is only one factor in determining the degree of the health of the animals. Treatment of diseased animals shall be authorized and documented. Warm-blooded animals require appropriate identification. The manner of identification is left to the discretion of the testing facility. The unique identification number, as required in the proposed rules,

has been deleted in the final ones. Feed and water shall be analyzed for contaminants known to be capable of interfering with
the study. If any pest control materials are used, the use shall
be documented.

Test and control article characterization (58.105) shall specify
identity, strength, purity, methods of synthesis, stability, batch
number, and storage conditions. This characterization shall be
done before the initiation of the study, and it is the responsibility of the management of the testing facility. In those cases
where a competitor's or supplier's product is used as a control
article, such a product will be characterized by its labeling.
For studies of more than 4 week's duration, reserve samples from
each batch of test and control articles shall be retained, for
the period of time provided below. Retention of a reserve sample
of water is required when it serves as the control article in a
nonclinical laboratory study. The reserve samples should be
stored under conditions that maximize their useful life.

Test and control article handling (58.107) shall be documented,
specifying the receipt and distribution of each batch.

The mixtures of articles with carriers (58.113) shall be analyzed for concentration, uniformity, and stability. For studies
of more than 4 week's duration, a reserve sample of each test or
control carrier article mixture shall be taken and retained for
the required period of time. All batches of test and control
article mixtures are to be retained even if they are prepared
daily. The Agency recognizes that the reserve sample retention
requirements are both extensive and expensive, however a petition
for changing the rule may be considered. This was officially
declared during the briefing sessions conducted by the Food and
Drug Administration on May 1, 2 and 3, 1979 in Washington, Chicago
and San Francisco.

Each study shall have an approved written protocol (58.120) that
shall contain, when applicable, at least the following information:

purpose of the study, identification of the articles, proposed starting and completion dates, identification of the test system, methods for the control of bias, description of the diet, route of administration, dose levels, methods for the control of the absorption of the test and control articles, type and frequency of measurements, list of records to be maintained, date of approval of the protocol by the sponsor, and statistical methods to be used. All changes in or revision of an approved protocol and the reasons therefor shall be documented, signed by the study director, dated, and maintained with the protocol. As regards the point on the degree of absorption comments raised were that this is usually unknown at the time of the preparation of the protocol. Food and Drug Administration said that, if absorption studies are conducted concurrently, this requirement can be fulfilled by amending the protocol.

The conduct of a nonclinical laboratory study (58.130) shall be done in accordance with the protocol. Specimens shall be identified by test system, study, nature, and date of collection. All data, except those that are generated as a direct computer input, shall be recorded directly, promptly, and legibly in ink. The document shall be dated and signed by the person entering the data. Where the input is via direct on-line recording, the magnetic media and the program would constitute raw data.

The final report of nonclinical laboratory study results (58.185) shall be signed by the study director, and shall include at least the following items: dates, objectives, statistical methods, article identification and stability, dosages, names of the scientists, summary and analysis of the data, location of specimens and raw data, description of all circumstances that may have affected the quality and integrity of the data, and the statement prepared and signed by the quality assurance unit.

There shall be archives (58.190) for orderly storage and expedient retrieval of all raw data, documentation, protocols, specimens, and interim and final reports.

The retention time (58.195) shall be as follows. Raw data, specimens, master schedule sheets, protocols, records of the quality assurance unit, summaries of training and job description, records of the maintenance of equipment shall be retained at least:

(1) two years following the date on which an application is approved by the Food and Drug Administration,

(2) five years following the date on which the results are submitted to the Food and Drug Administration,

(3) two years following the date on which the study is completed, when the results are not submitted to the Food and Drug Administration.

Specimens which are relatively fragile shall be retained only as long as the quality of the preparation affords evaluation.

The last part of the regulations concerns the disqualification of testing facilities. The purpose (58.200) of disqualification is to permit the exclusion from consideration of studies conducted by a testing facility which has failed to comply with the requirements of the good laboratory practice regulations.

The Commissioner (58.202) may disqualify a testing facility upon finding all of the following:

(a) the testing facility failed to comply with one or more of the regulations,

(b) the noncompliance adversely affected the validity of the nonclinical laboratory study, and

(c) other lesser regulatory actions have not been or will probably not be adequate to achieve compliance with the good laboratory practice regulation.

The following paragraphs concern several legal aspects, according to the following titles: notice of and opportunity for hearing on proposed disqualification (58.204), final order on disqualification (58.206), action upon disqualification (58.210), public disclosure of information regarding disqualification (58.213), alternative or additional actions to disqualification (58.215), suspension or termination of a testing facility by a sponsor (58.217), reinstatement of a disqualified testing facility (58.219).

CONCLUSIONS

The compliance with good laboratory practice regulations is mandatory for the applicants for a research or marketing permit for products regulated by the Food and Drug Administration.

The American Agency will consider petitions for changing some requirements. It is desirable that such petitions will be filed in order to modify the most excessive requirements, for example that concerning the daily retention of the reserve samples.

In my experience, the professional background of the inspectors is a very important prerequisite of a correct interpretation of the rules.

The good laboratory practice regulations may be considered a useful instrument for the reduction of the human error in performing the very complex toxicological studies, and a strong challenge for the harmonisation of the international acceptability of the nonclinical documentation. The safety studies are too costly and time-consuming to be repeated several times.

The compliance with the good laboratory practice has been differently dealt with in extra-USA countries. The governments of Canada, the United Kingdom and Sweden have already signed with the Food and Drug Administration a memorandum of understanding. The purpose of the understanding is to set forth cooperative working arrangements to develop standards or guidelines of good laboratory practices for nonclinical laboratories and to establish programs of inspection to implement those standards or guidelines. In France, Germany, Holland and Italy several proposals, generally less compelling than the American ones, have been prepared but no official documents have been published so far.

INTERACTION BETWEEN EPIDEMIOLOGY OF CANCER AND EXPERIMENTAL CARCINOGENESIS

BENEDETTO TERRACINI,

Professor of Cancer Epidemiology, University of Torino, Torino, Italy

Chemicals proved to be carcinogenic to man are fewer than substances reported to produce cancer in laboratory animals by at least one order of magnitude. There may be several explanations for this, among which: 1. interspecies metabolic differences, 2. other factors (such as viruses, hormonal imbalance etc) determining an excessive sensitivity of laboratory animals to chemical carcinogens, 3. insufficient implementation of epidemiological studies, 4. limitations in currently available epidemiological methods and 5. inadequacies of the epidemiological approach for investigating the role of specific risk factors in the genesis of a disease which is multifactorial in origin. The purpose of this paper is to discuss these possibilities. A most valuable source of information are the Monographs on the evaluation of carcinogenic risk of chemicals to man published since 1971 by the International Agency for Research on Cancer (1).

In reviewing the literature on chemicals and human cancer, a distinction must be made among: 1. chemically well defined agents for which a cause-to-effect relationship with cancer in man is either demonstrated or very plausible, 2. exposures associated with cancer for which the specific chemical(s) involved can only be suspected and 3. chemicals experimentally shown to be carcinogenic or mutagenic, for which information on effects on humans is inadequate or lacking. This paper deals with the first two categories.

In principle, an association between exposure to a specific chemical and cancer can be considered as causal when it is possible to rule out a bias in the design of the relevant studies and a role of exposures to other chemical or non chemical factors. Most epidemiological studies deal with complex exposures and cancer is a multifactorial disease: in the results of an epidemiological study suggesting an association between an environmental exposure and cancer, the first important issue is whether at least some of the cancers found in excess can be attributed to a specific chemical. The evidence of carcinogenicity of a chemical is strengthened when the association is biologically credible, externally valid (i.e. coherent with other results) and internally consistent (i.e. when a gradient exists between the extent of exposure and the relative risk). Reduction in cancer incidence following reduction of exposure adds further support to the causal nature of the association. In fact this requires a long period to be demonstrated: one among the few available examples is the decrease in incidence rates of bladder cancer in a dye manufacture industry after limitation of the exposure to benzidine (2).

WELL DEFINED CHEMICALS SHOWN TO BE CARCINOGENIC TO MAN

An acceptable list of chemicals causally related to cancer in man is shown in Table 1, together with an indication of the broad environmental sectors where such chemicals are present and a general qualitative assessment of the evidence of their carcinogenicity for laboratory animals (i.e. whether they have or have not produced cancer in at least one experimental system).

For most chemicals used as drugs or in the industry, the hunch of an association with cancer arose from clinical observations on small numbers of cases, subsequently confirmed by formal ad-hoc epidemiological studies. In the case of occupational cancers, often the original case reports related to occupations rather than to specific chemicals. A classic example is that of carcinogenic aromatic amines: Rehn was a surgeon who in 1895, within a short period of time, observed 4 cases of bladder cancer among workers engaged in the manufacture of dyes; he thought that this was unusual and suggested a cause-to-effect relationship (3). A large number of similar case reports were published in the following decades and as early as in 1921 the International Labour Organization (4) issued a warning against benzidine and 2-naphthylamine as probable causative factors of bladder cancer in the dye industry. However, the unequivocal demonstration that these aromatic amines are carcinogenic to man was obtained only in 1954 (5). In the case of chemicals entering the scene more recently, the time elapsing between the hunch and the demonstration of carcinogenicity was shorter, but the sequence of events was the same. The identification of specific carcinogens is obviously easier when the hunch is

developed by an alert industrial physician (or clinician, in the case of carcino
genic drugs) with some knowledge of the nature of the chemicals to which people
are exposed.

TABLE 1

CHEMICALS PROVED TO BE CARCINOGENIC FOR HUMANS

	Type of exposure	Carcinogenicity for laboratory animals
Aflatoxins	environmental (occupational?)	+
4-aminobiphenyl	occupational	+
arsenic trioxide	environmental drug occupational	− (adequacy?)
asbestos (4 amphiboles)	environmental occupational	+
benzene	occupational	− (adequacy?)
benzidine	occupational	+
cyclophosphamide	drug	+
bis (chloromethyl) ether	occupational	+
chloromethyl methyl ether	occupational	+
chlornaphazine	drug	+
diethylstilboestrol	drug	+
melphalan	drug	+
mustard gas	occupational	+
2-naphthylamine	occupational tobacco smoke	+
vinyl chloride	occupational	+

An exceptional situation in Table 1 is that of aflatoxins. These are the
only chemicals to which exposure occurs almost esclusively in the general (non
occupational) environment. The evidence of carcinogenicity to man relies on
epidemiological studies showing a positive correlation between average dietary

concentrations of aflatoxins in populations and their incidences of primary liver cancer (6). The stimulus to perform such studies derived from the observation that aflatoxins are powerful carcinogens for laboratory animals, particularly the rat (7). In the absence of ad-hoc studies in which individual exposures are estimated, a recent publication of the IARC includes aflatoxins among the chemicals which are probably (but not definitely) carcinogenic for humans (8).

All the chemicals included in Table 1 have produced cancer in laboratory animals with the exception of inorganic arsenic and benzene. Experimental investigations on the carcinogenicity of these chemicals have been considered as inadequate (8). A recent report of a small study in rats suggested that continuous administration of benzene by the oral route induces carcinomas of the Zymbal's glands and possibly leukaemias (9).

The correspondence between carcinogenicity for men and that for laboratory animals cannot be considered as a firm basis for a blind extrapolation in the opposite direction (i.e. from animals to man). However, it adds credibility to the causal nature of the association between exposure to a specific chemical and cancer in man, similarly to one of Koch's postulates regarding the etiology of bacterial diseases.

COMPLEX EXPOSURES SHOWN TO BE CARCINOGENIC TO MAN

Humans are exposed or expose themselves to complex mixtures; some of these have been found to be associated with cancer through acceptable ad-hoc epidemiological studies. However, on several of these circumstances, the specific substance(s) involved in the carcinogenic process has not yet been identified.

This situation is well exemplified by tobacco smoke, but it also applies to several occupational exposures and to some therapeutical practices. The carcinogenicity of tobacco smoke on the human species is shown beyond any doubt; however, for none of its components (10) there is an acceptable demonstration of carcinogenicity for man with the exception of 2-naphthylamine. The common assumption that the tar fraction has an important role in the effects of tobacco smoke is based on its carcinogenicity for laboratory animals, a part of which is due to the presence of polycyclic aromatic hydrocarbons (PAH). The great effort towards the consumption of low-tar cigarettes is based on this assumption (11, 12). However, for no PAH contained in tobacco smoke, including benzo(a)pyrene, there is an acceptable evidence that they produce cancer in man (13). The design of an epidemiological study aimed to obtain such evidence poses major problems. PAH are not produced or used on a commercial scale: they are formed as side-products in a large number of circumstances and in no situation the formation is limited to one of them. Therefore, it would be difficult to identify a group of people with the exclusive characteristic of being exposed to one polycyclic aromatic hydrocarbon, in order to compare its cancer experience to that of people unexposed to it.

However, and in spite of the above mentioned prudence about the extrapolation of evidence of carcinogenicity from laboratory animals to man, the attitude that identifies polycyclic aromatic hydrocarbons among the factors responsible for the carcinogenicity of tobacco smoke is commonly considered as acceptable. A corollary to this is that when exposure to complex environments or mixtures associated to cancer in man relates, among others, to chemicals proved to be carcinogenic in laboratory animals, it is plausible that such chemical(s) has a role in the association, although it does not necessarily explain the whole of it. This obviously applies to those chemicals whose carcinogenicity leaves little doubts, such as those for which IARC considers that there is sufficient evidence of carcinogenicity (*). When the experimental evidence is debatable, its relevance for the evaluation of risk to man is lower.

(*) According to IARC (8) sufficient evidence of carcinogenicity indicates that there is an increased incidence of malignant tumours: (a) in multiple species or strains, or (b) in multiple experiments (preferably with different routes of administration or using different dose levels) or (c) to an unusual degree with regard to incidence, site or type of tumour, or age at onset. Additional evidence may be provided by data concerning dose-response effects, as well as information on mutagenicity or chemical structure.

Occupational exposures

Some exposures to complex industrial environments have been shown to be carcinogenic to man, through acceptable ad-hoc epidemiological studies leading to the suspicion but not to the identification of the chemical(s) responsible for the association. Table 2 exemplifies some occupational exposures falling into this category.

Auramine, magenta and 1-naphthylamine are among the aromatic amines considered in the classic epidemiological studies of Case et al. (14). In these studies, a nominal roll of employees in the chemical industries in the U.K. after 1920, characterized as to whether they manufactured, used or purified specific aromatic amines, was compared with a list of people deceased because of bladder cancer in the same country during 1921-1949. For 2-naphthylamine and benzidine, Case et al. were able to identify groups of workers exclusively exposed to the specific aromatic amine, so that the association with cancer could be reasonably attributed to the latter. The same study demonstrated a carcinogenic risk for groups of workers exposed to either auramine, magenta or 1-naphthylamine. However, for none of these groups it was possible to rule out a role of the presence of other aromatic amines in the workplace, either used as intermediates in the manufacture of the relevant chemical or present as an impurity (such as 2-naphthylamine in 1-naphthylamine). Auramine is a well proven carcinogen for laboratory animals (15): this provides further suggestion but not a definite evidence that this compound had a role in the association shown by Case et al. Doubts on the carcinogenicity for man of 1-naphthylamine and magenta are even greater, in the absence of convincing evidence of carcinogenicity for laboratory animals (16).

TABLE 2

SOME OCCUPATIONS OR INDUSTRIAL MATERIALS ASSOCIATED WITH CANCER IN MAN, IN
WHICH THE CHEMICAL(S) UNDERLYING THE ASSOCIATION IS SUSPECTED BUT NOT
DEFINITELY PROVEN

	Suspected agent(s)	Carcinogenicity for laboratory animals
production of auramine	auramine	+
production of magenta	magenta	inadequate
production of 1-naphthylamine	1-naphthylamine 2-naphthylamine	inadequate +
production of chromates	Cr salts	+
production of isopropyl alcohol	isopropyl alcohol isopropyl oils	inadequate inadequate
nickel refining	Ni derivatives	+
exposure to cadmium dusts or fumes	Cd oxide	+
tar, soots, mineral oils	benzo(a)pyrene other PAH *	+ +
haematite underground mining	haematite radioactivity	− +

*polycyclic aromatic hydrocarbons

    The production of chromium salts, nickel refining, manufacture of isopropyl
alcohol by the strong acid method and exposure to cadmium derivatives in the
working environment are all associated with cancer in man, but they all entail
exposure to a variety of compounds. The first two activities determine the
contemporary exposure to more than one derivative respectively of Cr and Ni.
Since several of these are carcinogenic for laboratory animals (17, 18), it is
difficult to establish whether all or only some of them (and in the latter
case which ones) are responsible for the effect on humans. Studies relating to
Cd derivatives create a similar problem: in addition, the size of the
epidemiological investigations which have been reported (18) was relatively
small. Finally, the manufacture of isopropyl alcohol by the strong acid method

(which is now largely abandoned) was associated with cancer (19): since this method leads to the appearance of isopropyl oils as side products, it was thought that the latter were responsible for the association. Neither the alcohol nor the oils have been adequately tested in laboratory animals (19).

Exposure of chimney sweepers to soot was reported as a carcinogenic occupational hazard in 1775 by Sir Percival Pott (20). The carcinogenicity for the human species of tar and mineral oils was demonstrated in the nineteenth century or early in the present century. Cancer induction in laboratory animals by tar is a milestone in the history of cancer research (21). Soot, tars and mineral oils are mixtures containing several polycyclic aromatic hydrocarbons, many of which are powerful carcinogens for laboratory animals. The identification of the specific chemicals responsible for the carcinogenicity of soot, tars and mineral oils for men encounters the same difficulties as those mentioned above with regard to tobacco smoke.

Haematite represents a unique situation in Table 2. In one study, underground haematite miners, but not surface miners, were shown to have a high incidence of lung cancer (22). Epidemiological investigations regarding metal workers exposed to ferric oxide dusts in the workplace gave contradictory results; among these, in the studies suggesting an association with lung cancer it was not possible to rule out a role of other environmental factors (15). On the other hand, a relative large number of experimental studies in mice, hamsters and guinea pigs given ferric oxide intratracheally gave no evidence of carcinogenicity (15). In the study of Boyd et al. (22), underground haematite mining was associated to a high background radioactivity due to radon, which might explain at least a part of the excess of lung cancer. Therefore, there are serious doubts on the possibility that haematite itself is a carcinogen for men.

In conclusion, the situations reported in Table 2 share a common denominator: the design of the underlying epidemiological studies could not characterize the exposure in definite chemical terms. Suggestions regarding the chemical(s) responsible for the association with cancer derive from the extent and results of experimental studies.

Drugs

Problems created by the carcinogenicity of some therapeutical practices are by no means simpler. An association between therapy for a disease and subsequent development of cancer could be due to factors different from therapy itself. In the first place, both the original disease and cancer might share some common risk factors. Alternatively, a disease characterized by hormonal or immunological changes might enhance cancer development. In addition, the original disease might mask the existence of an underlying cancer. Finally, therapeutical practices other than the one under investigation might be overlooked.

A good example of control of exposures to other drugs and other counfounding factors is the demonstration that N,N'-bis(2-chloroethyl)-2-naphthylamine (chlornaphazine) is a bladder carcinogen for man. This drug has been used as an alkylating agent for polycithemia vera and Hodgkin's disease. Thiede et al. (23) compared the incidence of bladder cancer in patients with polycithemia vera among those treated respectively with P_{32} + chlornaphazine, P_{32} alone and other drugs. Only the first group showed an increased incidence of bladder cancer. The fact that the molecule of chlornaphazine contains 2-naphthylamine and that the drug is a carcinogen in laboratory animals (although the evidence is limited to the induction of lung tumours in mice) adds supportive evidence to the causal nature of the association.

Under other circumstances, the interpretation of the results of epidemiological investigations is more complicated. Some of these situations are reported in Table 3.

Reimer et al. (24) reported an excess of leukaemias among women with a previous ovarian cancer treated with several alkylating agents, among which chlorambucil and thiotepa. This is not a definite proof that these two chemicals are carcinogenic to man, although for both chemicals some case reports of association with cancer have also been published (25). In addition, there is indisputable evidence that both are carcinogenic for laboratory animals (25).

The association between analgesic mixtures, renal papillary necrosis and subsequent carcinoma of the renal pelvis is well demonstrated (26). Again, however, the role of each component of the mixtures cannot be ascertained. The

TABLE 3

SOME THERAPEUTICAL PRACTICES ASSOCIATED WITH CANCER IN MAN, IN WHICH THE DRUG(S)
UNDERLYING THE ASSOCIATION IS SUSPECTED BUT NOT DEFINITELY PROVEN

	Suspected drug	Carcinogenicity for laboratory animals
Alkylating agents for ovarian cancer	chlorambucil	+
	thiothepa	+
Abuse of analgesic mixtures	phenacetin	+?*
Anticonvulsants for epilepsy	phenobarbitone	+?*
	phenytoin	+?*

*+ ? = evidence of carcinogenicity but not falling into the category of
"sufficient" evidence

focus on phenacetin derives, among other factors, from the observation of a
carcinogenic effect on animals (26, 27). The latter, nevertheless, has not
been considered by IARC as sufficient evidence of carcinogenicity, as
previously defined.

With regard to the last situation indicated in Table 3, a recent study of
Clemmesen and Hjalgrim-Jensen (28) compared the occurrence of cancer among
several thousands epileptics treated with phenobarbitone and phenytoin to that
observed in non-epileptics, over a period of more than 10 years. The relative
risk for brain cancer was 2.8 (12 observed vs 4.3 expected) and that for liver
cancer was 3.9 (11 observed vs 2.8 expected). However, epilepsy might have been
a symptom of an underlying brain tumour. In addition, 8 of the 11 patients with
liver cancer had also been treated with thorotrast, a known liver carcinogen.
For both phenobarbitone and phenytoin studies aimed to detect carcinogenicity
in laboratory animals have been either inadequate or provided "limited"
evidence of carcinogenicity (26). Under these circumstances, an evaluation of
the carcinogenic risk to man of these two chemicals is most difficult.

These associations between therapeutical practices and cancer, as those
described in the previous section, point to the problems of the identification
of specific carcinogenic chemicals to man, not only when epidemiological

studies lead to debatable results but also when they demonstrate the existence of an association between a complex exposure and cancer.

OTHER CHEMICALS

IARC has recently reported (8) that among 442 chemicals or groups of chemicals for which a monograph has been prepared since 1971, only for less than 60 some information on long-term effects on humans had been published. In addition to the situations considered in Tables 1, 2 and 3, inadequate epidemiological studies have been reported for 15 chemicals (acrylonitrile, amitrole, beryllium and derivatives, chloroprene, DDT, dieldrin, dimethylsulphate, epichlorohydrin, ethylene oxide, isoniazid, lead compounds, N-phenyl-2-naphthylamine, PCBs, reserpine, trichloroethylene). For a further 10 substances (carbon tetrachloride, chloramphenicol, chlordane, dimethyl carbamoyl chloride, heptachlor, hexachlorocyclohexane, iron dextran, oxymetholone, styrene and triaziquinone) the scientific literature only contains some case reports. From a strictly statistical viewpoint, the latter are unsatisfactory. However, some of them are biologically plausible, such as the cases of leukaemias following pancytopenia among patients previously treated with chloramphenicol.

In addition, sufficient evidence of carcinogenicity for laboratory animals (as previously defined) has been collected for 142 chemicals (29, 30, 31, 32). Of these, 27 (including 11 PAH) are mentioned in Tables 1, 2 and 3; a further 9 are included among those mentioned in the previous paragraph. For the remaining chemicals with sufficient evidence of carcinogenicity, no case reports or epidemiological studies can be found in the open literature: most of them are somehow present in the human environment.

In 1978, epidemiological studies designed in order to investigate the carcinogenic effect on man of at least 71 chemicals were on the way (33, 34), i.e. 10 substances mentioned in Table 1, 7 included in Tables 2 and 3, 9 among those previously investigated under unsatisfactory conditions and 45 other chemicals.

MODELS OF AD HOC EPIDEMIOLOGICAL STUDIES FOR IDENTIFYING CHEMICAL CARCINOGENS

As mentioned above, for most chemicals included in Table 1, the first hunch on their carcinogenicity derived from case reports and this was followed by formal ad-hoc studies. The latter fall into two main models. In case-control studies, individuals characterized in terms of whether they bear or do not bear the disease under investigation are compared with regard to previous exposures to suspected risk factors. In cohort studies, groups of persons characterized as exposed or non exposed are identified at a time in which they are healthy and the subsequent frequency of pathological events is compared among groups. In the case of cancer, i.e. a disease whose latent period is measured in years, it is obvious that the interval between exposure and the occurrence of the disease plays a crucial role. Many chemicals to which nowadays groups of people are exposed have been present in the human environment for periods shorter than the average latent period of human cancer. This obviously decreases (or even reduces to 0) the sensitivity ot the epidemiological models for identifying carcinogenic chemicals.

Case-control studies

The potentialities of this model of epidemiological investigation have been recently reviewed (35). Case-control studies are powerful tools for relating cancer to previous events but their sensitivity and specificity in picking up associations between well identified chemicals and cancer are relatively poor. Identification and characterization of previous exposures rely usually on the individual's memory. For chemicals present in the general environment (air, food etc) awareness of specific exposures by individuals is practically nihil. Similarly, the persons being questioned usually are not in the conditions of providing precise information on chemicals to which they have been exposed in the workplace. However, they can provide items of information (such as occupational titles or previous diseases entailing certain therapeutical practices) which might indirectly lead to a characterization in terms of exposures. In the case of occupational titles, assumptions can be made on their correspondence with specific exposures. The demonstration - through case-control studies - of an association between bladder cancer and occupations related to the manufacture of azo-dyes (36, 37) suggests a carcinogenicic role of aromatic amines and azo-dyes, but could hardly lead to the identification of the specific carcinogenic chemicals. The model is more rewarding in the case of occupations assumed to entail exposure to a single carcinogenic agent: it has provided evidence of an association between cancer of the respiratory tract and occupational exposure to asbestos (38).

In case-control studies aimed to establish associations between drug consumption and cancer, information on previous exposures can be more precise when nominal records are available on drugs being prescribed. The suspicion of an association between breast cancer and reserpine (6) was greatly reduced through case-control studies in which adequate informative systems on drug consumption by individuals were available (39).

The potentialities of case-control studies for the detection of specific carcinogenic chemicals also rely on factors other than the specificity of the identification of previous exposures. These include the relative risk of illness associated with the exposure being investigated and the proportion of exposed people in the general population. When a risk factor is very rare in the general population (and/or among the controls) and slightly less so among the cases, it may be necessary to mount a very large study in order to obtain sizable figures to compare, even if the relative risk associated with the specific exposure is high. This is particularly so when the proportion of cases determined by the exposure is low. On the contrary, when the proportion is high, case-control studies may be a powerful tool for picking up associations. A well conducted case-control study (40) has first demonstrated the association between in utero exposure to diethylstilboestrol and cancer of the vagina in young women. This study related to a relative common and easily identifiable exposure and a cancer which in non-exposed persons is extremely rare.

Similar specific associations in the occupational field are those existing between scrotal cancer and mineral oil, liver hemangioendothelioma and vinyl chloride, pleural mesothelioma and asbestos. They all relate to tumours which are uncommon among non exposed people and to exposures which are relatively easy to recognize. When these conditions do not occur, case-control studies hardly lead to the recognition of previously unsuspected carcinogens for men.

Cohort studies

In cohort studies, exposed and non-exposed people are assembled before being followed up: non-exposed people are often identified to the general population. Information on exposure to chemicals does not necessarily rely on the individual's memory. Even in the case of historical studies - in which the cohorts are assembled a posteriori - it may be possible to characterize and estimate individual exposures. In addition, relative risks greater than 1 can be identified even when the proportion of cases attributable to the risk factor being investigated is low. Indeed, for most carcinogens for man included in Table 1, the proof of their carcinogenicity was derived from studies designed along this model.

Nevertheless, cohort studies do have some shortcomings. They are usually more expensive than case-control studies and require adequate informative systems for detecting the members of the cohorts reaching the end point (for instance, files of death certificates recorded nominally, cancer registries etc). Cohorts can be characterized as having been exposed to specific chemicals only on some occasions, such as in the case of drugs and industrial chemicals when environmental data regarding the workplace are satisfactory. Under other circumstances, they can only be characterized on a less precise basis such as the occupational titles. As in case-control studies, the latter may lead to a suggestion but not to an evidence that a specific chemical is involved in the association with cancer.

Cohort studies must have a critical size, under which they are not sensitive enough to detect an association. Such a size is greatly determined by the relative risk and by the incidence of the disease in the unexposed population. It can be estimated that in order to pick up a relative risk for bladder cancer of 2, in a cohort of men aged 40, living in an industrialized area and followed up for 20 years, the size of the cohort should be in the order of 1800. The identification of an association with a relative risk of 5 would require, given the same conditions, a cohort of about 400 people.

These figures are of the same order of magnitude of the size of the cohorts assembled in studies which led to the demonstration of the carcinogenicity for man of substances such as 2-naphthylamine (16), vinyl chloride (31) and asbestos

(38). They are, however, at least one order of magnitude greater than the size of the groups assembled in attempts to investigate the effects on man of other specific chemicals. For instance, the only two cohorts of workers characterized as being occupationally exposed to DDT, reported in the scientific literature, included less than 50 people each (these were, in addition, cross-sectional and not longitudinal studies) (41, 42).

CONCLUSIONS

Only a small number of chemicals so far have been shown or are suspected to be carcinogenic to man. An interpretation of this cannot ignore the following facts.

1. Particularly in the past, epidemiological studies on specific chemicals have been scarce, in relation to the real possibilities of undertaking them.

2. Observation and report of small series of cases of cancer associated with specific exposures have often been crucial for launching properly designed epidemiological studies which in turn provided evidence of carcinogenicity to man. Case reports by themselves cannot be considered as adequate evidence of the latter. However, on some occasions, the limited evidence provided by case reports is supported by a biological plausibility of the association.

3. In order to reach an adequate level of sensitivity, ad hoc epidemiological studies must have a critical size. Depending upon the circumstances and the type of the study, the critical size is determined by the relative and attributable risks, the prevalence of the exposure, the frequency of the disease under investigation in the general population, the extent and duration of the presence of the risk factor in the environment.

4. Such a critical size is more easily reached when factors being investigated are characterized with relatively broad criteria than in the case of specific, well defined chemicals.

5. The definition of exposures to individual chemicals is often insufficiently specific.

6. Adequate evidence of carcinogenicity for laboratory animals of a chemical increases the biological plausibility of the causal nature of a specific association resulting from an epidemiological study. It may also contribute to

the identification of che carcinogenic chemical(s) in the case of associations
between cancer and ill-defined exposures.

   The consideration of chemicals adequately shown to be carcinogenic in
laboratory animals and for which epidemiological studies have not been carried
out or gave unclear results is beyond the scope of this paper. It seems,
however, that the absence of evidence of carcinogenicity for man of a chemical
may be due to factors other than a lack of carcinogenicity. This should de
kept in mind when discussing preventive measures in relation to chemicals
"only" (but adequately) shown to be carcinogenic under experimental conditions

REFERENCES

 1. Tomatis L. et al. (1978) Evaluation of the carcinogenicity of chemicals: A
    review of the monograph program of the International Agency for Research on
    Cancer (1971 to 1977). Cancer Res. 38, 877-885.

 2. Ferber K. H. et al. (1976) An assessment of the effect of improved working
    conditions on bladder tumor incidence in a benzidine manufacturing facility.
    Am. Ind. Hyg. Assoc. J. 37, 61-68.

 3. Rehn L. (1895) Blasengeschwülste bei Fuchsin-arbeitern. Arch. Klin. Chir.
    50, 588.

 4. International Labour Office (1921) Studies and Reports, Series F, N° 1.

 5. Case R.A.M. et al. (1954) Tumours of the urinary bladder in workmen
    engaged in the manufacture and use of certain dyestuff intermediates in the
    British Chemical industry. I. The role of aniline, benzidine, alpha-
    -naphthylamine and beta-naphthylamine. Brit. J. Industr. Med. 11, 75-104.

 6. IARC Monographs on the evaluation of the carcinogenic risk of chemicals
    to man. (1976) Vol. 10: Some naturally occurring substances, Lyon, Interna-
    tional Agency for Research on Cancer (Aflatoxins pp. 51-72; Reserpine
    pp. 217-230).

 7. Lancaster M.C. et al. (1961) Toxicity associated with certain samples of
    groundnuts, Nature 192, 1095-1096.

 8. IARC Monographs on the evaluation of che carcinogenic risk of chemicals
    to man (1979) Supplement 1: Chemicals and industrial processes associated
    with cancer in humans. Lyon, International Agency for Research on Cancer.

 9. Maltoni C. and Scarnato C. (1979) First experimental demonstration of the
    carcinogenic effects of benzene. Long-term bioassays on Sprague-Dawley
    rats by oral administration. Med. Lavoro 5, 352-357.

10. U.S. Department of Health, Education and Welfare, Public Health Service
    (1971) The health consequences of smoking, a Report to the Surgeon General

11. Gori G.B. (1976) Low-risk cigarettes: A prescription. Science 194, 1243--1246.

12. Wynder E.L. and Stellmann S.D. (1979) Impact of long-term filter cigarette usage on lung and larynx cancer risk: A case-control study J. Nat. Cancer Inst. 62, 471-477.

13. IARC Monographs on the evaluation of the carcinogenic risk of chemicals to man (1973). Vol. 3: Certain polycyclic aromatic hydrocarbons and heterocyclic compounds, Lyon, International Agency for Research on Cancer.

14. Case R.A.M. and Pearson J.T. (1954) Tumours of the urinary bladder in workmen engaged in the manufacture and use of certain dyestuff intermediates in the British chemical industry. Part II. Further consideration of the role of aniline and of the manufacture of auramine and magenta (fuchsine) as possible causative agents. Brit. J. industr. Med. 11, 213-216.

15. IARC Monographs on the evaluation of the carcinogenic risk of chemicals to man (1972). Vol. 1. Lyon, International Agency for Research on Cancer (Haematite and iron oxide pp. 29-39, Auramine pp. 69-73).

16. IARC Monographs on the evaluation of the carcinogenic risk of chemicals to man (1974). Vol. 4: Some aromatic amines, hydrazine and related substances, N-nitroso compounds and miscellaneous alkylating agents. Lyon, International Agency for Research on Cancer (Magenta pp. 57-64, 1-naphthylamine pp. 87-96, N,N'-Bis(2-chloroethyl)-2-naphthylamine pp. 119-126).

17. IARC Monographs on the evaluation of the carcinogenic risk of chemicals to man (1973). Vol. 2: Some inorganic and organometallic compounds. Lyon, International Agency for Research on Cancer (Chromium and inorganic chromium compounds pp. 100-125).

18. IARC Monographs on the evaluation of the carcinogenic risk of chemicals to man (1976). Vol. 11: Cadmium, nickel, some epoxides, miscellaneous industrial chemicals and general considerations on volatile anaesthetics, Lyon, International Agency for Research on Cancer (Cadmium and cadmium componds pp. 39-74, Nickel and nickel compounds pp. 75-114).

19. IARC Monographs on the evaluation of the carcinogenic risk of chemicals to man (1977). Vol. 15: Some fumigants, the herbicides 2,4-D and 2,4,5-T, chlorinated dibenzodioxins and miscellaneous industrial chemicals. Lyon, International Agency for Research on Cancer (Isopropyl alcohol and isopropyl oils pp. 223-244).

20. Pott P. (1775) Cancer scroti Chirurgical Observations, London, Hawes, Clarke and Collins, p. 63.

21. Yamagiva K. and Ichikawa K. (1915) Ueber die Künstliche Erzeugung von Papillom. V. jap. path. Ges. 5, 142.

22. Boyd J. T. et al. (1970) Cancer of the lung in iron ore (haematite) miners. Brit. J. industr. Med. 27, 97-105.

23. Thiede T. et al. (1964) Chlornaphazin as a bladder carcinogen. Acta med. scand. 175, 721-725.

338

24. Reimer R.R. et al. (1977) Acute leukemia after alkylating-agent therapy of ovarian cancer. N. Engl. J. Med. 297, 177-181.

25. IARC Monographs on the evaluation of the carcinogenic risk of chemicals to man (1975). Vol. 9: Some aziridines, N-, S- & O-mustards and selenium. Lyon, International Agency for Research on Cancer (Thio-tepa pp. 85-94, Chlorambucil pp. 125-134).

26. IARC Monographs on the evaluatuon of the carcinogenic risk of chemicals to man (1977). Vol. 13: Some miscellaneous pharmaceutical substances. Lyon, International Agency for Research on Cancer (Phenacetin pp. 141-156, Phenobarbital pp. 157-182, Phenytoin pp. 201-226).

27. Isaka H. et al. (1979) Tumours of Sprague-Dawley rats induced by long-term feeding of phenacetin. Gann 70, 29-36.

28. Clemmesen J. and Hjalgrim-Jensen S. (1978) Is phenobarbital carcinogenic? A follow-up of 8078 epileptics. Exotoxicol. Environ. Safety 1, 457-470.

29. IARC Internal Technical Report N° 78/003 (1978) : Chemicals with sufficient evidence of carcinogenicity in experimental animals: IARC Monographs volumes 1-17. IARC Working Group Report. Lyon, International Agency for Research on Cancer.

30. IARC Monographs on the evaluation of the carcinogenic risk of chemicals to man (1978). Vol. 18: Polychlorinated biphenyls and polybrominated biphenyls. Lyon, International Agency for Research on Cancer.

31. IARC Monographs on the evaluation of the carcinogenic risk of chemicals to man (1979). Vol. 19: Some monomers, plastics and synthetic elastomers, and acrolein. Lyon, International Agency for Research on Cancer.

32. IARC Monographs on the evaluation of the carcinogenic risk of chemicals to man (1979). Vol. 20: Some halogenated hydrocarbons Lyon, International Agency for Research on Cancer (in press).

33. IARC Information bulletin on the survey of chemicals being tested for carcinogenicity N° 8 (1979). Lyon, International Agency for Research on Cancer.

34. Muir C.S. and Wagner G. Editors (1978). Directory of on-going research in cancer epidemiology 1978, IARC Scientific Publication n° 26. Lyon, International Agency for Research on Cancer.

35. Cole P. (1979) The evolving case-control study. J. Chron. Dis. 32, 15-27.

36. Cole P. et al. (1972) Occupation and cancer of the lower urinary tract. Cancer 29, 1250-1260.

37. Anthony H. M. and Thomas G.M. (1970) Tumours of the urinary bladder: An analysis of the occupations of 1030 patients in Leeds, England. J. Nat. Cancer Inst. 45, 879-895.

38. IARC Monographs on the evaluation of the carcinogenic risk of chemicals to man (1977). Vol. 14: Asbestos. Lyon, International Agency for Research on Cancer.

39. Aromaa A. et al. (1976) Breast cancer and use of Rauwolfia and other antihypertensive agents in hypertensive patients: A nationwide case-control study in Finland. Int. J. Cancer 18, 727-738.

40. Herbst A. L. et al. (1971) Adenocarcinoma of the vagina: Association of maternal stilbestrol therapy with tumor appearance in young women. New Engl. J. Med. 284, 878-881.

41. Ortelee M. F. (1958) Study of men with prolonged intensive occupational exposure to DDT. Arch. industr. Hlth. 18, 433-440.

42. Laws E.R. et al. (1967) Men with intensive occupational exposure to DDT. A clinical and chemical study. Arch. environ. Hlth. 15, 766-775.

ROUND TABLE

SURVEY ON CURRENT METHODS AND NEW APPROACHES TO THE EVALUATION OF MUTAGENIC
POTENTIAL

Speakers:

JOHN W. DANIEL (Life Science Research, Stock, Essex CM4 9PE, United Kingdom)

LEON GOLBERG (Chemical Industry Institute of Toxicology, Research Triangle Park,
North Carolina 27709, U.S.A.)

Discussants:

IVAN BARTOŠEK (Istituto di Ricerche Farmacologiche "Mario Negri", Via Eritrea
62, 20157 Milan, Italy)

JACK C. DACRE (Department of the Army, U.S. Army Bioengineering Research and
Development Laboratory, Fort Detrick, Frederick, Maryland 21701, U.S.A.)

IAN C. MUNRO (Health Protection Branch, Tunney's Pasture, Ottawa, Ontario KIA
OL2, Canada)

SHELDON D. MURPHY (The University of Texas, Health Science Center at Houston,
Division of Toxicology, Houston, Texas 77025, U.S.A.)

CHRISTIAN SCHLATTER (Institut für Toxikologie der Eidgenössischen Technischen
Hochschule und der Universität Zürich, Schorenstrasse 16, 8603 Schwerzenbach
bei Zürich, Switzerland)

MUNRO: The balance of this morning's session will be taken up with the
discussion of genetic toxicology and tests for mutagenesis, as well as a discussion for test procedures for assessing potential carcinogenicity. We are indeed
fortunate this morning to have Dr. Daniel with us, as well as Dr. Leon Golberg
from the Chemical Industry Institute of Toxicology, North Carolina. In between
these two speakers we will, I hope, have an interesting and formative discussion
on the subject of genetic toxicology.

The session will take place in the following manner. Dr. Daniel will first
describe some of the test procedures currently in use and will say a little bit
about their biological basis and, following that, Dr. Golberg will make a presen
tation regarding the application of these procedures in toxicity assessment.
This will be followed finally by discussion of both papers in panel form and we
hope at that stage that as many of you as possible could ask these experts questions so that we may gain a better understanding of the use of these tests in
modern toxicology.

Let us begin then with Dr. Daniel's presentation on short term tests.

DANIEL: A mutagen is any physical or chemical agent that increases the spontaneous rate of change in genetic material. The potential threat to human health posed by chemical mutagens is well recognised and many governments and international organisations have advocated measures designed to reduce the risk wherever possible of adding to the burden of those diseases which are either known or presumed to be of genetic origin.

It is not my intention to discuss the principles of either molecular biology or genetic toxicology, but to outline some of the various procedures that have been developed to assess the ability of chemicals to interact with DNA.

Mutations are classified as either gene mutations and which result from changes confined to a few or even a single nucleotide or chromosomal mutations which involve relatively large numbers of bases and which are recognised as changes in either chromosome structure, or number, or both.

There are two mechanisms whereby chemicals can induce gene mutations. Frameshift mutations involve either insertion or deletions of bases in DNA, while base substitution mutations are the result of modifications of existing bases. Examples of the former include 2-acetylaminofluorene, benzo(a)pyrene, acridine derivatives and 4-aminoquinoline, while cyclophosphamide, propylene oxide, ethylene oxide, epichlorhydrin, methyl methane sulphonate and other alkylating agents cause base substitution mutations.

There is no single experimental system that is sensitive to all mutagens and it is necessary therefore to submit the chemical to procedures capable of detecting gene mutations, chromosomal aberrations and primary effects on DNA.

Some of the principal systems that may be employed to detect induced gene mutations are listed in Table 1. The most widely used bacterial system is that based upon mutant strains of Salmonella typhimurium, developed by Dr. Bruce Ames and his colleagues at the University of California. The mutants require histidine for growth and a positive response is indicated by an increase in the number of colonies which grow on a histidine-deficient medium following exposure of the organism to the test material. Individual strains respond to either base substitution (strains TA 1535 and TA 100) or frameshift mutagens (strains TA 1537, 1538 and TA 98) and the sensitivity has been enhanced by the deletion of an excision repair gene (uvrB), a cell envelope lipopolysaccharide which increases the permeability of the cell wall and the insertion of a plasmid (pKM 101) in strains TA 98 and 100.

Although some chemical mutagens are capable of reacting directly with DNA it has become increasingly apparent that most require to be converted to electrophilic intermediates. These reactions are catalysed by $NADPH_2$-dependent enzymes located in the endoplasmic reticulum of mammalian cells and it is customary therefore to test the compound both in the absence and presence of a post-mitochondrial fraction prepared from rat liver, together with appropriate co-factors. Animals are normally pre-treated with either phenobarbitone, 3-methyl-cholanthrene or, particularly, the chlorinated biphenyl derivative, Aroclor 1254, to increase the activity of the microsomal enzymes.

Using this procedure it has been possible to demonstrate that many environmental chemicals are potential mutagens, although it is clearly impossible to attempt any estimate of risk assessment on the basis of such studies alone.

TABLE 1

PROCEDURES FOR THE DETECTION OF GENE MUTATIONS

Salmonella typhimurium (histidine reversion)

Escherichia coli (tryptophan reversion)

Host-mediated assay

Drosophila melanogaster (sex-linked recessive mutations)

Cultured mammalian somatic cells

Mouse specific locus assay

The test is employed extensively to assess not the mutagenic activity of chemicals, but rather their carcinogenic potential. This development, which will be reviewed in some detail by Dr. Leon Golberg, is the result of studies by Ames which indicated that some 90% of the known carcinogens examined induced reversion in the various strains of Salmonella typhimurium. The bacterial system does not respond to all types of neoplastic agents and it should not be assumed that the same quantitative correlation will apply on every occasion.

The tryptophan auxotrophs of E. coli WP2 detect base substitution mutagens only and the response is in general similar to that obtained with S. typhimurium strain TA 1535. Strains have been developed capable of detecting frameshift mutagens and forward mutations, but comparatively little is known of either their specificity or sensitivity.

The host-mediated assay is an attempt to avoid the need to include an activating system in the *in vitro* bacterial system. Bacteria are injected either intra venously or intraperitoneally into rats and mice that have been pre-treated with the test material. The organisms are recovered after an interval sufficient to allow cell division to have occurred and the number of revertant colonies are scored after plating on a medium deficient in the appropriate amino acid. Alter-

natively, the organisms may be incubated *in vitro* with partially purified metabolites isolated from the urine of treated animals.

Tests for gene mutations in cultured mammalian somatic cells *in vitro* are
based on the detection of mutations at, for example, the loci responsible for
the activity of the enzymes thymidine kinase (TK) and hypoxanthrene-guanine
phosphoribosyl transferase (HGPRT) or for resistance to oubain and 8-azaguanine.
Chinese hamster ovary cells (CHO) and Chinese hamster fibroblasts (V79) are used
to detect HGPRT-mutations, whereas a mouse limphome cell line (L5158Y) responds
to changes induced at both the TK and HGPRT loci. The addition of a metabolic
activating system is necessary for the full expression of mutagenic activity.

The fruit fly, Drosophila melanogaster, offers some advantages when compared
with the other systems in this category. It appears to be able to metabolise
chemicals in a manner but not necessarily at a rate similar to that of mammals
and it has proved possible to detect an increase in mutation frequency of as
little as 1 percent. It is in addition a test for heritable mutations for it
monitors changes induced in the germ cells. Male flies treated with the test
material are mated with virgin females. Siblings of the F_1 progeny are mated
and the F_2 generation examined for a specific male phenotype. When adult males
are treated all stages of spermatogenesis may be affected, whereas if larvae
are used the spermatogonium only will be susceptible.

There is no simple method for monitoring gene mutations in mammals. The mouse
specific locus assay measures rates of mutations at several recessive loci.
Treatment is restricted to the males which are then mated to virgin females.
Offspring are examined after 2 - 3 weeks for recessive genes that are readily
expressed as visible phenotypes. It is probable that the system detects point
mutations and although it has proved of considerable value in evaluating the
hazard from radiation, there are yet insufficient data in respect of chemical
mutagens.

Procedures capable of detecting chemicals that induce chromosomal abnormalities are listed in Table II.

A proportion of circulating red cells contain small chromatin fragments
(Howell-Jolly bodies) which have not been included in either of the daughter
nuclei at anaphase and are therefore not extruded from the erythroblast. Many
clastogens increase the frequency of the 'micronuclei' in polychromatic erythrocytes present in bone marrow preparations. The test is relatively simple to
conduct and it is possible to establish a dose response relationship for those
agents which cause the chromosomes to fragment. The test material is usually
administered on two occasions, separated by an interval of 24 hours, but there

is no reason why such investigations should not be included in either sub-acute or chronic toxicity studies.

TABLE II

PROCEDURES FOR THE DETECTION OF CHROMOSOMAL MUTAGENS

Micronucleus test
Metaphase analysis following *in vivo/in vitro* exposure
Dominant lethal test
Heritable translocations in Drosophila/rodents

An alternative and more complex procedure is the analysis at metaphase of bone marrow for structural and numerical chromosomal abnormalities. The test can be conducted *in vitro* with cell cultures exposed to the suspect mutagen both in the absence and presence of a metabolic activating system. Colcemid is added to accumulate cells in metaphase which are then harvested, fixed, stained and scored . It is advisable using this procedure to include both a solvent and a positive control.

The dominant lethal test has been widely used to detect genetic damage in male germ cells and which following mating with untreated females results in death of the fertilised ova. It is customary to treat the males throughout spermatogenesis which is 8 weeks in mice and 10 weeks in rats. Males are mated every seven days to two or more virgin females which are then sacrificed some 14 days after pregnancy is confirmed and examined for the number of implanta-- tions. As many chemicals induce genetic damage in only post-meiotic sperm it is possible to restrict the period of treatment of the males to four weeks. Although the test is relatively insensitivity and does not identify the nature of the genetic lesion, it does provide a basis for estimating the hazard asso- ciated with individual mutagens . The heritable translocation test is similar in principle, the end-point being the induction of semi-sterility in males of the the F_1 progeny.

The third category of tests (Table III) detects a variety of effects includ- ing primary interaction with DNA, but which not necessarily result in gross chromosomal aberrations.

Evidence for the production of DNA damage can be obtained from studies in cultured mammalian somatic cells and in bacteria. Unscheduled DNA synthesis is assessed by measuring the rate of incorporation of radioactive thymidine

TABLE III

SUPPLEMENTARY TEST SYSTEMS

Sister chromatid exchange

Unscheduled DNA synthesis

Sperm abnormalities (structural)

Gene conversion in yeasts

Primary DNA damage in bacteria

---

following exposure to the test material, whereas in studying sister chromatid exchange cells are grown in the presence of a thymidine analogue. This results in the formation of one chromatid with a single analogue substituent, while the second chromatid contains two such groups. Sister chromatid exchanges if present are detected microscopically after differential staining of the chromosomes. These two procedures are still under development and it would be premature to recommend either for routine application until their sensitivity has been further evaluated. Moreover, there is some doubt whether the procedures monitor for mutagenic activity. Primary DNA damage in bacteria results in increased lethality, particularly in those strains of organisms that are deficient in either the polymerase enzymes or those that affect the recombination of DNA.

Various combinations of tests have been suggested to examine the mutagenic activity of chemicals. Some degree of judgement is obviously required in the selection of such tests providing certain criteria are fulfilled. The consultative document prepared by the Department of Health and Social Security recommends an 'Ames'-test, the production of chromosome damage *in vivo* and *in vitro* and the induction of point-mutations in cultured mammalian cells. Supplementary tests may then be used to clarify or extend the initial observations should the need arise. This suggested approach replaces the concept of Tier-testing and answers at least some of the criticism that the latter engendered.

I have attempted to illustrate the range and type of systems that are currently recommended for the detection of chemical mutagens. The list is not intended to be comprehensive and it is to be anticipated that more sensitive procedures will be developed. As I have indicated, no single test procedure is capable of detecting gene mutations, chromosomal abnormalities and primary effects on DNA and it is necessary to examine the test compound in several systems.The identification of a substance as a mutagen on the basis of *in vitro* procedures does not provide information that can be used to assess the possible health effects for there are a variety of factors, including metabolism and the activity of DNA-repair processes that may reduce the ability of such an agent to produce genetic damage in man. It is far from clear how national authorities are going to regulate environmental mutagens on evidence afforded by such studies, particularly those for which the scientific basis is only poorly understood. Claude Bernard summarised the three stages of knowledge as: an observation is made; a comparison is drawn; a judgement is rendered. It is to be hoped that everyone recognises the importance of the second stage.

GOLBERG: Ladies and gentlemen, I hope you realise that both Dr. Daniel's presentation and my act are impromptu. In fact, they were organized last night and I just happened to have some slides with me which were suitable, but that was purely by chance. What I am going to say will be supplemented by my presentation tomorrow on natural toxicants.

I would like to begin with just one transparency on sister chromatid exchange (SCE), even though what Dr. Daniel said was correct, that is we do not fully understand the basis of SCE. Table 1 summarizes the papers that have been published in recent months describing SCE measurements both *in vitro* with cells like human fetal lung fibroblasts showing fluorescent light to be positive (and this is not a surprise), with bone marrow cells, and Chinese hamster ovary (CHO) cells, and also *in vivo* studies of human subjects exposed to various suspect chemicals.

The case of ozone is interesting in that *in vivo* exposure, followed by isolation of the human lymphocytes showed a negative result for SCE; but when ozone is used *in vitro* with the WI-38 diploid human fetal lung cells, it came out positive. Acetaldehyde, as you see, is positive both in CHO cells and in human lymphocytes; fortunately ethyl alcohol is negative, even though, of course, we know it is metabolized to acetaldehyde and many alcoholic drinks contain substantial amounts of acetaldehyde. Formaldehyde, which I will be touching on tomorrow is claimed to give a positive result in CHO cells (unpublished work). At the foot of Table 1, I indicate one of the potentially useful approaches, namely the application of transplacental mutagens in the pregnant animal resulting in DNA damage in the fetus, and then counting SCE in fetal mouse chromosomes.

I think what Dr. Daniel said was correct - and Dr. Schlatter made this point too - that one has to be very careful about using tests where you don't know the scientific basis. An example is the test based on sperm morphology

TABLE 1

INCREASED INCIDENCE OF SISTER CHROMATID EXCHANGE

Agent	System	Reference
Fluorescent light	Human fetal lung fibroblasts	1
Styrene	Mouse regenerating liver and bone marrow cells	2
Anesthetics (inhaled)	Chinese hamster ovary cells (CHO)	3
Urethane	Human lymphocytes	4
Ozone (*in vivo*)	Human lymphocytes (no increase in SEC)	5
Ozone (*in vitro*)	Diploid human fetal lung cells WI-38 (increase dose dependent)	5
Acetaldehyde	CHO cells (ethanol negative)	6
Acetaldehyde	Human lymphocytes	7
Formaldehyde	Human lymphocytes	8
Transplacental mutagens	Fetal mouse chromosomes	9

References: 1 - Monticone and Schneider, Mutat. Res. 59:215-221, 1979; 2 - Conner et al., Toxicol. Appl. Pharmacol. 50:365-367, 1979; 3 - Whiate et al., Anesthesiol. 50:426-430, 1979; 4 - Csukás et al., Mutat. Res. 67:315-319, 1979; 5 - Guerrero et al., Environ. Res. 18:336-346, 1979; 6 - Obe and Ristow, Mutat. Res. 56:211-213, 1977; 7 - Ristow and Obe, Mutat. Res. 58:115-119, 1978; 8 - Obe, G., Unpublished; 9 - Kram et al., Nature 279:531, 1979.

which was referred to before. We have used it, many people have used it apparently successfully, but the work of Dr. Malling has shown that you can have absolutely normal sperm which when submitted to histochemical studies reveal the lack of certain enzymes as a result of mutation, so even if they look normal morphologically, they are in fact mutated; and, on the contrary, you can have abnormal sperm whose abnormality is just the result of a translocation of mitochondria. When you look at them under the electronmicroscope, all that has happened is the mitochondria have shifted and the shape of the sperm looks abnormal, but functionally it is still probably capable of doing its job. Hence an approach that is based empirically on abnormal sperm morphology has to be dealt with very carefully.

Now, the first aspect of my presentation will concern this question of predictability of mutagenesis tests for carcinogenic potential. Dr. Daniel had that up as the first point and this subject has been a source of much misunderstanding. It is unfortunate that the very important issue of mutagenic potential has become confused with the idea that we have a very quick cheap way of assessing carcinogenicity. The illusion that has become widespread has to be dispelled as soon as possible, so the first part that I want to present concerns this question. What I have done is to choose a group of compounds other than the traditional standard carcinogens and standard mutagens which are usually used for validation and examination of mutagenesis tests. I have selected components of hair dyes because of the interest in this field in the last few years, so that many good workers have conducted a variety of mutagenesis tests, and the National Cancer Institute has also tested these compounds for carcinogenicity by the standard long-term bioassay. Hence we are now in the position to compare these two approaches and to assess how reliable the mutagenesis tests have proved to be as an index of carcinogenic potential. I think it is a fairly unique situation.

Before we pass on to those comparisons, let us just look at the definitions of the basic terms that we have to use (Table 2).

TABLE 2
EXPLANATION OF TERMINOLOGY

Short-term test outcome	Carcinogenicity (as judged by bioassay)	
	True Carcinogens	Non-Carcinogens
+	a	b
-	c	d

$$N = a+b+c+d$$

Sensitivity $= \dfrac{a}{a+c}$ (c = false negatives)

Specificity $= \dfrac{d}{b+d}$ (b = false positives)

Predictive value $= \dfrac{a}{a+b}$

Prevalence $= \dfrac{a+c}{N}$

These concepts are fundamental to the understanding of the question of predictive value. What you see there is carcinogenicity as determined by carcinogenesis bioassay. We have a population of true carcinogens (a+c) as judged by that assay and a population of noncarcinogens (b+d). In a particular short-term test we either get a positive result or we get a negative result, as indicated in Table 2. We define N as the total population of compounds, a+b+c+d, that have been investigated. The sensitivity of the test is the proportion of the true carcinogens which are found to be positive, that is, a/a+c. The sensitivity is greatly influenced by the number of false negatives c. The specificity of a short-term test is the proportion of true noncarcinogens which have been picked up by the test (d/b+d), and you will see that it is influenced by the number of false positives b. The predictive value is a/a+b, that is of the total number that have come out positive how many are true carcinogens? Finally, the prevalence is the proportion of true carcinogens in the total population of compounds. The reason for drawing your attention to these considerations is the fact that in the literature various people have claimed that their tests have been successful in predicting 90% of all the carcinogens in the group of compounds investigated, for instance in the Ames test. What is very rarely pointed out is the importance of the proportion of noncarcinogens that are found to be negative, that is the specificity of the test. Figure 1 relates prevalence to predictive value in three hypothetical situations, short-term tests A,B, and C. In the first test, that is test A, we have a sensitivity of 95% and a specificity of 95%, a relationship represented by curve A. In test B the sensitivity is much lower, that is the ability to pick up true carcinogens is lower but the ability to pick up true negatives, noncarcinogens, correctly is still very high. You see that we have an equally good test. What makes a test very bad is a low specificity, that is the poor ability to detect noncarcinogens. So the emphasis that has always been placed on the ability of a test to detect carcinogens, is misleading in that it omits a very important principle, namely that what is at least equally important is the specificity.

People who seek to validate tests start with a population which usually comprises a very high proportion of carcinogens, a prevalence of 50% or even 80% of carcinogens in their test population. But in real life, if you are working in industry, the prevalence of true carcinogens that you are screening for in the population of test compounds is usually very low, maybe only 5%. In Fig. 1, I have drawn a vertical line at 10%, which is a generous estimate of what you are usually working with. You can see that if you have a test that has a low specificity you are in real trouble, because the predictive value is only

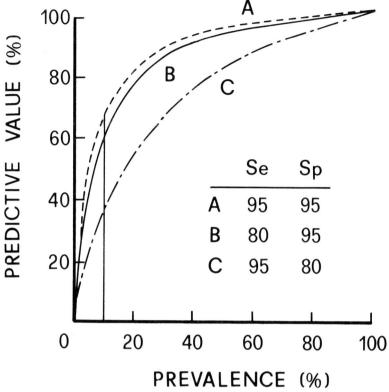

Figure 1

40%, whereas if the specificity is high and you have a reasonably good sensiti
vity too, then even at a 10% prevalence you have about 70% predictive value.
This issue is very critical when we come to look at the results obtained with
hair dye components.

As Dr. Daniel mentioned, one of the key aspects of mutagenesis testing is
the question of metabolic activation and this rather fanciful diagram that I
have drawn (Fig. 2) is really intended to make the point that we have metabolism at one end and predict the mechanisms and so on, and we have a cellular or
molecular target at the other end of the chain of events. With a true mutagen,
in order to elicit a mutagenic response everything has to work right all the
way along. It is a very complex system. What is particularly important in metabolism is the balance between metabolic activation and detoxication. Because
this balance is so critical, any attempt to standardize an approach using S9 as
a universal activating system is not scientifically tenable because the variety

352

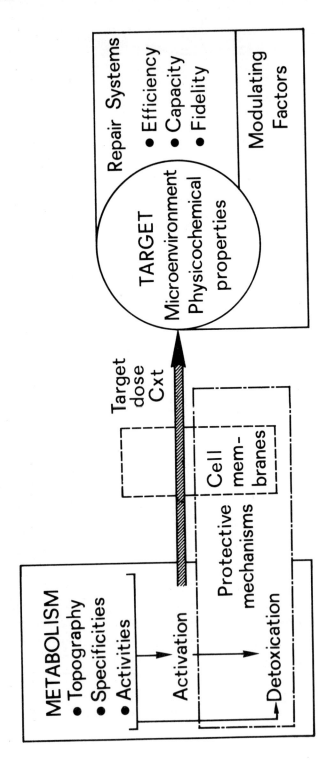

Figure 2

TABLE 3

COMPARISON OF RAPID TESTS WITH LONG-TERM TEST RESULTS

Test	Compounds※								
	m-PD	p-PD	2,4-DAT	2,5-DAT	2,4-DAA	4-NPD	2-NPD	2-N-4AP	N-PPD
Carcinogenicity: bioassay	-	-	+	-	+	-	+	+	-
Mutagenicity:									
Ames	+	+	+	+	+	+	+	+,-	+
Yeast	+	+	-		-	-,+	+		
Drosophila	-	+	+		+	+,-	+		
Mammalian Cells	+				-	+	+		
Chr. aberrations: human	±,-					-,+	+		
hamster						+	+		
S.C.E.	-					+	+		
DNA repair(UDS)	+,-	+	+			+,-	+	-	
Cell transformation	+	+	+		+	+	+		
Dominant lethal	-,+ weak +,-	-	-	-	-,-	weak +,-	-		
Micronucleus		-		-	-	-	-		
Sperm morphology					-	-			
Testis DNA synthesis	+	+	-						
Other bacteria						-,+	+		

※
m-PD, p-PD: m and p-phenylenediamine; 2,4-DAT, 2,5-DAT: 2,4- and 2,5-diaminotoluene; 2,4-DAA: 2,4-diaminoanisole; 4-NPD: 4-nitro-o-phenylenediamine; 2-NPD: 2-nitro-p-phenylenediamine; 2-N-4AP: 2-nitro-4-aminophenol; N-PPD: N-phenyl-p-phenylenediamine.

of compounds demands much greater flexibility. For instance, people have found that at least one form of insurance is to use a series of levels of S9, but even that is not the total solution to the problem. For instance, as was mentioned by Dr. Daniel, the very use of Aroclor 1254 presents a number of problems because it is not an inert material once it has stimulated the metabolic machinery. It, itself, has certain very peculiar properties which I don't have time to go into, but which can introduce complications. In addition to the mixed function oxidases, consideration of metabolism has to make allowance for the action of intestinal bacteria. The intestinal bacteria have very important metabolic and activating activities that are not reflected here at all. Hence carcinogenic aromatic nitro compounds may yield negative results in various short-term tests because these compounds are actually activated in the large intestine, and so cannot be expected to respond to activation by S9 or CHO cells, for example.

   With that introduction, let us go on to some of the results with components of hair dyes (Table 3). You will note that the Ames test is universally positive, despite the fact that only 4 of the 9 compounds are carcinogenic by bioas-- say. In the case of two compounds, 2,4-diaminotoluene (whose use in hair dyes has been discontinued) and 2,4-diaminoanisole, some short-term tests are positive and others negative. Only 2-nitro-p-phenylenediamine produced a high proportion of positive short-term tests; even in this instance the dominant lethal and micronucleus tests were negative. The compounds not found to be carcinogenic by bioassay yielded a fair proportion of positive tests in short-term tests. Even the test for neoplastic transformation was positive with m-phenylenediamine, p-phenylenediamine and 4-nitro-o-phenylenediamine, which are noncarcinogenic by bioassay. The lack of sensitivity of the dominant lethal test is confirmed by the uniformly negative results, and the micronucleus test is equally disappointing. All in all, even though the short-term tests may indicate genotoxic potential, many of them are seen to be poor predictors of carcinogenicity.

   The work of Purchase, Ashby, Styles and their colleagues at ICI in some respects emphasized the fact that the more tests that you do, the poorer your predictive capacity becomes. So what you really need to do, and I think that is where it will have to end also with government requirements, is to select a few tests appropriate to a particular class of compounds and not try to have a huge battery, because that just confuses the issue with a high proportion of erroneous results.

   I also have some tests carried out with the Ames procedure (Table 4) on a series of compounds whose carcinogenicity bioassay results were published by

TABLE 4

PREDICTIVE VALUE OF AMES TEST FOR CARCINOGENIC POTENTIAL

Compound	Ames test[a]	Carcinogenesis bioassay[b]		
		Rats (males)	Mice (CD-1) Males	Females
o-Phenylenediamine	+	+	+	+
o-Toluidine	-	+	+	+
m-Toluidine	-	-	±	-
p-Toluidine	-	-	+	+
2,4,5-Trimethylaniline	-	+	+	+
2,4,6-Trimethylaniline	-	+	+	+
2,4,6-Trichloroaniline	-	-	+	-
4-Chloro-o-toluidine	-	-	+	+
1-Chloro-2-nitrobenzene	-	+	+	+
1-Chloro-4-nitrobenzene	-	-	+	+
1-Chloro-2,4-dinitrobenzene	+	-	-	-
Benzoguanamine	-	-	-	-
2,5-Dimethoxy-4'-aminostilbene	-	+	+	-
Dicyclopentadiene dioxide	-	-	-	-

[a] Results kindly provided by Dr. C. Burnett.

[b] Weisburger et al., J. Environ. Pathol. Toxicol. 2:325, 1978.

Weisburger and her colleagues in 1978. These are the kind of organic compounds that industry uses and that are widely applied. The results of NCI carcinogenesis bioassays in male rats and in male and female mice are not always in accord, but usually they do agree with each other. Looking now at the results of the Ames test, with ortho-phenylenediamine, there seems to be general agreement. But with many other compounds, like ortho-toluidine, para-toluidine, the substituted anilines, there is just no concordance. Hecht et al.[1] recently studied these sorts of compounds, both as phenyl and biphenyl derivatives, using Ames' strains TA1535, 1538 an 100, with and without S9 activation. Aniline and p-toluidine were inactive, but the hydroxylamino and C-nitroso analogs of *o*-toluidine were mutagenic toward TA100 and TA1535, with activation. The aminobiphenyl derivatives could be activated to potent mutagens and some hydroxylamino and C-nitroso compounds were highly mutagenic without activation, in parallel with the carcinogenic activity of these compounds.

So, in essence the chemically-reactive form is often so unstable that it is very difficult to synthesize it or to use it. But where it is possible to make it, we do find that the Ames tests back up the carcinogenicity very well. This illustrates the fact that the fundamental problem in many cases is the activation. Just using the S9 fraction in a routine procedure may not produce the right kind of activation. As I mentioned, our own work has been concerned with 2,4-dinitrotoluene, which Dr. Dacre here has also studied, and which is a very powerful liver carcinogen. If you put it through the Ames test or CHO cells in culture, with S9 as the activation system, virtually nothing happens. But if you incubate with intestinal microorganisms you get a whole series of derivatives, some of which are azo, azoxy, hydroxylamino derivatives, and so on, and they are strongly positive in the Ames test. So we need to elaborate the whole approach to mutagenesis testing much more than has happened so far.

Now, in case any of you gain the impression that I am denouncing the Ames test and that I am saying it is no good, that is not true. The Ames test used appropriately is an extremely valuable procedure. What is happening now is that it is being applied by chemists and biologists as a quick tool to tell them whether they are proceeding in the right direction when looking for the metabolically active forms of a compound. One may cite an example from the elegant work by Dr. Casida's group.[2,3] They have studied a group of S-chloroallyl thiocarbamate herbicides like diallate and triallate. They followed the course of the various metabolic changes by means of Ames tests, and ended up by showing that the ultimate mutagen is 2-chloroacrolein. The beauty of this work is the demonstration that, as so often happens, the moeity that does the damage is really quite a small and relatively simple molecule; so, starting with all these complex molecules, you end up with 2-chloroacrolein as the ultimate mutagen. If all these compounds and their metabolites had to be tested in lifespan studies carried out in rodents, in order to work out the mechanism of activation, it would take the rest of our lives. Here, in the matter of a month or two, you get the total answers. It is this kind of brilliant approach which I think is going to give us a fantastic insight, in the coming years, into the manner of activation, the mechanism of toxic effects and particularly the mechanism of expression of mutagenic potential of compounds.

At the beginning, I talked about the importance of prevalence; that is, if you take a population of compounds and just screen them blindly, your problem is that the proportion of carcinogens in that population may be very low. So, ideally, what you should do before you apply mutagenesis tests is to enrich the population by substantially increasing the proportion of likely carcinogens. This is a very serious problem for the world at large, because we have - it is estimated - 70,000 compounds that have never been tested, or maybe even more. Just testing them blindly by routine application of short-term tests is going to get us into very serious trouble because the prevalence of true carcinogens or mutagens is probably very low. So there has to be some way to enhance the prevalence, in other words to set priorities. In the past this was done by chemical intuition; people looked at the structure and said: well, there is an epoxide ring, or there is a potential for metabolically forming an epoxide ring. That is a potentially hazardous compound, let's test it. What has been happening in recent years is the application of computerized procedures for selecting the compounds that have the greatest toxic potential. What I am going to illustrate is the work on pattern recognition by computer, which is one approach among several used to select compounds that are most important from the point of view of early testing. The pharmaceutical industry has used this kind of technique in trying to devise new drugs, or to go from an established drug structure to new areas; but the predictive methods have not been widely applied to toxicology, at least not very effectively.

A paper by Jurs, Chu and Yuan, which appeared just a few months ago[4] is a very interesting attempt in that direction. What was done was to take from the IARC, that is the volumes published by the International Agency for Research on Cancer, their conclusions on carcinogenesis tests - yielding a total of 130 compounds which have been accepted by IARC as carcinogens, 79 as noncarcinogens and a few others which either are weak or about which there is some doubt (Table 5). You will see that these compounds cover a wide variety of chemical types. The authors asked themselves the question: what kind of predictability of carcinogenic potential can we achieve with the assistance of a computer without using Ames tests or any other biological approach?

What you do in this kind of pattern recognition - and I am not an expert in it, but I will try to explain it as best I can - is to have various kinds of descriptors that you program in (Table 6). These descriptors can be topological, that is various characteristics of the molecule and the way in which you can move across the molecule from one end to the other, the so-called connection table. Or they can be geometrical, that is properties of the molecule that are

TABLE 5

HETEROGENEOUS DATA SET OF CHEMICAL CARCINOGENS*

	+	-	Weak	?
Aromatic amines	23	10	1	10
Alkyl halides	13	2		4
Polycyclic aromatics	23	6	3	4
Esters, epoxides, carbamates	11	7	5	5
NO₂ aromatics and heterocycles	14	3		3
Miscellaneous	5	7		8
Nitrosamines	19	2		1
Fungal toxins and antibiotics	3	1	2	1
Miscellaneous	2	2	1	6
Misc N compds	8	1		
Azo dyes and diazo compds	9	2	2	4
Naturally occurring compds		36		
Totals	130	79	14	46

*Jurs et al., J. Med. Chem. 22:476(1979)

TABLE 6

MOLECULAR STRUCTURE DESCRIPTORS

Type	Source
Topological	Molecule: topological representation (connection table)
Geometrical	Molecule: three-dimensional model
Physicochemical	Measurement, mathematical model, linearly-correlated calculable descriptor

three dimensional. Or they can be physicochemical measurements like lipophili-city. For many years we have known that this is a very very important character-istic from the point of view of toxicity. There are various mathematical mod-els involved and other types of descriptors.

Table 7 shows us what Jurs et al. actually used as ADAPT system descriptors for this population of compounds. They had four descriptors that were made up of the characteristics of the atoms and the bonds or what are called the basis rings in these molecules. Then there was the chemical environment within the molecules. For instance, if you had a keto group, what was connected to either side of it. If you had an imino group, what was linked to either side. Whether there was X-nitro or methyl linked to something else, and so on. All these were put in, to a total of thirteen descriptors. Molecular connectivity, that is the branching of the structure and the ways in which one can travel across the molecule by various paths provided three descriptors.

These ADAPT descriptors listed in Table 7 are largely structural, chemical and mathematical. What I think holds tremendous promise for the future would be to fit into these descriptors an understanding of metabolic activation, of various properties of the molecule from a biochemical point of view. Jurs and his colleagues are chemists and I don't think they really grasp the kind of insight that we as toxicologists could bring to bear to improve the descriptor characteristics. But, anyway, let's take what they have used and see how well they did.

TABLE 7
ADAPT DESCRIPTORS

No. used	Type	Nature
4	Fragment	No. of N, Cl atoms, double bonds, basis rings
13	Environment	Code of immediate surroundings of substructures (eg. X-C(O)-X, X-NH-X, $X-NO_2$, CH_3-X, C_6H_5-X)
3	Molecular connectivity	Measure of branching of the structure (paths 1, 2, 4)
1	Geometric	Smallest principal moment of inertia (PMI)
5	Combined	No. of ring atoms/no. of basis rings; $X-C(O)-NH_2$, $X-C(O)-NHX$, $X-C(O)-NX_z$ etc.
26		Largest PMI x intermediate PMI = "area"

Applying various mathematical analytical approaches (Table 8), their percentages of correct results for these 209 compounds were as follows: for the 130 carcinogens, the method of iterative least squares yielded 93.1%. For the noncarcinogens - and, of course, I stressed to you earlier the question of specific ity, what proportion of noncarcinogens do you really find to be negative -

their best result was as high as 94.9%. I don't think there is any single test in mutagenesis that will give you a specificity as good as that. So, when you look at the claims made for the Ames test and so on, this is really as good, if not better, without ever using a test tube, or a petri dish or an organism.

TABLE 8
PATTERN RECOGNITION RESULTS
(209 compounds, 26 descriptors)

PR TECHNIQUE	Correct results(%)	
	Carc. (130)	Noncarc. (79)
Bayes (quadratic)	88.5	94.9
Bayes (linear)	76.9	82.3
Learning machine	83.1	63.3
Iterative least squares	93.1	82.3
K nearest neighbor (K=1)	62.0	73.7

They did another interesting thing. By dividing their compounds into sets of ten, they carried out thirty trials to see how well they could do with six carcinogens and four noncarcinogens in each prediction set. In this way they got 90% correct for the carcinogens and 78.3% for the noncarcinogens, which is still a respectable performance.

TABLE 9
PREDICTIVE ABILITY[*]

	Number predicted	Number correct	% correct
Carcinogens	180	162	90.0
Noncarcinogens	120	94	78.3
Total	300	256	85.3

[*] 30 Trials on 10 prediction sets, each containing 6 carcinogens and 4 noncarcinogens chosen at random; 17 compounds excluded.

The message that I want to convey to you is as follows: if you have a single compound that your company has produced, you might find it useful to have a program like this in order to judge how your compound performs and what its potential for hazard might be. For the future, where we have to test large numbers of compounds, we would be well advised to set priorities on the basis of computerized pattern recognition or similar systems, so that we enrich the population that we then submit to our biological tests. We should not carry out large batteries of mutagenesis tests at random; I think we shall have to develop appropriately selective, rational batteries on a small scale. You will see some of the applications of this approach tomorrow, in the case of natural toxicants. For the moment, I hope that I have given you some food for thought. Thank you.

DISCUSSION

MUNRO: Thank you very much, Dr. Golberg, for a very interesting and provocative presentation. If you would kindly join me here with Dr. Daniel at the table, we will open both papers for discussion. We have approximately 25 minutes and I hope in that period we can excite a considerable amount of discussion. Are there any questions? I will start off the questioning by asking either Dr. Daniel or Dr. Golberg what they would consider to be the minimum manipulation, if you will, of the Ames test before you can be satisfied that you have a truly negative result? One could think, for example, of the use of S9 as an added means in some cases of increasing the sensitivity of the assay. One can think in terms of substrains of main organisms. One can think in terms of use of other organs, say, even from the rat or in fact from other species. And the questions has long bothered me as to when does one stop manipulation of the assay in terms of its application as a prescreen tool?

GOLBERG: My philosophy in this is as follows: the Ames test is intended to be a short term test. If you are going to do as much work in elaborating it as you would with a long term test, you might as well forget about it. I think that there has to be a certain minimum effort put in. As I mentioned earlier, I think you need to use various levels of S9 and to try to establish dose-response curves for both toxicity and mutagenicity of the test compound. But if it comes up negative under those circumstances, you would be better advised, I think, to move on to some of the other tests; and, particularly, to get as soon as possible to a mammalian test involving exposure of a whole animal to the compound and thus metabolism and activation. Then one applies various criteria of genotoxic effect in the whole animal. I feel we will always, no matter what procedures are developed for toxicology - at least in the foreseeable future - we will always be doing tests on whole animals such as the subchronic test that was described yesterday. That is a must. We have those exposed animals. They contain in them, if we only know how to look, evidence establishing whether the compound has had a mutagenic effect or not. It is up to us to derive that evidence from the animal. Sperm abnormality seemed at one time to provide a promising and useful information. As I mentioned, I am not so sure about that now; but there are other measurements to be made, such as cytogenetic analysis, sister chromatid exchange counts, a variety of things that one can use that animal for quite apart from the aims that were described yesterday in the subchronic test. It seems to me that is the way to go.

MUNRO: Thank you. Are there other questions? Could you please use a microphone when you raise a question because this discussion is being recorded.

MURPHY: Yes, I have one question to be addressed to Dr. Daniel. Your comments regarding the battery test developed in the U.K. of what to do with the data is a familiar one. I recall a year or two ago sitting on an EPA science advisory board when they came up with a list of battery tests and several of us insisted that if we were going to publish this in a Federal Register, they would also have to publish how to interpret it. I don't know quite honestly how this came off but what would you say should be the regular criteria or do you have any suggestion as to what criteria you think should stimulate a regulatory action or what would be the nature of the regulatory action with respect to attitude, whether there is a threshold or not and so forth.

DANIEL: I really don't believe there is a simple answer to that question - unless one subscribes to the opinion that all chemicals which induce mutations in two or more test systems should be proscribed. I would be reluctant to make any assessment based on just *in vitro* studies and would seek confirmation from experiments in the whole animal. In the integrated scheme I outlined on Monday it is possible to examine for possible chromosomal damage during a conventional sub-acute toxicity study. It is frequently claimed that the dominant lethal assay is too insensitive, that it fails to detect mutagens with the frequency of other systems. Perhaps our defence mechanisms are so sophisticated that the problem is less critical than we imagine. I am frequently asked to identify any chemical that has been demonstrated to produce a heritable disease in the population. One may have one's suspicions, but that is not quite the same thing. I can only suggest that no attempt be made to regulate environmental mutagens until more information is available.

I am of course not referring to the use of such procedures for predicting carcinogenic potential. That in my opinion is a related, but quite separate, issue and every attempt should be made to avoid the confusion that frequently appears even in the scientific literature.

MUNRO: Dr. Golberg, do you have any comments to add to that question?

GOLBERG: We don't really have evidence of any compound producing heritable genetic effects in man. However, there is a suspect therapeutic combination, the so-called PUVA therapy which is used for the treatment of psoriasis and consists of administering 8-methoxypsoralen, followed by exposure to ultravio-let light. Already some patients have developed skin cancer as a consequence of this treatment. It has been suggested that some patients may have undergone actual genetic effects that have been manifested in the germ cells, but the really concrete evidence has not been published. It would be very interesting if this actually happened to be the first instance of such an effect.

MUNRO: Thank you. Other questions?

MURPHY: Well, neither of our speakers commented on tying this in with pharmacokinetics in the germ cell. Is that a conceivable approach, one used perhaps in a short term mutagenicity test coupled with pharmacokinetic data specifically in finding out the distribution of compounds availability to the germ cell. And on the basis of that find out the regulatory position. For at least ten years now the FAO/WHO has looked at this and said: well, there is no harm in doing these tests but we don't know how to interpret them.

GOLBERG: I have a slide, that I unfortunately had put in among those to be shown tomorrow, which deals with the question of demonstration of genetic effects not necessarily on germ cells but also on somatic cells of man. In that slide I do stress the need to determine how much of the material gets to germ cells, the time and dose relationships, and all the connected parameters of those measurements. I agree with you. I think it is very important. The fact that we cannot apply all that information yet is just a consequence of our failure to generate enough of it hitherto.

MUNRO: Are there other questions or comments?

DACRE: Dr. Golberg, you have shaken my confidence to some extent in the use of the S9 fraction. We have used, of course, other activators, phenobarbital. Any suggestions on what other activators might be used to overcome some of these deficiencies which you mentioned?

GOLBERG: If induction of cytochromes P450 and P448 is desired, most of the compounds you can think of to try as inducing agents are toxic or dangerous; for instance, dioxins would do a good job but you wouldn't want them around. I hope it will be possible to find something that doesn't have the undesirable properties of Aroclor 1254, or else to persuade people to use it at lower doses. I think that you can achieve maximum activation at very much lower doses than are being used at present and thus avoid these undesirable effects of the Aroclor itself.

DANIEL: There is a further point. You can optimise the response and obtain a maximal increase in the number of revertant colonies. There is probably no inducer that is applicable for all classes of chemical compounds. The use of Aroclor 1254 is probably an acceptable compromise, although little attempt, if any, is made to select the appropriate inducing agent. Japanese workers have advocated the use of phenobarbital and benzoflavone with some justification based on analysis of the components of the microsomal electron transfer system.
There is a question I would like to direct to Dr. Golberg. I am struck by the association in the Ames test between cytotoxicity and mutation frequency. Is cytotoxicity a further expression of genetic damage, not wholly perhaps, but in part. Experience with the cell transformation bio-assay system indicates a similar association. Would you care to comment.

GOLBERG: Yes, I agree with you. I have a slide that I will show tomorrow on the effects on sunlight doing exactly what you say. The number of Chinese hamster ovary cells drops off as the mutation rate rises and I agree that the cytotoxicity could be a manifestation, and often is, of mutagenic activity. But I need hardly mention that there are thousands of compounds which are cytotoxic without being mutagenic. A preliminary cytotoxicity test provides a measure of the toxic capacity of the compound under those conditions before starting the

Ames test but I am not sure how valuable that information would be. In practice what you have to do is to manipulate your dosage and duration of exposure in such a way as to reveal mutagenic potential if it is there, despite the killing off of a large proportion of the population of bacteria, or cells, or whatever the test system is.

MUNRO: Are there other questions or comments?

BARTOŠEK: I would like to ask you what is your opinion about the possible use of Corwin Hansch's approach to correlate the structure and toxicity or carcinogenesis?

GOLBERG: I have been an admirer of Corwin Hansch for the last 25 years and his approach, which started with lipophilicity as a basis for structure activity correlation has been applied very widely. To-day many of the systems aimed at structure activity correlation use lipophilicity as one criterion among many, for example in the additive molecular thermodynamic or linear free energy model. This was the point I was trying to make here, that I think there are a lot of biochemical and biological properties that could be fitted in to improve predictability over a very wide range of chemical structures. As a matter of fact, I should mention that we are arranging a conference in America on this subject because we think it has such tremendous potential. We hope to get an update on all the new approaches there.

DANIEL: Could I add something to what Jack Dacre has said? The Japanese guidelines for the 'Ames'-test require the addition of both NADPH and NADH. I can only assume that the NADH-cytochrome b_5 component increases the sensitivity of the activating system. This would accord with the data presented by Dennis Parke on Tuesday.

MUNRO: Are there any other questions or comments?

SCHLATTER: It has been shown in drosophila that chromosomal damage is always accompanied by point mutations but that normally chromosomal damages is only induced by the administration of high-dose levels whereas point mutations also occur at low-dose levels. Now my question is: is the same also true for mammalian systems? If so, one could conclude that every substance which shows positive results in cytogenic assays or in dominant lethal tests would also induce point mutations at low-dose levels.

GOLBERG: I really don't believe that. There was published some years ago by Dr. Shaw a list of what she called clastogenic compounds which caused chromosome breaks *in vivo* and they included ethanol, which I don't believe is a compound capable of producing point mutations; but, seriously, the list included compounds like ethyl acetate, acetone and so on, and I just cannot believe that those compounds will produce point mutations under any circumstances. So it may apply in Drosophila with certain compounds but I doubt very much whether you can generalize beyond that. One of the problems with chromosomal aberrations, while we are on that subject, is the fact that they are a very valuable epidemiological tool, but the fundamental difficulty you have is the establishment of what is a normal incidence level in a normal human population. Prof. Sram of Czechoslovakia and a number of Russian workers have carried out cytogenetic analysis of peripheral lymphocytes and have shown for example, that bis-chloromethyl ether and epichlorohydrin will give an increase in the chromosomal aberrations in exposed populations. But if you look at all their work and put it all together you find they are operating in the range from about 1.5% to 4% of chromosomal aberrations. In some studies their matching control population has over 2% of aberrant cells.The difference between the exposed and the controls is often within this very narrow range. Accordingly they have found positive results with dimethyl formamide, in spite of the fact that, as far as I know, in all the mutagenic tests it is negative. The percentage of aberrant cells was 3.82, 2.74 and 1.59 in December-January, April-May and September-October for exposed subjects and 1.61% in controls. This illustrates the difficulty we have, and it has existed for many years. That is where I hope that analysis of sister chromatid exchange might be of help.

MUNRO: We have time for one more short question. If not, then I would like to thank the speakers for this morning's session for very interesting and provocative and education lectures and I would like to thank each one of you for your partecipation ensuring the success of this session. Thank you.

REFERENCES
1. Hecht et al. (1979) J. Med. Chem., 22, 981-987.
2. Casida et al. (1979) Science, 205, 1013-1015.
3. Casida et al. (1979) J. Agric. Food Chem., 27, 1060-1067.
4. Jurs et al. (1979) J. Med. Chem., 22, 476-483.

ROUND TABLE

AN EXAMPLE OF ENVIRONMENTAL TOXICOLOGY: THE DIOXIN EVENT

Chairmen:

RODOLFO PAOLETTI (Istituto di Farmacologia e Farmacognosia, Via Andrea del Sarto 21, 20129 Milan, Italy)

ANTONIO SPALLINO (Ufficio Speciale per Seveso, Via S. Carlo 4, 20030 Seveso, Milan, Italy)

Discussants:

FLAMINIO CATTABENI (Istituto di Farmacologia e Farmacognosia, Università degli Studi, Via Andrea del Sarto 21, 20129 Milan, Italy)

VITO FOA' (Clinica del Lavoro "L. Devoto", Università degli Studi, Via S. Barnaba 8, 20122 Milan, Italy)

UMBERTO FORTUNATI (Ufficio Speciale per Seveso, Via S. Carlo 4, 20030 Seveso, Milan, Italy)

SILVIO GARATTINI (Istituto di Ricerche Farmacologiche "Mario Negri", Via Eritrea 62, 20157 Milan, Italy)

SIMONETTA NICOSIA (Istituto di Farmacologia e Farmacognosia, Università degli Studi, Via Andrea del Sarto 21, 20129 Milan, Italy)

GIORGIO WEBER (Istituto di Anatomia Patologica, Università degli Studi, Via Laterino 8, 53100 Siena, Italy)

PAOLETTI: Ladies and gentlemen, in July 1976 there was an unexpected event in this Region, the Region of Lombardy. It was the dispersion of the highly toxic compound dioxin over a heavily populated area called the city of Seveso. This was an ecological event, unexpected and never recorded before in an industrialized country and after that period an intensive investigation has been started with the help of Italian and foreign scientists, under the control of a special office.

Today I have asked Dr. A. Spallino, who is in charge of this office, and several scientists who have contributed towards these investigations, to report to you what the status of the Seveso event is like three years after the original observations. I would like to ask Dr. Spallino to start this session.

SPALLINO: It seems to be of interest to know a bit more about the public intervention in this area of Seveso after the dioxin event. On July 10, 1976, very little was known on the effect of large amounts of dioxin in a highly populated area of unknown dimensions on animals and particularly on men. For about ten days the company,where the event started,did not disclose information on the chemical properties or chemical entities released during the dioxin event; this was only known to Italian analysts when they were asked to go to Zurich where the company had the laboratories, but only ten days after the event.

On July 24, fourteen days after the event, the first maps with about 44 determinations of dioxin in vegetables and on the ground have been given to the local government and at about the same time the same determinations, carried out by the local analytical laboratories, also became available.

The definition of the area contaminated by dioxin required after this period a very intensive effort by the local analytical laboratories in order to be able to measure the compounds with the maximum sensitivity, at that time one billion of grams (today the sensitivity in ten times higher) and in a sufficient number of samples.

On July 24, the Mayors of Meda and Seveso, the two towns affected by dioxin, released the first orders for the population to be removed from that area, and the area affected was about twice as large as that covered by the original map developed by the analysts of the chemical company, where the dioxin event started. In twenty-four hours, several hundred people had to leave their homes, activities and belongings without really knowing the possible danger related to the chemical compound dioxin, which was unknown to most of the people at that time. This was a very unusual event in the history of an industrialized community.

There is a very interesting difference between natural disasters and ecologi cal disasters of this type, because the population are not ready to these sudden changes in their life and so they asked the local administration, the government and the scientists for information and for advice that usually these organizations and even science are not ready to give.

On July 26 the first families were evacuated and the evacuation was completed early in August with the total removal of about 700 people from the area.

Today, most of the area has been decontaminated and so the majority of these 700 people are back home after three years, and the control has been continued as scientists will report to you later.

One important aspect today of the Seveso situation is how to reimburse this large section of the population affected by the event, and the Special Office, set up by the government and directed by myself, has arranged with the counterpart - the company where the Icmesa event took place - to establish joint committees and to decide on a cooperative basis how to reimburse the different groups of the population affected by the event.

Four millions of dollars to be devoted to reconstruction of homes in the de-
contamined area are paid by the company responsible for the event.

Until now the chemical company has reimbursed around 13 millions of dollars
to individuals affected by the event, but an undisclosed amount of money, certainly larger than this, should be given directly to the local government for
expenses involved in these operations and again to individuals to complete the
reimbursement in the near future.

The responsible organizations to take care of this event were the Central
Government of Italy, through the Ministry of Health, the Region of Lombardy
where Seveso and Meda are located and the Municipal Administrations of the two
cities. The Italian Government through two differnt laws in 1977 and 1978 has
provided the necessary financial support, but all the organization and the
coordination of scientific research has been taken care by the Region of Lombardy in collaboration with local Universities, with the Mario Negri Institute
and with the Universities located in other parts of the country. The Municipal
Administrations have collaborated in pointing out the priorities in the intervention.

It is obvious that both Municipal Administrations and the local Regional
Government,which have been organized and set up to respond to regular flow of
requests but not to emergencies such is this, had a very difficult time particu
larly because of the psychological tension that underlined any type of request
under these circumstances. It is quite interesting that two organizations coope
rated in this event: the Municipal Administrations which are centuries old in
Italy - quite old fashioned in their organization - and the Regional Governments
which are on the contrary quite new, because, as many of you may know, the Regional subdivision of the country only became effective in the seventies.

Now some figures concerning the number of people affected by the dioxin
event: the zone to be evacuated contained about 730 people, the surrounding
zone, called zone "B", 4699 people; the area immediately adiacent to these affected areas, 31,000 people. These 40,000 people were part of several municipal
subdivisions. The total population directly or indirectly affected in these
towns were about 120,000 people.

This episode has also shown some deficiencies in the Italian scientific organization, for istance the epidemiology is certainly not sufficiently developed in this country, and it has been extremely difficult to obtain young well-
trained epidemiologists from the Italian Universities. At the beginning Milan,
Padua and Palermo have helped and now the University of Genoa is also taking
part in this investigation.

Another aspect of how difficult is to obtain the support of analytical laboratories is that at the present time there are only four analytical laboratories in Italy able or willing to study and to analyze samples of dioxin. It is also interesting to observe that the four analytical laboratories that have been interested over this period of three years in examining the dioxin samples have been more interested to develop more sofisticated and sensitive methods than to really reduce the time lag for the analysis. This has been a phenomenon which has been observed over this period of time.

Now we can move from the purely technical area to a more socio-political area. In fact, the Seveso event had also stirred up a major political turmoil, because the possible effect of dioxin on the fetus had implications on the national debate on the abortion law; the fact that dioxin was produced and released by a multinational company working in this territory was a very important fact in the ideological and political discussion over the Icmesa event and so on. As you see, a toxic event may have far reaching consequences.

In spite of this fact, all the difficulties - lack of sufficient scientific structures, political difficulties as the social service and reconstruction and normalization of the economy - are now almost completely achieved, and for this reason the Special Office set up by the Government for Seveso will end its activity in this area by the end of this year. The Office is still active for public health and for some specific purposes but no longer for the main purposes of reconstruction and help to the local economy.

From the economical point of view, the situation is also very intricated because we are dealing with mixed population active in farming, small business, small factories. It may be calculated that the three areas affected, or closed to the areas affected by dioxin, contain something like 4,000 vegetable gardens and that all these gardens must be controlled continuously and they are still under control; and a number of small companies which are over 1,000 and of course further activities such as the production of honey, and even the honey, had to be controlled all the time because bees can fly over 5 miles, and they could go to the contaminated areas. This just gives you an example of how many controls and how frequently the area should be controlled and what effort should be done from the analytical point of view to keep all this complex area with 120,000 people under continuous control.

Concerning the health problems, the Lombardian Region has medical consortia, so called, combining several towns with a local organized medical system. These consortia were already existing before the Icmesa dioxin episode, but were absolutely insufficient for that purpose. For this reason, the Regional Government has potentiated financially this local-medical organizations, particularly in view of the necessary preventive medical efforts in different areas such as gynecology and so on. Unfortunately, the difficulty here is not so much in providing financial support but in finding sufficiently well-trained medical doctors and medical assistants, to carry on such an enormous task as the control of all the population on an individual basis.

Two efforts, in terms of fall out from this episode - a better organization of the epidemiological studies and collection and analysis of information must be underlined, both concentrated on the area because the Government thinks that at least something should remain from this episode, an organized structure for the area responsible for health control and for the collection and retrieval of data concerning public health.

At the present time the economy of the area is almost completely normalized; the social fabric of this area is back to normal and these of course are the most important achievements of the Special Office set up in Seveso.

There are several points which should be stressed,a sort of lesson we can draw from the Seveso episode. Number one is that usually we have very little knowledge of industrialized areas, so when we collect the data after a critical experiment, a very well designed experiment on the Seveso area, we are at loss because we cannot compare these data with so called normal areas similar to Seveso. This, I think, pinpoints a missing link in our epidemiology and analytical sciences.Number two is that the time necessary for research and the time requested for the intervention are quite different, so that public power should do whatever is possible for intervention without relying on ongoing research; that's the second message. The third is that the man-made disasters - technological disasters - require legislation and public means quite different from the nature of disaster, both for technical reasons and psychological reasons. So, special laws should be designed and forced in industrialized countries, par ticularly for man-made disasters.

PAOLETTI: I would now like to ask Dr. F. Cattabeni who has been involved in the analytical procedure for the determination of TCDD from the very beginning to report on the work of himself and his colleagues.

CATTABENI: When the local authorities requested our help, the main goal was to define in the quickest possible way the map of contamination due to TCDD. And it was immediately apparent that there was a need for analyzing hundreds of samples in a short time, in order to restrict the heavily contaminated area from human exposure.

I wish here to give some insight on how the whole methodology was developed. The analytical methods are usually developed beforehand, knowing the levels of sensitivity to be reached and without political and social pressures. But this was not the case of Seveso. The analytical work started when the issue was already very hot. In fact the Icmesa company, as was mentioned before, did not immediately reveal the identity of the toxic compound and it took about one week before it became apparent that TCDD was in fact the most dangerous compound present in the so-called "cloud" which came out from the trichlorophenol plant. At that time - that is after the company revealed the presence of this compound - animal and human pathology already revealed the severity of the contamination. In this context the analytical methodology was developed. The problem of analyzing environmental samples implied the need of an analytical method which was at the same time sensitive and specific. In fact the more specific the method is, less clean up is necessary and, therefore, the time required for the analysis is shorter. In this respect the combined technique of gas chromatography and mass spectrometry is extremely helpful. This technique was confined up to that time only to research laboratories and had never been used for routine analysis and in particular to monitor environmental contamination.

This is probably the first time that mass fragmentography, the quantitative application of gas chromatography-mass spectrometry, was utilized to analyze thousands of environmental samples.

Low resolution gas chromatography and low resolution mass spectrometry were used and these analytical techniques proved to be of the utmost utility. Environmental samples were collected, extracted with dichloromethane and the extract evaporated and reconstituted with a small volume of solvent and analyzed[1]. This obviously took a rather short time.

Table 1 summarizes the procedure utilized at the time of the emergency period which started about July 22 and ended about August 6. About one thousand samples were collected in an area of about 300/400 hectares. Obviously, the analysis of such a great number of samples was possible because of the collaboration of different Institutes: Laboratorio Provinciale di Igiene e Profilassi, Istituto Superiore di Sanità and Istituto di Farmacologia e Farmacognosia, Università di Milano. It must be pointed out that during the emergency period the clean up procedure was very simple because the analytical technique utilized to measure TCDD was mass fragmentography, which offers a high degree of specificity.

Work was carried out twentyfour hours a day in eight-hour shifts and the approximate sensitivity at that time of the development of the method was in the order of 0.1/0.5 ppb. This sensitivity level was good enough to have the first idea of the extension of the contamination. The highest level found was 50 ppm, which, taking into account the toxicity of TCDD, is an extremely high level.

TABLE 1

EXTRACTION PROCEDURE UTILIZED FOR THE ANALYSIS OF TCDD DURING THE EMERGENCY PERIOD (22 July - 6 August, 1976)

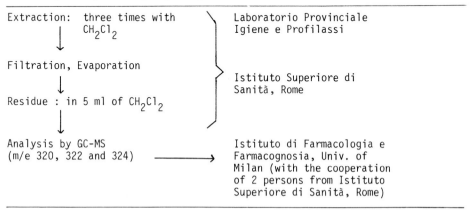

Extraction: three times with
CH_2Cl_2

Filtration, Evaporation

Residue : in 5 ml of CH_2Cl_2

Analysis by GC-MS
(m/e 320, 322 and 324)

Laboratorio Provinciale
Igiene e Profilassi

Istituto Superiore di
Sanità, Rome

Istituto di Farmacologia e
Farmacognosia, Univ. of
Milan (with the cooperation
of 2 persons from Istituto
Superiore di Sanità, Rome)

The analytical results obtained by the restless work, started on July 22, gave the possibility to the local authorities - with the help of toxicologists - to divide the area into three different zones on the basis of the levels of TCDD contamination: zone A, with a contamination > 50 $\mu g/m^2$, zone B with a contamination < 50 $\mu g/m^2$ and > 5 $\mu g/m^2$ and zone C (or R) with a contamination < 5 $\mu g/m^2$.

The extremely high toxicity of TCDD requested that the levels of sensitivity were decreased by at least a factor of 100 in order to reach the levels of 1 ppt. To increase the sensitivity to these levels, much more sophisticated clean up procedures were required and this methodology was developed starting at the beginning of August. Moreover such an increase of sensitivity implies longer time for the analysis and the only way to overcome the lack of time was to increase the number of persons and institutions collaborating in this project.

Table 2 describes the analytical procedure developed for the first systematic mapping of zone B and the Institutes which have and still are collaborating in analyzing environmental samples of TCDD.

The analytical procedure involved extraction and purification of the samples with column chromatography. This was performed exclusively at Laboratorio Provinciale di Igiene e Profilassi of Milan. Only for the instrumental analysis the sample extracts were divided up and given to the four different laboratories. In order to ensure that the response of each instrument was compatible with that of the instruments placed in the other laboratories, a quality control was developed. With the analytical procedure described, the sensitivity reached was in the order of parts per trillion. All the technical details on the whole analytical procedure developed and now in use have been recently published in extense[2].

TABLE 2

LABORATORIES INVOLVED AND THEIR ROLE IN THE FIRST SYSTEMATIC MAPPING OF TCDD CONTAMINATION IN ZONE B

INSTITUTE OR LABORATORY IN CHARGE

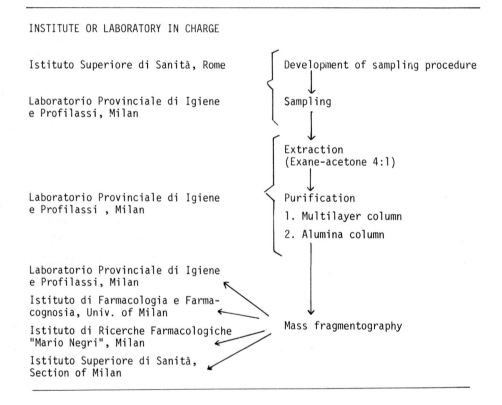

In conclusion, the environmental contamination by TCDD over a large and

populated area, requested the set up of a rapid and reliable method for monitoring this extraordinarily high toxic compound in thousands of samples. This was
obtained mainly through the use of mass fragmentoghraphy, which is considered
one of the most sensitive and specific techniques available today.

However, the analysis of thousands of samples (20,000 up to now) has been
made possible also through the collaboration of several institutions: Laboratorio Provinciale di Igiene e Profilassi, Istituto Superiore di Sanità, Istituto
di Ricerche Farmacologiche "Mario Negri", Istituto di Farmacologia e Farmacognosia (Università di Milano).

Finally it must also be pointed out that such a sophisticated analytical
technique has been successfully applied for the environmental monitoring of
TCDD because the technique was previously utilized for many years in basic research by the scientists involved in this program.

PAOLETTI: Now let us move on to the biological problems. Professor Garattini with his group at the Mario Negri Institute has been involved in this investigation on the biological effect of dioxin right from the start. I think he
will now report on the results.

GARATTINI: This is a short review of the studies we have carried out since
July 1976 on TCDD*. Two main aspects will be reported:
1) Distribution of TCDD in the Seveso area studied through contamination of do-
   mestic animals
2) Characterization of some aspects of the toxicological effects of TCDD
1) The first conspicuous evidence of environmental toxicity soon after the
event was animal mortality. On August 31 1976 (50 days after the accident) there
were around 3,000 dead animals out of a total of 81,000. Mortality was very high
among farmyard rabbits (2,062 out of 24,885) and other small animals (1,219 out
of 55,545). The contaminated area was soon divided into three zones (A,B and R)
according to the amount of TCDD found in the soil (fig. 1). Rabbit mortality
was higher in zone A (31.9%) than in B (8.8%) or R (6.8%) and there was some
even outside zone R.

Measurements of TCDD in samples of animals which had died or been slaughtered
for safety reasons started quite soon with the aim of monitoring the
accumulation of TCDD in living organisms and checking whether and to what extent

*This work has been carried out by the group of research on TCDD from Mario Ne-
gri Institute with the collaboration of the Provincial Veterinary Service.

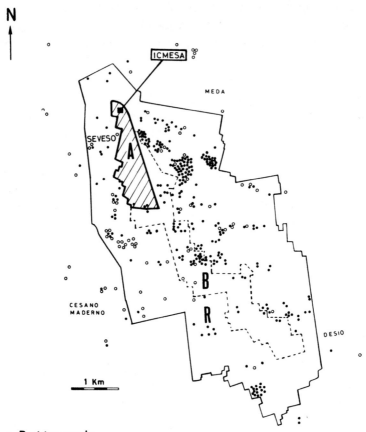

N

Positive sample

Negative sample

67 positive and 2 negative samples were
collected in zone A (no identified location)

Fig. 1.   Distribution of positive (= presence of TCDD) and negative (= absence
of TCDD) assays for TCDD in rabbit liver in the area of the accident (July –
October 1976).
On the basis of soil analyses for TCDD three zones were mapped out, referred to
as: A = TCDD levels in soil from n.d. to 5,477 µg/sq.m; B = TCDD levels in soil
from n.d. to 43.8 µg/sq.m; R = zone of respect n.d. to 5 µg/sq.m; n.d. < 0.75
µg/sq.m.   TCDD was analyzed by gas chromatography / mass spectrometry after
extraction and purification of the sample[3].

the chemical mapping of the soil reflected the bioavailability of TCDD for living organisms.

Rabbit liver was selected as the most sensitive and quantitative index of
toxicity[4]. Rabbit liver analysis (July - August 1976) showed the presence of
TCDD in 97, 92 and 75% of the rabbits from zone A, B and R respectively. 27% of
the samples from the surrounding area were positive (maximal TCDD value per
g/liver was 633 ng/g), indicating the presence of TCDD outside the limited
area. Fig. 1 shows the distribution of the positive and negative samples in
the three areas. In its general lines rabbit liver analysis confirms the division of the polluted areas into 3 zones, with A being the most contaminated and
R the least contaminated area.

However, the presence of similar concentrations of TCDD in the liver of rabbits from zones A and B (fig. 2) and the high variability observed even between
groups of animals living very close to each other documented the presence of
various sources of variability (uneven pattern of TCDD distribution in soil,
different exposure times of the animals to the contaminant, commercial uncontaminated food versus contaminated grass eaten by the various groups, etc.).

Later determinations of TCDD in wild animals again showed varying degrees of
contamination related to the amount of TCDD present in the soil and also to the
living and nutritional habits of the various species[5]. Milk collected in July-
August 1976 from cows living inside and outside the polluted area was also
found to be contaminated, with a maximum concentration of 7 μg/liter[5]. An inten
sive cows milk monitoring program started in March 1978. 28 farms from zone A
and surrounding areas were checked and only one (repeatedly checked) was found
positive with levels of TCDD ranging from 20 to 32 μg/l. Later it was found
that part of the fodder given to these cows had been harvested in zone R.
Thereafter these cows were fed on fodder purchased in uncontaminated areas and
after a few months TCDD became undetectable.

A few months after the accident test plots of rabbit were distributed in
fenced areas of zone B and R with the purpose of monitoring over a long period
of time the bioavailability of TCDD from soil (some decontaminated) to living
organisms. In 1978 only 2% of the animals living in test plots were found positive for TCDD. The amount of TCDD in their livers did not exceed 0.25 ng/g.
Rabbits from 119 farms located outside zone R were also examined and 5 out 119
were slightly contaminated.

At the same time of these experiments, others were carried out in laboratory
animals under controlled conditions. Cold or tritiated TCDD was used in this
series of studies according to the sensitivity and type of sample to be exami-

378

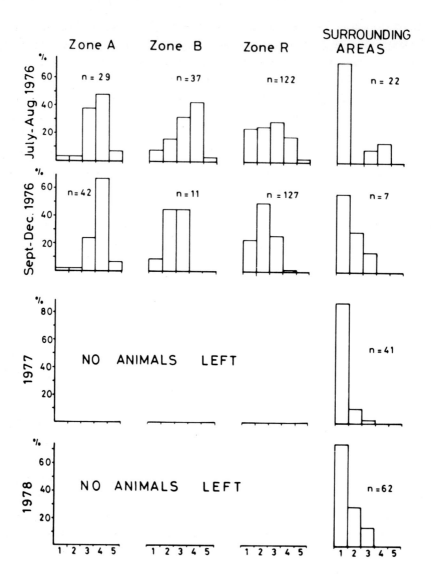

Fig. 2. Distribution of TCDD concentrations in rabbits liver from various zones.
Distribution of TCDD levels in rabbits liver from zones A, B, R and surrounding area divided in months or years. All animals from zone A, B, and R were
killed by december 1976 except those in test plots which are not included here.
Bars show in what percentage of rabbits (n = number tested) TCDD concentrations
were found in liver. The concentrations in ng/g are:
1 - < 0.25; 2 - > 0.25 < 2.5; 3 - > 2.5 < 25; 4 - > 25 < 250; 5 - > 250.

ned. The two methods of analysis were comparable as checked on occasional samples. The distribution of TCDD in various rabbit and mouse organs was examined at different intervals after a single or repeated doses of TCDD. Tissue distribution in both species confirms that the target organ for TCDD accumulation is the liver where the concentration was higher than in any other organ. The liver contained up to about 50% of the dose administered. In the rabbit TCDD concentrations in the liver were 20 times higher than in adipose tissue and 1,000 times higher than in blood or skin. The elimination half-life from the liver was around seven days. When ^{3}H-TCDD was administered every other day for 30 days a steady state was soon reached. There was a direct relationship between the dose administered and the tissue level. Experimental steady state values were very similar to theoretical values. 500 ng/kg given every other day for 30 days resulted in a steady state value of 20 ng/g in the liver (calculated value was 25 ng/g). In the mouse ^{3}H-TCDD concentrations in the liver were twice higher than those in adipose tissue and 500 time higher than those in the blood (Table 1). The half-life for elimination of the toxic compound from the liver was about 13.5 days.

Studies on the subcellular distribution of ^{3}H-TCDD by differential centrifugation of liver homogenates in isotonic medium showed that whereas 7 days after administration most TCDD was recovered in the high speed supernatant (100,000xg) fraction, at 14 days most of the TCDD was associated with the fractions containing cell fragments.

The accumulation of ^{3}H-TCDD in the liver also depends on the physical state of the substance and/or the vehicle in which it is given by oral route. When comparable amounts of ^{3}H-TCDD either adsorbed on finely ground soil or dissolved in oil were administered by gavage to mice, less ^{3}H-TCDD was recovered in the liver of mice given the soil.

TCDD has been described as the most potent inducer of hepatic ala synthetase in chick embryos[7]. Experiments were carried out to check whether in the rat long-term treatment with TCDD induced a change in the amount and pattern of excretion of porphyrins. Table 2 shows that the pattern of distribution of copro, hexa, hepta and uroporphyrins is modified by TCDD and that the alteration is similar to that induced by other polyhalogenated aromatic hydrocarbons.

Another important target for TCDD is the immunological system. Atrophy of the thymus, suppression of cell mediated immunity and, in the few published data available, a minimal effect on humoral responses are reported[8,9,10] . Our group[11,12] found that TCDD markedly suppresses the primary humoral response to thymus dependent (sheep erithrocytes) and independent (type III pneumococcal

TABLE 1

DISTRIBUTION OF TCDD IN VARIOUS MOUSE TISSUE

ng equivalent of ^{3}H-TCDD per g/tissue

TISSUE	DAY 1	DAY 7	DAY 14	DAY 21
Liver	36.3 ± 12.5	26.8 ± 4.5	17.9 ± 4.9	6.2 (5.1-7.4)
Adipose tissue	26.0 ± 7.3	9.9 ± 3.2	5.7 ± 1.4	3.1 (2.6-3.5)
Kidney	2.00 ± 1.21	0.56 ± 0.10	0.32 (0.19-0.46)	0.29(0.26-0.31)
Lung	1.60 ± 0.14	0.60 ± 0.14	0.43 ± 0.14	0.18(0.17-0.20)
Heart	0.65 ± 0.16	0.19 ± 0.06	0.12 ± 0.03	0.07(0.07-0.08)
Spleen	3.00 ± 1.90	0.19 ± 0.05	0.19 ± 0.06	0.13(0.09-0.16)
Brain	0.44 ± 0.14	0.14 ± 0.04	0.11 ± 0.02	0.06(0.05-0.07)
Blood	0.06 ± 0.01	0.05 ± 0.01	0.05 ± 0.01	0.02 ± 0.01

Radioactivity in tissues of C 57Bl/6 J mice was determined 1, 7, 14 and 21 days after oral administration of tritium labelled TCDD 1 mC, 633 μg/kg dissolved in acetone:oil (1:6) Radioactivity values are mean ± S.D. of triplicate or duplicate determinations. Radioactivity was measured by liquid scintillation after dissolving the sample (Soluene ^{R}). Chromatography (thin layer chromatography on silica gel G, solvent system cyclohexane:ethylether, 16:1) of occasional samples of different tissues at different time points did not reveal any radioactivity product other than authentic TCDD.

TABLE 2

CHANGES IN THE PATTERN OF URINARY PORPHYRINS IN PORPHYRIA CAUSED BY HEXACHLORO-
BENZENE (HBC) AND OTHER POLYHALOGENATED AROMATIC HYDROCARBONS IN RATS

PORPHYRIN	CONTROL	HBG[a]	TCDD[b]
PROTO	+	+	
Tricarboxylic	+	+	
COPRO	+++++	++	+++++
PENTA	+	+	
HEXA	-	+	+
HEPTA	+	+++	++
URO	++	+++++	++++

a) data from Doss, Schermuly and Koss 1976[13]
b) TCDD (1μg/KG) dissolved in corn oil was given per os once a week for 6
months to groups of 5 rats. Porphyrins were determined in the urine collected
for 24 hours every 30 days. Porphyrins were separated by thin layer chromatography and analyzed by spectrophotometry[14].

polysaccharide) antigens in C 57 Bl / 65 mice (Tables 3 - 4). The minimal effective single dose is 1.2 μg/Kg which is still active after 42 days. When
TCDD is given once a week for 4 weeks the minimal effective dose is 0.5 μg/kg.
The response is back to normal 55 days after the last dose. In animals treated
with TCDD spontaneous macrophage mediated and NK cell mediated cytotoxicity
were not altered on a per cell basis but the numbers of macrophages and lymphoid
cells were low[12]. Impairment of these humoral and cellular immune mechanisms
might play a role in the lowered resistance to bacterial infection[15] of mice
given TCDD[16] and in the carcinogenic and cocarcinogenic activity of this chemical.

TABLE 3

EFFECT OF A SINGLE DOSE OF TCDD ON PRIMARY HUMORAL RESPONSE TO SRBC (SHEEP ERYTHROCYTES)

Day after treatment	TCDD (μg/kg)	PFC / 10^6 splenocytes	PFC / spleen
7	0	204(173-240)	27,334(24,106-30,900)
	0,1	130(119-189)	20,414(18,694-24,108)[****]
	1,2	94(77-114)[****]	10,514(8,698-12,709)[****]
	6,0	29(21- 41)[****]	3,723(2,666- 5,199)[****]
	30,0	11(9- 12)[****]	915(765- 1,095)[****]
42	0	1,028(938-1,127)	83,086(73,215-94,257)
	1,2	458(367-572)[**]	51,844(45,153-59,526)[****]
	6,0	152(115-201)[****]	16,795(11,865-23,774)[****]
	30,0	128(90-167)[****]	12,226(10,247-14,586)[****]

[**]$p < 0.05$ by Dunnet's test
[****]$p < 0.01$ by Dunnet's test

TCDD was given i.p. to C57Bl/6 mice (6 per group). 4 x 10^8 SRBC were injected i.p. 7 or 42 days after treatment and the test was performed 5 days later by Jerne's technique. Plaque forming cells (PFC) are mean ± (1 s.e.) after logarithmic transformation of the data.

TABLE 4

EFFECT OF REPEATED DOSES OF TCDD ON PRIMARY HUMORAL RESPONSE TO SRBC

Day after last treatment	TCDD (μg/kg)	PFC / 10^6 splenocytes	PFC / spleen
7	0	338(292-392)	43,216(39,534-47,241)
	0,1	254(229-282)	36,946(34,221-39,888)[****]
	0,5	125(109-144)[****]	15,886(14,044-17,969)[****]
	2,5	85(74- 98)[****]	9,285(8,387-10,269)[****]
55	0	269(232-311)	36,593(32,133-41,673)
	2,5	288(259-319)	35,589(32,304-39,208)

[****]$p < 0.01$ by Dunnet's test

TCDD was given weekly per os, for 4 weeks, to 6 C57Bl/6 mice per group. 4x10^8 SRBC were injected i.p. 7 or 55 days after the last dose and the test was performed 5 days later by Jerne's technique. PFC values are mean ± (1 s.e.) after logarithmic transformation of the data.

PAOLETTI: Many of the effects shown by Dr. Garattini in his presentation, of course, can be studied at molecular level and Dr Nicosia will report on this aspect of TCDD action.

NICOSIA: 2,3,7,8-Tetrachloro-dibenzo-p-dioxin (TCDD) is the most toxic of all the substances known so far, with the exception of a few high molecular weight natural toxins[17]. Its toxicity is particularly evident when considering the LD_{50} in guinea pig; the severe lethality of TCDD prompted many investigators to test the effects of this dioxin on the most fundamental process of life.

For instance, DNA synthesis in rat regenerating liver has been checked and has been found to be unchanged by TCDD[18].

The oxidative phosphorylation of liver mitochondria, and therefore the production of ATP, in rats is not modified after TCDD treatment[19] even with lethal doses[20]. In a more sophisticated experiment, where the levels of the pyridine nucleotides in the oxidized and reduced forms were measured, some decrease of NAD and NADP content was noticed in TCDD-treated rats versus pair-fed controls[20]. However, NAD/NADH ratios in cytosol and mitochondria, which reflect more closely the redox state of the cell, though different from the ratios in the pair-fed controls, were very similar to those in *ad libitum* fed animals[20]. Therefore, the alteration in redox state of the cell cannot be the cause of the extreme toxicity of TCDD.

The dioxin has been reported to inhibit mitosis in endosperm cells of African Blood Lily[21]; however, no effect has been recognized on the mitotic process of a number of mammalian cell lines[22].

TCDD does not affect the absorption of nutrients from the gastrointestinal tract, as the severe weight loss in dioxin-treated animals seems to suggest. In fact, animals receiving either ^{14}C-glucose or ^{14}C-alanine or ^{14}C-oleate produce the same amount of $^{14}CO_2$ whether they have been pretreated with TCDD or not.[20]

In addition, protein and lipid synthesis generally is not impaired in TCDD-treated rats[23] and the fatty acid composition of liver, plasma and adipose tissue does not differ significantly from that of pair-fed controls[20].

Therefore, it appears that the most important processes of the living cells are not affected by TCDD. However, very recent results obtained in our Department[24] show that TCDD *in vitro* can affect the biosynthesis of rat myelin.

In fact, the incorporation of ^3H-leucine and ^3H-glycerol into central nervous system myelin is significantly increased by the addition of TCDD at 2 ng/ml

Other data obtained very recently in our Department demonstrate that TCDD interferes also with cholesterol metabolism[25]. TCDD-treated rats show cholester ol plasma levels significantly higher than control rats; the increase is to be ascribed mainly to a higher cholesterol content of the HDL (high density lipo-protein) fraction.

These very recent results shed new light on some aspects of TCDD toxicity, but they cannot explain the extreme lethality of this dioxin. This applies also to a number of other toxic effects of TCDD, which, though severe, cannot be the only cause of death.

For instance, TCDD causes extensive hepatic damage in a number of mamma-lians[26]; but this toxic effect is less severe in guinea pig, for which the LD_{50} is the lowest, than in other animals such as rat.

The pattern of TCDD toxicity somewhat resembles a state of hypothyroidism, and actually this dioxin decreases the plasma level of thyroxine by increasing its excretion[27]. However, the high toxicity of TCDD is not due to its effect on thyroid function, since injections of triiodothyrorine (T_3) only slightly increase the survival time; this increase can be attributed to a higher food intake and not to a direct protective effect of T_3[20].

Impairment of the immune system occurs in many species after exposure to TCDD[28], but it is not the cause of the acute lethality. In fact, the dioxin is as lethal to germ-free rats as it is to control animals[29]. Some of the possible molecular mechanisms for this aspect of TCDD toxicity have been investigated. Neal and coworkers[20] have hypothesized that the effect on the lymphoid tissues might be mediated by an increased biosynthesis or activity of glucocorticoids. TCDD can actually raise the level of circulating hydroxycorticosteroids, but this apparent increase of adrenal function is not the mechanism of its toxicity since adrenalectomy does not reduce mortality[20]. Neither can TCDD mimick gluco-corticoid action by binding to the same receptor, as it cannot displace ³H-dexa methasone from its binding sites[20].

Finally, it is well known that TCDD is a very potent inducer of some microso-mal enzymes[19,30]; however, other inducers of the same enzymes such as 3-methyl-cholanthrene (3-MC) are not nearly as lethal as TCDD. Therefore, once again this toxic action of dioxin is not the relevant one to the high mortality rate it can induce.

It is interesting, however, to discuss in detail this aspect of TCDD toxici-ty, because it is the only one for which a mechanism at molecular level has been described.

Poland *et al.*[31] have identified in mouse liver cytosol a receptor that binds TCDD specifically, reversibly and with high affinity ($K_D = 2.7 \times 10^{-10}M$). This receptor is responsible for enzyme induction, as demonstrated by a structure-activity study of a number of dibenzo-p-dioxins[31]; such a study has demonstrated a close correlation between the relative binding affinity of the different dioxins to the TCDD receptor and the relative biological potency in terms of induction of aryl hydrocarbon hydroxylase (AHH).

As mentioned earlier, 3-MC can induce the same enzyme, even if it is 30,000 fold less active than TCDD[32]. It is well known, however, that only certain inbred strains of mice such as C57BL/6J are responsive to 3-MC, while other strains such as DBA/2J are not[33,34]. When responsive and non responsive strains are administered TCDD, AHH induction occurred in all the strains; the ED_{50}, however, was 10-fold higher in the so-called non responsive strains than in responsive ones[35]. This has been interpreted by the authors as meaning that a mutation in "non responsive" mice caused the receptor to have a much lower affinity for both TCDD and 3-MC. Such an hypothesis was confirmed by investigating the binding of TCDD to the cytosolic receptors obtained from responsive and non responsive animals[31]: the affinity of TCDD for its binding sites is definitely higher in the responsive strains.

Recently , Poland *et al.*[36] have discovered that non responsive strains are also less susceptible to some of the toxic effect of TCDD, such as thymus involution, than the responsive animals, while hybrids are intermediate. The data indicate that the molecular events responsible for this aspect of TCDD toxicity segregate with the locus for AHH induction. In addition, the binding affinity of different dioxins to the cytosolic receptor correlates well with their toxicity .

According to Poland and coworkers[36], the available evidence points toward the possibility that the toxicity of TCDD and related compounds is mediated through the identified cytosolic receptor. The TCDD-receptor complex migrates into the nucleus[37] where it would interact with the genetic material, and therefore trigger a number of different responses, one of which is the AHH induction.

While this hypothesis is definitely fascinating, there are data indicating that the real situation might be more complex, since the inducibility of AHH in hepatic cell culture lines seems to correlate with the increase in the number of cytosolic receptors more than with their presence[38].

In addition, it cannot be ruled out that the other aspects of TCDD toxicity could be mediated by a different type of receptor, for instance a membrane bound receptor, as it has been demonstrated for other chlorinated compounds[39].

PAOLETTI: Now Professor Weber is going to show the morphological aspects of the liver of animals affected by TCDD. Professor Weber is the professor of

Pathology of the University of Siena and has been in contact with our group while carrying out this morphological research.

WEBER: I am simply showing you some slides concerning the liver research. These are rats which have been injected with TCDD in the Seveso laboratories by members of Paoletti's group and have been examined at Siena by myself together with Drs. P. Luzi, L. Resi and P. Tanganelli. The technical help by E. Capaccioli is aknowledged. The rats used are about fifty. The livers show important lesions which were studied fifteen, thirty and sixty days after the day of the single injection of TCDD (20 micrograms / kg 5 P). The light microscopy observation discloses lesions which are quite different from the lesions that can be appreciated with the transmission electron microscope. This should be fully understood by an interdisciplinary group because very frequently scientists, who are not directly concerned with morphology, are not accustomed to consider that, for the preparation of morphological experiments, different approaches may be necessary. So we have to collect samples for histology and ultrastructural research and this requires different methods of collecting, fixing, including and finally observing samples of the tissue and therefore collaboration may be difficult in some instances.

At light microscopic observation in a semithick section of an Epo-Araldite embedded, osmic acid fixed fragment of a rat liver collected 15 days after TCDD injection. This section shows you that the nuclei are not similar to the ones of normal control livers. They are very blown up and clear, very poor in chromatine. The liver structure is very heavily modified, many liver cells are necrotic and others are charged with small lipid droplets whereas the whole of the cell is blown up. At fifteen days heavy regressive lesions are already present.

The pictures observed at the microscope are similar to the ones obtainable after administration of CCl_4, largely used in experimental studies for the induction of liver cirrhosis. Our findings, at this stage, are not very different to what other Authors have seen after the administration of dioxin, for instance Jones and Butler[40] in England few years ago or Gupta and coll.[41] in the United States.

Many lipid inclusions are present after 30 days, together with many fatty cells. Those cells are very frequently observed and whole lobules are composed only of fatty and or necrotic hepatocytes. Near the portal space there are lots of inflammatory cells. The picture is very similar to the ones obtained after injections or inhalations of carbon tetrachloride.

In other cases, the hepatic lesions may even be more pronounced. Most of the cells are not stained, but one can see also well stained cells even if in a small number (so excluding any artifact).

The liver sections after 60 days show a regeneration of the liver cells. The hepatocytes are in the large majority stained but some of them show the presence of lesions well evident in the cytoplasma. A huge number of cisternae are present in the liver cell cytoplasma. Nearby well stained cells, other cells which are not or faintly stained are present. Necrotic lesions are going on even in the regenerationg liver after sixty days.

I should like to underline that nobody has studied such long term lesions up to this moment and it must really be stressed that lesions are still present in the regenerating liver cells.

A trasmission electron microscopic picture shows the liver cells of a control rat which has been caged in Seveso but not injected with dioxin. The nucleus, the glycogen amounts and the endoplasmic reticulum and borders of this cell are very nitid.

Fifteen days after a single injection of TCDD, the cells are deeply altered. The shape of the nucleus is modified. The number of the lipid droplets is very high. The mytochondria are almost packed together by those huge droplets, and among them almost no endoplasmic reticulum is evident.

The following figure shows what happens in other districts of the cell. There is no distinction between two contiguous cells, their borderline is confused. ATPase has been found strongly decreased by English Authors[42] under such conditions. And again areas where lipid droplets and mytochondria are packed all together and areas which are empty of organelles can be found (fig. 1).

After thirty days, in the peripheral zone of the hepatocyte a huge increase of the smooth endoplasmic reticulum,which is a sign of the "enzymatic induction", on which previous authors have spoken,is seen. The "enzymatic induction" is really at a very high level at the thirtieth day in the peripheral portions of the hepatocytes (fig. 2). In other observations, the amount of the smooth endoplasmic reticulum is incredibly huge. It means "enzymatic induction" and this is indeed one of the most important morphological signs of the lesions which are caused by the TCDD, both by oral administration or, as in our experiments, by intraperitoneal injection.

After sixty days there is an important modification and not only important for a morphologist: this liver cell looks like a plasmacell (fig. 3). It is quite unusual to find liver cells with such a huge endoplasmic reticulum. Experiments are now under way in order to investigate further liver changes

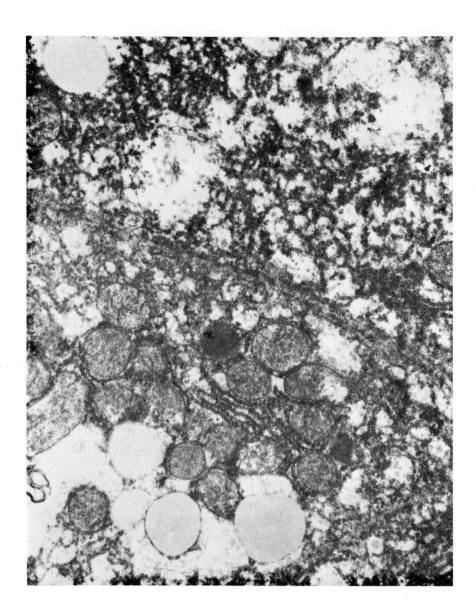

Fig. 1. Rat liver 5A (II Gr.)
Two weeks after a single dose treatment with TCDD.

three, six and twelve months after a single administration of TCDD.

In other experiments, we have been impressed by the huge quantity of those structures and also by the cells that in some way are regenerating. The glycogen

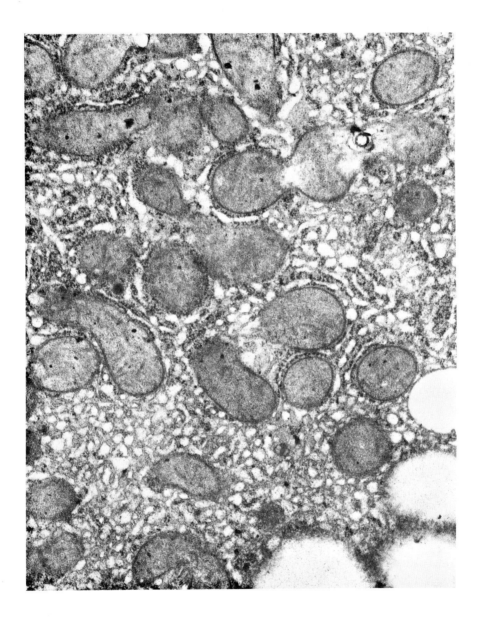

Fig. 2. Rat liver 5B (III Gr.)
Four weeks after a single dose treatment with TCDD.

is to be found in the cytoplasma, but the mytochondria are still huge and swol-
len, some deep change is taking place in these cells. But what? In a semithick
section it is possible to see cells which are regenerating but they are suffe-

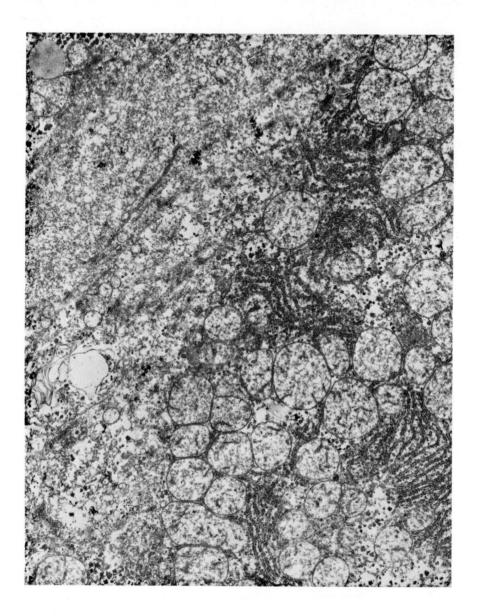

Fig. 3. Rat liver 9C (IV Gr.)
Eight weeks after treatment with TCDD.

ring and some of them are dying again.

We are also studying the thymus gland, the spleen, the brain of those animals which have been injected with TCDD and the results will be ready in some

months.

PAOLETTI: Of course toxicology like pharmacology is a science of microsome, mice and man and we have heard about microsome and mice. Dr. V. Foà will report on man.

FOA': I shall report only some results obtained by monitoring the workers engaged in the area and not all the human data so far collected. As you know the Institute of Occupational Health of the University of Milan has been involved, since the very first day after the accident, both with personal interventions in the medical-epidemiological commissions created at the moment as well as in the coordination of the activities of occupational health services or the physicians involved in the medical control in the area concerned, and also as supervisor in organizing in the Desio Hospital, the service of occupational health established at the moment of the accident. In addition to this we are involved in the neurological follow-up of the workers, which were involved in the dioxin accident, that is the ICMESA workers, workers belonging to other industries in the same area or engaged in decontamination operations, such as laboratory technicians who are collecting samples. Of all the overmentioned activities, started in '76, the Institute is presently performing only the neurophysiological monitoring of the exposed subjects because both the services of the municipality and of the hospital have grown now and are walking on their own legs. A number of accidents, producing exposure to dioxin, with neurological or/and psychiatric symptoms in workers who were involved, was the background on which the neurological monitoring program was built with at least a yearly control for five consecutive years. Later we can discuss the results obtained but for the moment I have to say that nearly all the ICMESA workers examined have normal clinical findings but on the contrary there were a great number of subjects with impaired neurophysiological parameters. At this point, I prefer to discuss this experience to evaluate if, among the methods in modern toxicology, neurophysiological studies on peripheral nerves are to be considered as reliable and useful parameters for monitoring people exposed to neurotoxic substances and to suggest recommended health-based permissible levels both for occupational and for environmental exposure to neurotoxic agents. Before entering into this discussion, let me present the results obtained in a study of this type carried out within the framework of the Seveso surveillance program.^{::}

::The study was carried out by Gilioli R., Cotroneo L., Genta P.A.

So far 35 technicians examining the samples coming from the polluted area and 35 sex and age matched controls received a thorough neurophysiological investigation. Of course the hazardous nature of the chemical was well appreciated by those concerned and careful laboratory precautions were taken to avoid personal contamination at least after the first emergency period. This investigation consisted in conventional electromyographic studies, in a study of motor conduction velocity for fast and slow conducting fibres of the ulnar and common peroneal nerves, in a study of sensory conduction velocity of the ulnar nerve and an automatic study with a new technique of the motor unit parameters. And the results with needle electromyography show a difference between the controls and the technicians but this difference as far as regards fibrillation was not significant. More interesting was what happened with conduction velocity studies, where we found a significant difference between controls and technicians for motor conduction velocity both for the fast and slow fibres.

The finger to wrist sensory conduction velocity of the ulnar nerve showed a highly significant difference ($p < 0.001$) between controls and the technicians, whereas duration and amplitude of the sensory potential did not show any significant difference (fig. 1).

The study of the motor unit parameters (MUP) gave these results: MUP duration in m. abductor of V finger (fig. 2) showed a highly significant difference ($p < 0.001$) between technicians and controls and also at the same level of significance for amplitude. Similar results were found in the m. tibialis anterior (fig. 3) even though MUP amplitude was not significantly different.

We can now draw some considerations in the light of these results. The highly significant reduction of the sensory conduction velocity studied, and the highly significant increase in the duration and in the amplitude of the motor unit potential of the nerves, have the same meaning, that is a tendency towards neurogenic involvement. Of course the history collected and the examination performed permitted to rule out the most common causes of peripheral neuropathy (diabetes, alcohol, potentially neurotoxic drugs, ecc.). These subjects, in the first period after the accident-probably had a certain degree of exposure to dioxin found in the samples. However, more recently the levels of dioxin from the samples tended to decrease and moreover the technicians used solvents, mainly n-exane (in order to extract dioxin from the samples) which are potentially neurotoxic agents. These data hold an interest on a group level, whereas on the individual level these neurophysiological findings are not clearly in favour of a real damage to the nerves fibres. We will not, therefore, speak of a proved damage to the individual but only of a shifting of functional parameters which, being evident in the exposed group, may be inter-

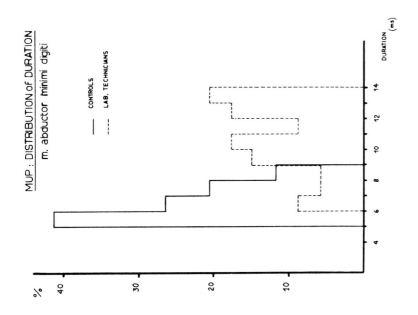

MUP : DISTRIBUTION of DURATION
m. abductor minimi digiti

CONTROLS
LAB. TECHNICIANS

Fig. 2.

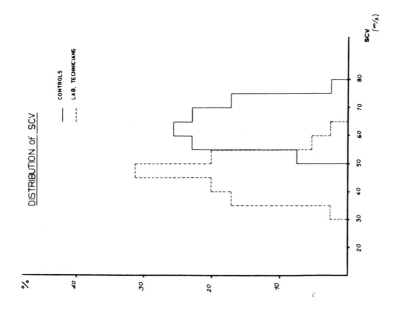

DISTRIBUTION of SCV

CONTROLS
LAB. TECHNICIANS

Fig. 1.

394

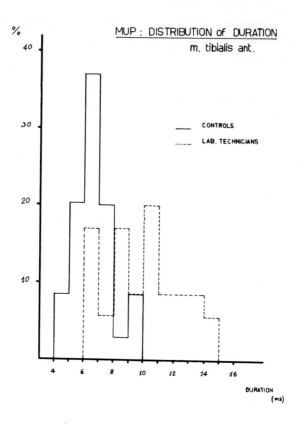

Fig. 3.

preted as an early sign of the action of the neurotoxic agent under investigation. It seems to me, therefore, very difficult to attribute to one neurotoxic
agent alone the aethiology of this neurogenic involvement because TCDD in soil

and n-hexane used to extract it from the samples, may all play a role in causing the peripheral neurogenic signs found.

At this point, we have to come back to our question: i.e. are the neurophysiological parameters useful to suggest recommended health-based permissible levels for exposure to neurotoxic agents?

We believe that the dose or the concentration in a work room which can give, on a group basis of workers, a shifting of the neurophysiological parameters, must be considered not harmless also in the absence of any clinical sign. There fore, this dose or concentration, utilized as a safety standard for work places, has to be lowered because there is evidence of a harmful effect.

This point is under worldwide discussion now because these methods are consi dered too sensitive and because we don't know until now which is the meaning of an impairment of such a parameter, without any clinical sign, in respect to health expectations of a man during his life. Even if this area is still contro versial, I might suggest that, in the methods of a modern toxicology, we have to measure also neurophysiological and behavioral parameters, before concluding if a substance may be used or not in total safety.

PAOLETTI: Now the last speaker will be Dr. N. Fortunati, an officer of the Regional government who is in charge of the organization of research in this area.

FORTUNATI: I was called by Mr. Spallino to organize the research department for the Lombardy regional office for Seveso. Through the law n. II/488 publi shed on July 14, 1977, the regional government established what the office should accomplish in a short period of time.

Firstly, I must say that there is a gap between the time of research, necessary long, and the need to face the every-day problems of the Seveso population. This being stated, I would like to mention some of the investigations so far carried out. One of the most important research efforts that has been made was to try to establish a relationship between TCDD on the soil and TCDD in vegetables. One of the problems we had to face in the region (where the population continued to live and where limitations had been enforced in the use of gardens and of products of the soil) was to establish a limit in the pollutant existing in the soil, a limit within which we could allow the use of vegetables. For this purpose the University of Milan has been charged to carry on part of the research program which is still going on now, with Carbon 14 and/or Tritium labelled dioxin. The results have been clear: the vegetables absorb measurable

amounts of dioxin and therefore, for the time being, the population living in
the Seveso area are prohibited to sell or to use vegetables grown in the B zone
and in the R zone.

Another research that will be carried on in 1980 by the Institute of Agricul
tural Chemistry, University of Milan, in the botanic field has the object to
find out exactly what is the final destination of the dioxin which has been
absorbed; in fact apparently part of the dioxin is transferred to vegetables
and then leaves them. We don't know if it leaves the vegetables by sublimation,
if it is transformed into some metabolites or if it is destroyed by the UV
light.

Another investigation tries to determine a chemical mean to destroy the dioxin still contained in the reactor in the ICMESA plant, where the contamination
originated. This experiment will be carried on, at least in part, at the Ispra
International Laboratory for Atomic Research.

Very few organizations in Italy want to have anything to do with highly polluted samples and to run the risk of contaminating their laboratories. This is
one of the problems that we are facing every day in managing and organizing
research, involving TCDD measurements.

The attempt of refining the methods of analysis, especially concerning the
vegetables, object of the research previously explained, is of great interest.
A certain number of rabbits grown up in the ICMESA plant (the only place where
we are free to use contaminated animals) have been fed with vegetables raised in
fields with low TCDD contamination. The purpose is to find out whether there is
any relationship between soil contamination, grass or carrots or potatoes given
to the animals and rabbit livers. If we find that there are negative and consistent results for the soil, grass and the rabbit livers, we might come to the
conclusion that the area is free and can be returned to the owners for unre-
stricted utilization.

Beyond what I have just said, there are minor researches which are going on
involving university laboratories. I am at disposal of anybody willing to examine the activity developed by the Regional office for Seveso.

PAOLETTI: We are at the end of the reports on the dioxin event. As you see,
many data have been collected, many investigations have been made over a period
of three years. The main question however still waits for a definitive reply.
What are the long lasting effects of dioxin after an acute dose or prolonged
exposure in the human species?

REFERENCES

1. Adamoli, P. et al. (1978) Ecol. Bull.,27, 31-38.

2. Di Domenico, A. et al. (1979) Analyt. Chem.,51, 735-740.

3. Fanelli, R. et al. Submitted to Bull. Envir. Contam. Toxicol.

4. Fanelli, R. et al. (In press) Arch. Environ. Contam. and Toxicol.

5. Fanelli, R. et al. Submitted to Experientia

6. Fanelli, R. et al. Submitted to Bull.Envir. Contam. Toxicol.

7. Poland, A. and Glover, E. (1973) Science, 179, 476-477.

8. Vos, J.G., Moore, J.A. and Zinkl, J.G. (1973) Environ. Health Perspect.,
5, 149.

9. Moore, J.A. and Faith, R.E. (1976) Environ.Health Perspect., 18, 125.

10. Mc Connell, E.E., Moore, J.A., Haseman, J.K. and Harris, M.W. (1978) Toxicol. Appl. Pharmacol., 44, 335.

11. Vecchi, A. et al. Submitted to Chimico-Biol. Interac.

12. Mantovani, A. et al. Submitted to Biomedicine.

13. Doss, M. et al. (1976) Ann. Clin. Res.,8, suppl. 17, 171-181.

14. Doss, M. (1970) Z. Klin. Chem. u. Klin. Biochem., 8, 197-207.

15. Thigpen, J.E., Faith, R.E., Mc Connell, E.E. and Moore, J.A. (1975) Infect.
Immun., 12, 1319.

16. Kouri, R.E. et al. (1978) Cancer Res., 38, 2777.

17. Poland, A. and Kende, A. (1976) Fed. Proc.,35, 2404-2411.

18. Greig, J.B., Taylor, D.M. and Jones, J.D. (1974) Chem. Biol. Interact.,8,
31-39.

19. Lucier, G.W., McDaniel, O.S., Hask, G.E.R., Fowler, B.A., Sonawane, B.R.
and Faeder, E. (1973) Environ. Health Perspect.,5, 199-209.

20. Neal, R.A., Beatty, P.W. and Gasiewicz, T.A. (1979) Ann. N.Y. Acad. Sci.,
320, 204-213.

21. Jackson, W.T. (1972) J. Cell Sci., 10, 15-25.

22. Beatty, P.W., Lembach, K.J.,Holscher, M.A. and Neal, R.A. (1975) Toxicol.
Appl. Pharmacol.,31, 309-312.

23. Cunningham, H.M. and Williams, D.T. (1972) Bull. Environ. Contam. Toxicol.,
4, 45-51.

24. Petroni, A. and Galli, C., in publication.

25. Poli, A. Franceschini, G. and Sirtori, C.R. (1980) Biochem. Pharmacol.,
in press.

26. Fowler, B.A., Lucier, G.W., Brown, H.W. and McDaniel, O.S. (1973) Environ.
Health Perspect.,5, 141-148.

27. Bastomsky, C.H. (1977) Endocrinology,101, 292-296.

28. Vos, J.G., Moore, J.A. and Zinkl, J.G. (1973) Environ.Health Perspect, 5,
149-162.

29. Greig, J.B., Jones, G., Butler, W.H. and Barnes, J.M. (1973) Food Cosmet.
Toxicol.,11, 575-595.

30. Greig, J.B. and De Matteis, F. (1973) Environ. Health Perspect.,5, 211-219.

31. Poland, A., Glover, E. and Kende, A.S. (1976) J. Biol. Chem.,251, 4936-4946.

32. Poland, A. and Glover, E. (1974) Mol. Pharmacology,10, 349-359.

33. Nebert, D.W. and Gielen, J.E. (1972) Fed. Proc.,31, 1315-1325.

34. Nebert, D.W., Gonjon, F.M. and Gielen, J.E. (1972) Nature New Biol.,236, 107-110.

35. Poland, A. and Glover, E. (1975) Mol. Pharmacol.,11, 389-398.

36. Poland, A., Greenlee,W.F. and Kende, A.S. (1979) Ann. N.Y. Acad. Sci.,320, 214-230.

37. Greenlee,W.F. and Poland, A. (1979) Fed. Proc.,38, 425.

38. Guenthner, T.M. and Nebert, D.W. (1977) J. Biol. Chem.,252, 8981-8989.

39. Singhal, R.L. and Kacew, S. (1976) Fed. Proc.,35, 2618-2623.

40. Jones, G. and Butler, W.A. (1974) J. Path.,112, 93-97.

41. Gupta, B.N., Vos, J.G., Moore, J.A., Zinkl, J.G. and Bullock, B.G. (1973) Environ. Health Perspect., September, 141.

42. Greig, J.B. and Osborne, G. (1977) Ecol. Bull., 27.

AUTHOR INDEX

R.L. Baron   191

I. Bartošek   341

F. Cattabeni   367

A. Cosco   295

J.C. Dacre   341

J.W. Daniel   71, 341

G. Della Porta   159

T.A. Dragani   159

P.S. Elias   169

G. Falconi   311

V. Foa'   367

U. Fortunati   367

S. Garattini   367

A. Gerard   35

L. Golberg   341

K.R. Hill   55

N. Loprieno   107

W.K. Lutz   207

O. Marelli   295

R.G. McConnell   223

A. Mondino   259

I.C. Munro   125, 341

S.D. Murphy   277, 341

P.M. Newberne   223

A. Nicolin   295

S. Nicosia   367

A.K. Palmer   139

R. Paoletti   367

D.V. Parke   85

F. Sarra   295

C. Schlatter   207, 341

A. Spallino   367

B. Terracini   321

R. Truhaut   1

G. Vettorazzi   9

G. Weber   367